Diagnostic Virology in Primary Care

Case vignettes for general practitioners and trainees in medical microbiology

Written by: Dr Brendan Crowley MSc MD DTM FRCPath FFPath(RCPI)

Edited by: Professor Anna Maria Geretti MD PhD FRCPath

All royalties to LauraLynn Ireland's Children's Hospice

Copyright © Brendan Crowley, 2019

First Published in Ireland, in 2019, in co-operation with
Choice Publishing, Drogheda, County Louth, Republic of Ireland.
www.choicepublishing.ie

Paperback ISBN: 978-1-913275-02-0
eBook ISBN: 978-1-913275-03-7

A CIP catalogue record for this book is available from the National Library.

Acknowledgements

I am very grateful to the many people whose help allowed this book to come to fruition. Thanks to Deirdre Devine at Choice publications for her support and to Anthony Edwards for designing the front cover. I am most grateful to my team including the following medical scientists in virology: Yvonne Lynagh, Carmel Roche, Kate O'Driscoll, Lorraine Clancy, Alma Clancy, Fiona O'Rourke, Martina Windsor, Vanessa Mulligan, Christian Coates, Ruth Rumgay, Denyce Browne, Patrice Keane, Michael O'Meara and Ger Reid. A special word of thanks to Bairbre Ni Laoi, Anne Walsh and Linda Dalby who contributed significantly over the years to the development of the molecular virology and serology laboratory. I want to thank all of my Consultant colleagues and laboratory management for their support in developing the clinical virology service. I am most grateful to Deirdre Mulvee and the secretarial staff for their support.

I acknowledge my mentors in Virology, Professor Conor Keane, Professor Tony Hart, Professor Barry Duggan. I am very grateful to three Presentation Brothers who taught me in secondary school in Cork City, Brothers Colmcille, Bede and Dominic.

I wish to pay special tribute to Professor Anna Maria Geretti whose expert guidance and enthusiasm made writing this book enjoyable. I am very grateful to Dr Philip Mortimer, retired Consultant Virologist, for his very helpful contribution and for writing the back cover. A word of thanks to other colleagues who made useful suggestions on specific chapters in the book: Professor Ed Guy, Professor P Griffiths, Dr M Edelstein, Dr A Stockdale and Dr D Freedman.

I am forever grateful to my parents Jack and Judy. This book is dedicated to my wife Deirdre and son David. Their love and support of me made the writing of this book possible.

CONTENTS

FOREWORD

One day, during my first month as a trainee in clinical virology, the senior medical registrar called in to the Virology department in a state of great distress. He had been feeling tired over the last couple of weeks and then that morning he had seen a faint rash on his torso. Could we take a look? Had he caught a nasty virus? Was this measles? A quick consultation and a blood sample followed, and two hours later a diagnosis of infection with parvovirus B19 was delivered to the registrar, alongside a full debrief about the virus and guidance on potentially vulnerable contacts. Since those early days and over the many years of clinical practice that followed, certain characteristics of this area of specialism have proved true for me again and again. *It's not just any old virus!* Making a prompt, specific diagnosis of a viral aetiology is not only scientifically satisfactory, but also extremely helpful in guiding counselling, use or avoidance of medications and interventions, and appropriate referrals. Sometimes a prompt, specific diagnosis simply provides reassurance for the patient and their treating clinician. In many cases, it ensures vulnerable contacts can be adequately protected. Frequently, it provides surveillance data that merge with country-wide statistics to inform and preserve public health. *The field evolves at a fast pace.* The medical applications of virology are in constant motion, ready to take advantage of, and in many cases driving both technological advances that improve diagnostics and new understandings that advance drug development. However, *the field is often seen as off-limits to non-specialists.* That early experience as a trainee taught me that clinical virology is typically perceived as complex to master, and the challenges can appear both interesting and difficult. The range of diagnostic tests and their use and interpretation is often bewildering for the non-specialist, and there never seems to be enough time to dive into the large textbooks or make sense of multiple but often disparate online resources. If this sounds familiar, this book will prove a perfect companion to a busy day of practice.

When Dr Brendan Crowley asked me whether I would like to read the draft chapters of his book and provide feedback on the work in progress, I could immediately see the need and benefit. A highly valued colleague of many years, Brendan and I share a common passion for clinical virology and a strong desire to make the subject less intimidating for the non-specialist and trainees in medical microbiology and public health medicine. This is a book with a mission: not just to summarise the main features of viral infections, but to attempt to translate a vast field of knowledge and experience in succinct, practical guidance. The book is organised in chapters that cover specific viruses and broader syndromes, keeping firmly in mind the scenarios that are most likely to occur in general practice. The content spans common presentations such as gastroenteritis, skin rashes, influenza and infectious mononucleosis, while also giving consideration to specific populations, including pregnant women and travellers. The structure of the book allows the reader to dip in each chapter individually according to need. Clinical vignettes are drawn from everyday practice and prove effective in framing the discussion around the essential points. Each chapter briefly describes key scientific and clinical data as a background to the more practical aspects: the most common differential diagnoses, which test to use and how to interpret the results, and how to manage the patient in terms of treatment, infection control, and if indicated, application of public health measures to family and other contacts.

I am grateful for Brendan's efforts towards explaining the topic of virology and its practice in primary care. I enjoyed reading each chapter of the book, and I feel sure that trainees in medical microbiology and colleagues in general practice, for whom the book was primarily conceived, will find it an essential guide to clinical virology, and a valuable tool for good clinical decision-making.

Anna Maria Geretti
MD PhD FRCPath
Professor of Virology and Infectious Diseases
United Kingdom

LABORATORY-BASED DIAGNOSIS OF COMMON VIRAL INFECTIONS SEEN IN GENERAL PRACTICE

CLINICAL SYNDROME	Virus	Specimen required
GASTROENTERITIS	Norovirus	Send faeces sample
	Rotavirus	Send faeces sample
	Adenovirus	Send faeces sample
	Calicivirus	Send faeces sample
	Astrovirus	Send faeces sample
CLINICAL SYNDROME	**Virus**	**Specimen required**
GENITAL INFECTION	Herpes simplex virus (HSV)	Send viral swab for HSV 1 & 2 DNA
CLINICAL SYNDROME	**Virus**	**Specimen required**
HEPATITIS (ACUTE)	Hepatitis A (HAV)	Serum for anti-HAV IgM / IgG
	Hepatitis B (HBV)	Serum for HBsAg and other HBV markers
	Hepatitis C (HCV)	Serum for HCV Antibody and HCV Core Antigen
	Hepatitis E (HEV)	Serum for anti-HEV IgM / IgG
	Cytomegalovirus (CMV)	Serum for anti-CMV IgM / IgG
	Epstein Barr Virus (EBV)	Serum for EBV VCA IgM / IgG
CLINICAL SYNDROME	**Virus**	**Specimen required**
INFECTIOUS MONONUCLEOSIS-LIKE ILLNESS	EBV	Serum for EBV VCA IgM / IgG Alternatively, send plasma for Monospot test - interpret with haematological findings such as absolute lymphocytosis and/or atypical lymphocytosis
	CMV	Serum for anti-CMV IgM / IgG
	Toxoplasma gondii	Serum for anti-*T. gondii* IgM / IgG
	HIV 1 & 2	Serum for HIV 1 & 2 Antigen / Antibody

CLINICAL SYNDROME	Virus	Specimen required
MUMPS	Mumps	≤ 7 days since onset of parotitis send oral fluid for mumps virus RNA. More than 7 days since onset of illness, send serum for anti-mumps virus IgM / IgG
CLINICAL SYNDROME	Virus	Specimen required
RESPIRATORY TRACT VIRAL INFECTIONS	Influenza A & B	Send viral swab from nose & throat for Influenza A & B RNA
	Respiratory Syncytial Virus (RSV)	Send viral swab from nose & throat for RSV RNA
	Parainfluenza Virus (PIV)	Send viral swab from nose & throat for PIV RNA
	Human Metapneumovirus (HMPV)	Send viral swab from nose & throat for HMPV RNA
	Adenovirus	Send viral swab from nose & throat for Adenovirus DNA
CLINICAL SYNDROME	Virus	Specimen required
VESICULAR SKIN LESIONS	Enterovirus	Send viral swab from lesion for Enterovirus RNA
	Herpes simplex virus (HSV)	Send viral swab from lesion for HSV 1 & 2 DNA
	Varicella-zoster virus (VZV)	Send viral swab from lesion for VZV DNA
CLINICAL SYNDROME	Virus	Specimen required
MACULOPAPULAR RASH	Parvovirus B19 (slapped cheek)	Send serum for anti-B19 IgM / IgG
	HHV6 (exanthemsubitum)	Send oral fluid for HHV6 DNA
	Enterovirus	Send oral fluid for Enterovirus RNA
	Measles	Oral fluid for measles RNA or viral throat swab for measles virus RNA and serum for anti-measles virus IgM / IgG
CLINICAL SYNDROME	Virus	Specimen required
LUMPS & BUMPS	'Farmyard pox'	Clinical diagnosis. Otherwise, contact laboratory
	Molluscum contagiosum (MC)	Clinical diagnosis. Otherwise, contact laboratory
	Warts	Clinical diagnosis. Otherwise, contact laboratory

CLINICAL SYNDROME	Virus	Specimen required
TRAVEL-RELATED ARBOVIRAL INFECTIONS	Dengue (DENV)	Serum for anti-DENV IgM / IgG
	Chikungunya (CHIKV)	Serum for anti-CHIKV IgM / IgG
	West Nile fever (WNF)	Serum for anti-WNF IgM / IgG
	Zika (ZIKV)	If symptomatic or within 4 weeks of last possible exposure, send plasma & urine for ZIKV RNA and serum for anti-ZIKV IgM / IgG If more than 4 weeks since last possible exposure, send serum for anti-ZIKV IgM / IgG only

GASTROENTERITIS (VIRAL)

- Norovirus
- Rotavirus

NOROVIRUS

What is norovirus infection?

Globally, noroviruses are the commonest cause of acute gastroenteritis, in all age groups *(1)*. They are synonymous with 'Norwalk-like viruses' and 'winter vomiting virus'. While infections are reported throughout the year, activity peaks during the winter months. In Ireland, there are frequent notifications of norovirus outbreaks from nursing homes, community hospitals and long-stay units *(2)*. The incidence of illness is highest among those aged < 5 years *(3)*. However, norovirus-related morbidity and mortality are significant in those aged over 65 years. Immunocompromised individuals may develop chronic norovirus infection *(4)*.

What vocabulary is used when describing clinical and epidemiological features of norovirus?

Noroviruses have a single-stranded RNA genome and belong to the family *Caliciviridae*. They are classified in the *Norovirus* genus which, on the basis of molecular analysis, is divided into genogroups and genotypes. Human infection is associated with viruses belonging to three genogroups (designated GI, GII and GIV) each of which is further subdivided into many genotypes by amino acid analysis of two proteins, the major viral capsid protein (VP1) and RNA-dependent RNA polymerase (RdRp) *(5)*. Thus, for example, noroviruses belonging to genogroup II and genotype 4 are designated as GII.4. Genotypes can be further sub classified into variants: GII.4, which is the commonest circulating genotype globally, has at least seven variants.

CASE VIGNETTE

A 66-year-old woman phoned her GP to say that she and her 70-year-old husband had sudden onset of vomiting and diarrhea, mainly non-bloody diarrhoea, six days previously. Her illness had now settled but her husband, who had chemotherapy 10 weeks ago for a haematological malignancy, still had watery diarrhoea. The couple developed symptoms 36 hours after the visit of their 18-month-old grandson who had a bout of vomiting and diarrhoea while at their home.

How were the two cases managed?

LABORATORY DIAGNOSIS

How was norovirus infection confirmed?

Diagnosis of norovirus was confirmed by detection of viral RNA in faecal samples using a real-time reverse transcription polymerase chain reaction (rRT-PCR) assay. Further molecular analysis showed infection with norovirus GII.4. Viral gastroenteritis may be difficult to distinguish from bacterial infection on clinical findings alone *(1)*. Molecular assays are the current gold standard for confirmation of bacterial and viral gastrointestinal infections because of their excellent performance characteristics. In the case of noroviruses, these assays differentiate genogroups GI and GII *(4)*. Novel variants may, however, emerge due to genetic drift, and may be missed by some molecular assays, hence the need to distribute proficiency panels regularly to laboratories to ensure accurate detection of emergent noroviruses *(6)*.

What other enteric pathogens were tested for in this case?

Molecular testing was performed for other viral pathogens causing similar clinical features including Rotavirus A, Sapovirus, Astrovirus and Adenovirus F40/41. Molecular assays were also done for bacterial pathogens including *Campylobacter* spp, *Salmonella* spp, *Shigella* spp, shiga toxin-producing *Escherichia coli* and *Clostridium difficile* toxin B gene but no other viral or bacterial enteric pathogen was identified.

CLINICAL PRESENTATION

What is the typical course of norovirus infection?

Two thirds of norovirus infections manifest clinically as mild to severe diarrhoeal illness while the rest are asymptomatic *(7)*. After an incubation period of 12 to 72 hours, there is usually a sudden onset of watery diarrhoea and/or vomiting and abdominal pain, almost always accompanied by fever, headache, myalgia and malaise. In otherwise healthy individuals, the illness typically resolves in two to three days *(8)*. In the very young and elderly however, particularly those with underlying comorbidities, complications may occur including severe dehydration, acute renal failure and cardiac dysfunction *(4)*.

Why did the elderly couple in this case have more prolonged illnesses?

Age and immune status predisposed to severity of norovirus infection in this couple. Both patients were aged over 65 years, a group associated with higher norovirus-related morbidity and mortality *(9)*. It is thought that age-related decline in immune function accounts for more prolonged infection. Similarly, immunocompromised individuals may develop chronic symptomatic norovirus infection (> 4 weeks' duration). Resolution of chronic norovirus infection seems to coincide with appearance of strain-specific blocking antibody in serum during immune reconstitution *(10)*.

What is the relationship between clinical presentation and pathogenesis of norovirus infection?

Noroviruses infect cells in the small intestine causing histopathological changes including villous blunting, crypt cell proliferation and inflammatory cell infiltration: diarrhoea is due to malabsorption *(11)*. Severe symptoms are more likely in those with robust antiviral immune responses as indicated by higher proinflammatory cytokine levels in serum of those with clinical illness compared to the levels among those infected asymptomatically *(12)*.

TREATMENT

Was an antiviral agent available to treat norovirus infection in this elderly couple?

No antivirals are currently licensed for treatment of norovirus infection. Management is primarily supportive and aims to restore hydration. The 70-year-old immunocompromised gentleman was hospitalised for intravenous rehydration and correction of electrolyte imbalance, and all immunosuppressive drugs were stopped until recovery. Use of oral nitazoxanide (see below), was considered but his diarrhoea settled within a few days of admission, probably due to immune reconstitution.

What potential antiviral therapeutic options are available?

Anecdotally, nitazoxanide, an anti-parasitic drug licensed for treatment of *Cryptosporidium* spp and *Giardia lamblia*, has been used for treatment of chronic norovirus illness in immunocompromised persons, with favourable results in some cases *(13, 14)*. Furthermore, a systematic review showed nitazoxanide to be beneficial in treatment of viral gastroenteritis, including norovirus infection, in immunocompetent children. However, further evaluation of its safety and effectiveness is required *(11, 15)*. Recently, favipiravir, an oral agent used to treat influenza, gave some symptomatic relief when used to treat chronic norovirus infection in an immunocompromised host *(16)*. Oral ribavirin and oral human serum immunoglobulin appear to have therapeutic potential in the treatment of norovirus in immunocompetent and immunocompromised hosts, but more data are needed to evaluate these options *(1, 17)*.

TRANSMISSION AND INFECTION CONTROL

What was the most likely route by which the elderly couple acquired norovirus?

Noroviruses are transmitted most commonly by the faecal-oral or vomitus-oral routes either indirectly through contaminated hands, fomites or environmental surfaces, or by direct contact with infected persons or ingestion of aerosolised virus generated during vomiting *(4)*. The 18-month-old grandson, who had vomiting and diarrhoea 36 hours before onset of illness in his grandparents' home, was the likely source of infection. A less likely source in this case was food borne transmission from food contaminated at source, especially shellfish and fresh fruits like raspberries, and then consumed undercooked or raw. An infected food handler may contaminate food after it has been cooked *(18)*.

What infection control advice was given to the elderly couple?

Both were advised that they were infectious during the symptomatic period and for at least 48 hours after resolution of illness. Visitors were discouraged unless it was absolutely necessary. Both patients were advised to wash their hands frequently with soap and running water for at least 20 seconds, and told not to prepare meals for others. Because noroviruses can persist in the environment, advice was given on disinfection of surfaces likely to be contaminated such as toilets, door handles, remote controls, and kitchen utensils and surfaces, using sodium chlorite (chlorine bleach) at a concentration of 1,000 ppm to 5,000 ppm (dilution of household bleach 1:50 to 1:10) *(4, 19)*.

Why are noroviruses so infectious?

It is estimated that the dose of norovirus needed to cause infection in humans (infectious dose) is low, ranging from only 18 to 2800 viral particles *(20, 21)*. During the first five days after symptom onset, huge viral loads are shed in faeces and vomitus probably corresponding to the period of peak infectivity *(22)*. Furthermore, some infected cases may shed the virus before onset of illness. Moreover, noroviruses remain stable and potentially infectious in the environment for several days after contamination. Their relative resistance to many common disinfection protocols facilitates persistence on surfaces *(23, 24)*.

SUSCEPTIBILITY AND IMMUNITY

Why was this elderly couple susceptible to infection with norovirus strain GII.4?

Susceptibility to norovirus infection is determined by host genetics and any pre-existing immunity. Most people infected with norovirus are genetically susceptible to infection with common circulating viral strains like GII.4 because these viruses bind to histoblood group antigens (HBGAs) on gut mucosal epithelium to establish infection and cause disease *(11)*. A functional fucosyltransferase 2 enzyme (encoded by *FUT2* gene) partly controls expression of HBGAs: individuals producing this enzyme are known as secretor-positive and are innately susceptible to infection *(25)*. In contrast, nonsecretors (i.e. persons in whom expression of HBGAs on gut epithelium is absent due to mutations in the *FUT2* gene) are resistant to infection with many strains of noroviruses. However, protection against norovirus infection is incomplete in nonsecretors because some less commonly circulating viruses can still infect the gut epithelium by binding to cell receptors other than HBGAs *(26)*.

Do antibodies to noroviruses prevent infection?

Yes, the presence of strain-specific antibodies, which block binding of virus to HBGAs, decreases the risk of infection when secretor-positive individuals are exposed to that particular strain of virus *(27, 28, 29)*.

Why were the two elderly persons infected when they had already been exposed to noroviruses throughout their lifetimes?

Following infection with a viral genotype or GII.4 variant, immunity develops which is genotype-specific. Therefore, immunity against other genotypes, even those within the same genogroup, or against emerging variants of GII.4, is limited, even negligible *(27, 30)*.

How long does immunity to the infecting strain of norovirus usually last?

Norovirus-blocking antibodies appear about one week after infection. Protection persists for at least six months and it may last as long as nine years *(4)*.

REFERENCES (*useful reviews)

1 K.Bányai *et al.*, *Lancet.* **392**, 175 (2018)*

2 Health Protection Surveillance Centre; Infectious Intestinal Diseases; April 2018

3 G. Phillips *et al.*, *Am. J.Epidemiol.* **171**, 1014 (2010)

4 C.V.Cardemil, U.D.Parashar, A.J. Hall.*Infect. Dis.Clin. N. Am.* **31**, 839 (2017)*

5 A.Kroneman *et al.*, *Arch.Virol.* **158**, 2059 (2013)

6 B.L. Rooney *et al.*, *Virol. J.* **11**,129 (2014)

7 C.I. Gallimore *et al.*, *J.Clin.Microbiol.42*, 2271 (2004)

8 R.I. Glass, U.D. Parashar, M.K. Estes. *N. Engl. J. Med.* **361**, 1776 (2009)*

9 F. Mattner *et al.*, *Clin.Microbiol. Infect.* **12**, 69 (2006)

10 B.M. Knoll *et al.*, *Infection.* **44**, 551 (2016)

11 R.L.Atmar, S. Ramani, M.K. Estes. *Curr.Opin. Infect. Dis.* **31**, 422 (2018)*

12 K.L. Newman *et al.*, *Clin. Exp.Immunol.* **184**, 347 (2016)

13 K. Bok, K.Y. Green. *N. Engl. J. Med.* **368**, 971 (2013)

14 K.Haubrich, S. Gantt, T. Blydt-Hansen.*Pediatr.Transplant.***22**, e13186 (2018)

15 E.M. Tan *et al.*, *Int. J. Travel Med. Glob.Health.***5**, 107 (2017)

16 C. Ruis *et al.*, *N. Engl. J. Med.***379**, 2173 (2018)

17 L.K. Brown *et al.*,*Rev. Med.Virol.*doi; 10.1002/rmv.1926 (2017)*

18 A.J. Hall *et al.*, *Emerg. Infect. Dis.***18**, 1566 (2012)

19 A.J. Hall *et al.*, *MMWR Recomm. Rep.* **60**, 1 (2011)

20 P.F. Teunis *et al.*, *J. Med.Virol.* **80**, 1468 (2008)

21 R.L. Atmar *et al.*, *J. Infect. Dis.* **209**, 1016 (2014)

22 R.L. Atmar *et al.*, *Emerg. Infect .Dis.* **14**, 1553 (2008)

23 J.Barker, I.B. Vipond, S.F. Bloomfield.*J. Hosp. Infect.* **58**, 42 (2004)

24 E. Duizer*et al.*,*Appl. Environ.Microbiol.* **70**, 4538 (2004)

25 R. Currier *et al.*, *Clin. Infect. Dis.* **60**, 1631 (2015)

26 J. Nordgen *et al.*, *PLOS Pathog.* **12**, e1005385 (2016)

27 M. Malm *et al.*, *J. Infect. Dis.* **210**, 1755 (2014)

28 R.L. Atmar *et al.*, *Clin.Vaccine Immunol.* **22**, 923 (2015)

29 A. Reeck *et al.*, *J. Infect. Dis.* **202**, 1212 (2010)

30 M. Saito *et al.*, *Clin. Infect. Dis.* **58**, 483 (2014)

ROTAVIRUS

What is rotavirus infection?

Rotavirus (RV) is the leading cause of acute gastroenteritis in children < 5 years of age worldwide. It is estimated that over 200,000 deaths annually are RV-related, mainly in developing countries in Africa and Asia, and despite availability currently of two licensed rotavirus vaccines *(1)*.

What should the GP know about the virology of RV?

RV is a non-enveloped double-stranded RNA (ds RNA) virus of the family *Reoviridae*. The RNA genome has 11 segments, each of which encodes at least one protein, including structural viral proteins (designated VP) that have a role in forming the structure of the virus, and non-structural proteins (designated NSP) that either have a role in viral replication or act as an enterotoxin *(2)*. Ten RV species (A – J) have been identified so far on the basis of molecular and antigenic differences in structural viral protein 6 (VP6) *(3, 4)*. However, RV species A (designated RVA) is the commonest circulating group of RV in humans and is the focus of this review. This viral species is further classified into many genotypes based on molecular analysis of RNA segments encoding two proteins found on the viral surface, VP7 (termed G for glycoprotein) and VP4 (termed P for protease cleaved protein). Both VP7 and VP4 are represented in rotavirus vaccines and induce neutralising and protective antibody responses *(4)*. Almost 90% of clinical infections with RVA are attributed to six combinations of G types and P types with the following nomenclature: G1P[8], the commonest strain globally, G2P[4], G3P[8], G4P[8], G9P[8] and G12P[8] *(4, 5)*.

EPIDEMIOLOGY

Who usually presents to the GP with RVA infection?

It is mainly young children who present with RVA infection. Nearly every child in developing countries and developed nations will have had an episode of RVA-related gastroenteritis by 5 years of age. In general, susceptibility to RVA-related disease is highest among those aged < 24 months, though in neonates < 12 weeks old infection is usually subclinical or mild. This is probably due to protection from maternally-acquired antibody *(4)*. Children are typically infected several times with RVA in early life, with progressive development of broader immunity to other strains of the virus after each episode of symptomatic or asymptomatic reinfection *(6)*. In fact, it is rare for children to be hospitalised more than once for severe RVA infection *(7)*. Therefore, RVA infection in older children and adults is usually mild or subclinical. Severe disease may however occur among the elderly and immunocompromised individuals *(1)*. Outbreaks of RVA-related gastroenteritis also occur among young children attending créches and on paediatric wards in hospitals (16 were notified in Ireland in 2017) *(8)*. Furthermore, outbreaks of RVA disease can occur occasionally among elderly residents in congregated living settings, such as nursing homes and community hospitals/long-stay units. Episodes of intrafamilial spread of RVA have been reported.

What is the mortality rate due to RVA disease?

In general, RVA-related fatalities are rare in developed countries. Most (> 90%) of fatal RVA infections occur among young children in sub-Saharan Africa and Asia, probably related to limited access to health care for rehydration therapy and significant comorbidities like malnutrition *(4, 9)*.

Is RVA-related gastroenteritis seasonal?

There are between 1,500 and 2,300 notifications of RVA infection annually in Ireland with peak numbers of cases notified typically between March and May each year, similar to seasonality observed in other developed countries. In contrast, RVA infections occur throughout the year in tropical countries *(10)*.

CASE VIGNETTE

A 30-month-old girl was brought to the GP by her mother because of a 48-hour history of vomiting, non-bloody diarrhoea, fever and lethargy. Although vomiting persisted, it became less frequent; however herdiarrhoea worsened, increasing to 12 episodes daily. There was no recent history of travel abroad. The child had not been immunised against RVA. On physical examination, she was febrile (38.5°C) and had evidence of mild-to-moderate dehydration. The GP suspected viral gastroenteritis and recommended oral rehydration immediately. Nevertheless, 20 hours later she was referred to hospital for intravenous rehydration after which she was discharged home. Her four-year-old sister also developed diarrhoea 72 hours after illness onset in the index case which was laboratory-confirmed as RVA infection. Her 10-year-old brother, an adoptee from Mexico, remained asymptomatic.

What can the GP learn from this case?

LABORATORY DIAGNOSIS

How was RVA infection confirmed?

Viral infection was rapidly confirmed by detection of RVA antigen in stool samples using an immunochromatographic assay (similar to a pregnancy test). This type of rapid diagnostic test is usually accurate during active infection when the amount of virus shed in stool is very high ($\geq 10^{10}$ viral particles/g of faeces) *(11)*. The result was later confirmed by real-time reverse transcription polymerase chain reaction (rRT-PCR).

Sequence analysis in this case identified the virus as the commonest strain of RVA circulating in humans, G1P [8].

What other enteric pathogens were tested for in this case?

No other viral or bacterial enteric pathogen was identified on routine diagnostic testing of faeces. Molecular testing was performed concurrently on the stool sample for other viral pathogens causing similar clinical features including Norovirus, Sapovirus, Astrovirus and Adenovirus F40/41. In addition, molecular assays were also done as part of routine diagnostics for common bacterial pathogens including *Campylobacter* spp, *Salmonella* spp, *Shigella* spp, shiga toxin-producing *Escherichia coli* and *Clostridium difficile* toxin B gene.

CLINICAL FEATURES

Was the course of clinical illness typical of RVA-related gastroenteritis in children?

While prolonged vomiting and non-bloody diarrhoea suggested viral infection rather than a bacterial aetiology, laboratory testing was needed to confirm RVA infection. The clinical manifestations of RVA infection vary from a mild, transient diarrhoeal illness to severe gastroenteritis. Illness usually begins after an incubation period of 24–72 hours with acute onset of fever and vomiting usually followed 24 hours later by non-bloody diarrhea *(12)*. Sometimes respiratory illness is present which may reflect coinfection with respiratory viruses *(13)*. Gastrointestinal symptoms resolve typically within a week *(14)*.

Which RVA-related clinical complications may be seen in general practice?

Prolonged vomiting and diarrhoea in otherwise immunocompetent young children may lead to severe dehydration (> 10% loss of body weight) accompanied by electrolyte imbalance. Convulsions may occur with high fever and abnormal electrolytes. A recent study showed that RVA infection in children was associated with a higher likelihood of hospitalisation compared to gastroenteritis caused by other viral pathogens. Encephalopathy was a feature in a small proportion of cases (6%) in the study *(15)*. Other infrequent complications associated with RVA infection in children include shock, encephalitis, intussusception, features of Kawasaki disease and transient biochemical hepatitis *(12)*.

In which groups is severe RVA disease likely to be seen in general practice?

Although the illness course may be severe in any child, severe RVA disease has been associated with prematurity, low birth weight and malnutrition *(16)*. In children with profound cellular immune deficiencies like severe combined immunodeficiency disorder (SCID) and recipients of solid-organ and haematopoietic stem cell transplantation, a prolonged and severe course of illness may occur *(12)*.

PATHOGENESIS

How does RVA cause vomiting and diarrhoea?

Malabsorption and secretory mechanisms are involved in causing RVA-related clinical disease. The virus replicates rapidly in enterocytes lining the small intestine leading to their destruction. Impairment of dissacharidases in cells lining intestinal villi leads to accumulation of undigested sugars in the gut lumen thereby causing osmotic diarrhoea (4). In addition, viral non-structural protein 4 (NSP4) is a putative enterotoxin that activates the enteric nervous system. This, in turn, increases intestinal motility and also induces secretory diarrhoea by stimulating crypt cells in villi to secrete sodium chloride and water into the gut lumen (1, 17). Vomiting is thought to be caused by viral stimulation of enterochromaffin cells in villi leading to release of 5-hydroxytryptamine which activates vagal afferent nerves and the vomiting centre in the brainstem (18).

MANAGEMENT

How did the GP approach management of the index case?

The GP assessed the hydration status of the 30-month-old child and diagnosed mild-to-moderate dehydration on the following clinical grounds: her general appearance was restless and she was irritable to touch; her tongue was dry; her eyes were slightly sunken and shed few tears; skin pinch test was decreased with prolonged capillary refill time. He recommended oral rehydration solution (ORS) immediately. However, 20 hours later he referred her to hospital for intravenous rehydration due to parental concerns about their child's persistent diarrhoea, even though the GP observed that her hydration status had improved. Referral for intravenous or enteral rehydration is generally limited to those with severe dehydration (> 10% loss of body weight) that is refractory to oral rehydration therapy, abnormal neurological findings including seizures and encephalitis, and hypovolaemic shock, or ileus (12, 19, 20, 21, 22).

Is any antiviral available currently to treat a case like this?

No, although use of oral nitazoxanide has been proposed, it is not recommended currently for the routine treatment of RVA infection as further confirmatory data are needed (4). However, nitazoxanide has potential as an effective therapeutic option in management of acute RVA infection in immunocompetent children and possibly in immunocompromised hosts (23, 24, 25, 26).

TRANSMISSION AND INFECTION CONTROL

What were the likely routes of spread of RVA between siblings in this case?

Transmission of RVA between the two sisters was probably by the faecal-oral route, for example through contaminated fingers or contaminated fomites like toys. The virus is highly contagious, only needing ingestion of a low number of viral particles (10^2 to 10^3) to cause disease in susceptible persons *(27)*. In addition, it is hypothesised that aerosolisation of viral particles during vomiting is a potential route of RVA transmission and may explain the ubiquity of the virus among children in both developed and developing countries regardless of standards of sanitation, as well as contributing to spread in institutions *(1)*.

What advice should be given to prevent viral spread within the household?

Household transmission of RVA is common *(28)*. Recommendations are similar for rotavirus and for norovirus: infected children are infectious during the symptomatic period and for at least 48 hours after resolution of illness. Visits to the house should be discouraged. Frequent hand washing with soap and running water for at least 20 seconds is advised, particularly before eating meals. Advice should be given on disinfection of surfaces likely to be contaminated such as toilets, door handles and toys using soap and water followed by sodium chlorite (chlorine bleach) at a concentration of 1,000 ppm to 5,000 ppm (dilution of household bleach 1:50 to 1:10) *(29)*.

PREVENTION BY VACCINATION

What are the reasons for the 10-year-old boy in this case having remained asymptomatic?

It is likely that the combination of previous vaccination against RVA in Mexico and cumulative immunity protected him against clinical disease. Vaccination against RVA is the most important means of protection against severe disease. He was fully vaccinated as an infant while resident in a Mexican orphanage, and he was probably reinfected with RVA several times during his lifetime. This would have induced further development of heterotypic immunity against RVA.

For information on vaccination schedule in Ireland, contraindications and side-effects, including risk for intussusception, see

http://www.hpsc.ie/hpsc/A-Z/VaccinePreventable/Vaccination/

What types of RV vaccines are available currently?

Two live attenuated RV vaccines (RVVs) are currently licensed in Ireland. Rotarix (GlaxoSmithKline), is an attenuated human RVA carrying genes encoding one strain of VP7 and VP4, G1 and P [8], respectively. This monovalent vaccine (RV1) is used in the national immunisation programme. Rotateq, which is made by Merck, is a pentavalent vaccine (RV5). Each viral component is composed of 10 cow RV genes with one of five human RVA genes produced by reassortment. One of the reassortant vaccine viruses carries the gene encoding one variant of VP4 of human RVA, P[8] while each of the other four reassortants carries a gene encoding a variant of VP7 of RVA, G1, G2, G3 and G4 *(30)*.

Are current RVVs effective in developed countries?

The efficacy of RVVs in clinical trials in developed countries was shown to be excellent, as high as 95%, in protecting against severe disease *(31, 32)*. In the United Kingdom, introduction of RV1 vaccine in 2013 was associated with decreased incidence of acute gastroenteritis, particularly in communities with significant socioeconomic deprivation *(33)*.

Should infants be given RVVs if pregnant women and immunocompromised persons live in the same household?

Yes, vaccination of infants should be encouraged. Any potential risk from exposure of pregnant women or immunocompromised hosts to the vaccine, an attenuated (weakened) viral strain, is preferable to natural infection with RVA which causes clinical disease. RVV is shed in faeces for up to 14 days post-vaccination *(34)*. Pregnant women and immunocompromised contacts should, in particular, observe strict hand hygiene precautions when changing nappies of infants in the 14 days post-RVV. RVVs are not teratogenic.

Can immunocompromised children be immunised with RVVs?

While it is contraindicated in children with severe combined immunodeficiency syndrome (SCID), its benefit may outweigh any theoretical adverse effect for those with other immunocompromised disorders, and therefore an individual benefit-risk assessment should be done by the child's paediatrician *(35)*. Immunisation with RVVs is recommended in HIV-positive infants in whom it has been shown to be safe *(36)*.

Is there a need to give an RVV to an infant who had a past laboratory-confirmed RVA infection?

Yes, natural infection with RVA only induces partial immunity, therefore immunisation will further stimulate broader immunity when administered according to the recommended schedule.

REFERENCES (*useful reviews)

1 S.E. Crawford *et al.*, *Nat. Rev. Dis. Primers.* **3**, 17083 (2017)*

2 R. Dóró *et al.*, *Expert Rev. Anti Infect.Ther.***13**, 1337 (2015)*

3 J. Matthijnssens *et al.*, *Arch.Virol.* **157**, 1177 (2012)

4 K. Bányai *et al.*, *Lancet.* **392**, 175 (2018)*

5 N. Santos, Y. Hoshino. *Rev. Med.Virol.* **15**, 29 (2005)

6 F. Velázquez *et al.*, *N. Engl. J. Med.* **335**, 1022 (1996)

7 K. Johansen *et al.*, *Scand. J. Infect. Dis.* **40**, 958 (2008)

8 Health Protection Surveillance Centre; Annual Epidemiological Report; August 2018

9 J.E. Tate *et al.*, *Clin. Infect. Dis.* **62**Suppl 2, S96 (2016)

10 M.M. Patel *et al.*, *Pediatr. Infect .Dis. J.* **32**, e134 (2013)

11 J. Kaplon *et al.*, *J.Clin.Microbiol.***53**, 3670 (2015)

12 U.D. Parashar, E.A.S. Nelson, G. Kang. *BMJ.***347**, f7204 (2013)*

13 C.D. Brandt *et al.*, *J.Clin.Microbiol.***23**, 177 (1986)

14 M. Gurwith *et al.*, *J. Infect. Dis.* **144**, 218 (1981)

15 K.Karampatsas *et al.*, *PLOS One.* **13**, e194009 (2018)

16 H.I. Huppertz, N. Salman, C. Giaquinto. *Pediatr. Infect. Dis. J.* **27**Suppl 1**,** S11 (2008)

17 M. Lorrot, M Vasseur.*Virol. J.* **4**, 31 (2007)

18 M. Hagbom *et al.*, *PLOS Pathogen.* **7**, e1002115 (2011)

19 A. Guarino *et al.*, *J.Pediatr.Gastroenterol.Nutr.***59**, 132 (2014)

20 C.K. King *et al.*, *MMWR Recomm. Rep.* **52**, 1 (2003)

21 WHO http://whqlibdoc.who.int/publications/2005/9241593180.pdf;

22 J. Van den Berg, M.Y. Berger. *BMC Fam.Pract.* **12**, 134 (2011)

23 E.M. Tan *et al.*, *Int.J. Travel Med. Glob.Health.* **5**, 107 (2017)

24 J.F. Rossignol *et al.*,*Lancet.* **368**, 124 (2006)

25 C. Teran, C. Teran-Escalera, P Villarroel. *Int. J. Infect.***13**, 518 (2009)

26 S. Mahapatro *et al.*, *J. Trop. Med.* **2017**, 7942515 (2017)

27 R.L. Ward *et al.*, *J. Infect. Dis.* **154,** 871 (1986)

28 M. Senecal *et al.*, *Can. J. Infect. Dis. Med.Microbiol.* **19**, 397 (2008)

29 R.M. Burke *et al.*, *Morb.Mortal. Wkly. Rep.* **67**, 470 (2018)

30 P.H. Dennehy. *Clin.Microbiol. Rev.* **21**, 198 (2008)*

31 T.Vesikari *et al.*, *N. Engl. J. Med.* **354**, 23(2006)

32 G.M. Ruiz-Palacios *et al.*, *N.Engl. J. Med.***354**, 11 (2006)

33 D. Hungerford *et al.*, *BMC Med.* **16**, 10 (2018)

34 E.J. Anderson. *Lancet Infect. Dis.* **8**, 642 (2008)

35 L. Rubin *et al.*, *Clin. Infect. Dis.* **58**, 309 (2014)

36 A.D. Steele *et al.*, *Pediatr. Infect. Dis. J.* **30**, 125 (2011)

GENITAL INFECTION (COMMON VIRAL CAUSES)

- Anogenital Warts
- Herpes Simplex Virus

ANOGENITAL WARTS

What are anogenital warts?

Anogenital warts (also known as genital warts or condylomata acuminata) are benign proliferative lesions on the skin and mucous membranes of the genitals and anus caused by infection with human papillomaviruses (HPVs).

What is the natural history of anogenital warts?

Infection is acquired when micro abrasions in the skin and mucous membranes of the anogenital area allow HPV-infected epithelial cells from an infected individual to infect the basal cell layer in skin and mucous membranes of the sexual contact. This usually occurs during vaginal and anal intercourse but also during oral sex resulting in HPV infection of the mouth and throat (1). Perinatal transmission of HPV from an infected mother to her neonate resulting in disease can also occur, albeit rarely (2). The incubation period for anogenital warts is usually about3 months although it may vary from 2 weeks to 18 months (3, 4). Spontaneous regression of these lesions occurs in many cases in the absence of treatment in the first year after diagnosis (5). Resolution of lesions is thought to be mediated by HPV-specific T cells, although there is increasing evidence that the virus may persist in a latent form in basal epithelium of skin and mucous membranes with periodic reactivation, particularly in the elderly and immunosuppressed individuals (6).

Which types of HPV are associated with anogenital warts?

HPV types can be classified as 'low-risk' or 'high-risk' depending on their potential to become cancerous. 'Low-risk' types of HPV, mainly HPV-6 and -11, are the main causative agents of anogenital warts (7). In addition, HPV types 6 and 11 are potential causes of warts in extra-genital sites such as the conjunctiva, nose, mouth and larynx (2, 8). However, 'high-risk' HPV types, including HPV-16, -18, -31, -33 and -35, which have oncogenic potential, may co-infect anogenital warts together with HPV types 6 and 11 (9). While HPV infection causing condyloma acuminate is predominantly self-limiting, individuals with a history of anogenital warts were found to have a significantly increased risk of anogenital and head and neck cancers on 10-year follow-up (10, 11). This excess risk of neoplasia may relate to behavioural factors, like excess alcohol intake and smoking, but also persistent infection with co-infecting 'high-risk' types of HPV which, after regression of anogenital warts, may lead to neoplasia (2, 11).

EPIDEMIOLOGY

What is the epidemiology of anogenital warts?

HPV infection, both symptomatic and asymptomatic, is the most common sexually transmitted infection globally (12). It is estimated that the annual incidence of anogenital warts is 1% in sexually active populations with an estimated lifetime risk of 10% *(13)*. The prevalence of HPV is highest in adults < 25 years of age and then declines until around 50 years of age, but is then followed by a second peak which may be due to renewed sexual activity with new partners resulting in infection with HPV types to which the individual was not previously exposed *(13)*.

What has been the impact of the introduction of HPV vaccination on HPV prevalence?

In general, data suggest that the introduction of female HPV vaccination has had a beneficial effect by decreasing the incidence of genital HPV infections, precancerous cervical lesions and anogenital warts in young women and men *(14)*. The incidence of cervical cancer will probably decline in the future since both the cause (HPV infection) and occurrence of high-grade cervical intraepithelial neoplasia are decreasing significantly due to the impact of HPV vaccination programmes *(14)*. Six years after the introduction of the quadrivalent HPV vaccination programme (protects against HPV types 6, -11, -16, -18) in the United States, the prevalence of those four HPV types decreased by 64% and 34% among females aged 14 to 19 years and 20 to 24 years, respectively *(15)*. A similar trend in HPV prevalence following introduction of HPV programmes was observed in the United Kingdom and Australia *(16, 17)*. Moreover, Australia is the first country to report a significant decline in the incidence of juvenile-onset recurrent respiratory papillomatosis, attributed to the effectiveness of its national quadrivalent HPV vaccination programme *(18)*.

CLINICAL FEATURES

What are the typical clinical presentations of patients with anogenital warts?

Patients usually present with otherwise symptomless skin lesions which vary from small, flat-topped papules to large exophytic masses on the skin of the genitals and anogenital mucosa *(19)*. Small lesions (1 – 5 mm diameter) usually occur in clusters but may form plaques which are seen in immunocompromised hosts and diabetics *(20)*.

Warts are usually flesh-coloured but sometimes appear reddish-brown (pigmented) *(21)*. The lesions are typically found on the penis shaft in circumcised males and in the preputial cavity of those who are uncircumcised. Other locations of warts include the urethral meatus, scrotum, groin, perineum and perianal skin. In females, genital warts usually occur in the labia, pubis, clitoris, urethral meatus, perineum and perianal skin *(20)*. Internal warts can be found in mucous membranes of the vagina, urethra, ectocervix, mouth and anal canal *(21)*. Warts in the anal canal present mainly in those who had receptive anal intercourse or a history of receptive anodigital insertion *(22)*. Patients with warts frequently suffer emotional distress and a sense of stigma, which may result in socio-sexual dysfunction. Pain, bleeding, dyspareunia or interference with defaecation and urinary obstruction may also occur *(19)*.

What uncommon clinical conditions occur with anogenital warts?

Juvenile-onset recurrent respiratory papillomatosis is an uncommon condition due to infection with HPV types 6 or 11 following vertical transmission to the neonate at birth *(23)*. Verrucous lesions on the larynx recur frequently and may even extend to the lower respiratory tract with fatal consequences *(24)*. Bowenoid papulosis is an uncommon premalignant condition of anogenital warts which presents as reddish-brown papules on skin in the anogenital area and is associated predominantly with HPV 16 infection *(20)*. A rare, low-grade, differentiated form of squamous cell carcinoma, thought to be associated with both low-risk and high-risk HPV types, presents as giant verrucous lesions (known as Buschke and Lowenstein tumours) in the anogenital area *(25)*.

What other conditions should be considered in the differential diagnosis of anogenital warts?

There are many dermatoses which need to be considered as well as premalignant and neoplastic lesions. The following are some of these conditions, both infectious and noninfectious, with some distinguishing features *(19)*: molluscum contagiosum usually appears as pearly flesh-coloured lesions with a central umbilication *(26)*; smooth purple papules or plaques are typical of lichen planus *(27)*; small (about 1mm diameter) pearly penile papules typically seen on the glans penis are normal *(20)*; condylomata lata due to treponemal infection may have verrucous features and are seen on moist mucous membranes *(19)*; Fordyce spots are flesh-colored spots found on the scrotum and vulva *(20)*; smooth, annular plaques are suggestive of granuloma annulare *(28)*; seborrhoeic dermatosis is characterised by keratotic plugs and brown pigmentation *(19)*; vulvar intraepithelial neoplasia may appear as a pigmented irregular plaque on the vulva; squamous cell carcinoma may appear verrucous *(19)*.

DIAGNOSIS

How are anogenital warts diagnosed?

Diagnosis of anogenital warts is made by visual inspection under bright light and, if the lesions are small, examination should be aided with a magnifying lens or colposcope where the characteristic papillary form with punctate capillaries can be seen *(20)*.

There is a role for histopathological examination of biopsy material to confirm the diagnosis of condyloma acuminatum if the lesion has atypical features including pigmentation, induration, fixed to underlying structures or ulceration *(2, 19)*.

Furthermore, biopsy should be considered if the diagnosis is uncertain, particularly in immunosuppressed individuals, or if lesions are refractory to appropriate treatment *(2, 21)*. There is no recommendation for HPV typing as it has no impact on management of anogenital warts. Testing of patients for other sexually transmitted infections is mandatory.

TREATMENT

Do all patients with anogenital warts request treatment of the lesions?

Anogenital warts cause emotional distress so nearly all patients are likely to request treatment, even if the lesions are asymptomatic. Warts are rarely itchy or painful. While warts can resolve spontaneously within 1 year of onset, HPV transmission to sexual partners may still occur when lesions have cleared due to subclinical shedding of HPV-infected cells (29, 30).

What treatment modalities are available for patients with anogenital warts?

Topical, surgical and ablative approaches are used to treat anogenital warts. However, no single therapy for anogenital warts is regarded as the gold standard since therapies vary in their effectiveness (31). Selection of a treatment modality depends on the number, size, site and morphology of the lesions as well as the adverse effects of the therapies and needs of the individual (19, 20). Individuals with condylomata acuminata who are pregnant, immunosuppressed or children should be referred to a specialist physician (20). Topical treatments can be safely applied by patients such as imiquimod, podophyllotoxin and sinecatechins. Physician-applied treatment is commonly cryotherapy, but may include trichloroacteic acid and surgical removal as well as electrosurgery, laser, curettage and scissors excision (20, 31). Irrespective of treatment modality, clinical evidence indicates that after primary clearance of lesions, recurrence of warts within 6 months of treatment may appear at a frequency of 30% to 70%, including warts at sites different to those treated initially, reflecting failure of lesion-directed therapies to treat subclinical infection in surrounding tissue (31).

Which treatments are commonly used for management of anogenital warts?

Imiquimod is an immunomodulator i.e. it induces a local cell-mediated immune response by stimulating production of interferon and other cytokines locally. It is available as a 5% cream which is applied by the patient to lesions on alternate nights for three nights until the warts resolve (2). Although imiquimod is not regarded as teratogenic, more data are needed before its use is recommended in pregnancy. Podophyllotoxin acts by inhibiting cell division within warts causing tissue necrosis (31). It is available in the form of a 0.5% solution or 0.15% cream. It is applied to warts twice daily for three days then stopped for four days. This weekly cycle is repeated for weeks. Podophyllotoxin is more successful in treatment of non-keratinised warts. Furthermore, podophyllotoxin is contraindicated in pregnancy and its use should be stopped in other patients who develop ulceration. Sinecatechins are chemicals in extract of green tea leaves used for treatment of anogenital warts. They may have important antiviral and antitumour properties (32). Recent evidence suggests that use of sinecatechins and imiquimod sequentially may achieve rapid and sustained clearance of anogenital warts (10).

Chemical cautery using trichloroacetic acid (TCA) 80% - 90% solution is useful for small numbers of non-keratinised lesions including vaginal and anal warts. It is important to avoid application of excess TCA due to corrosion of non-infected tissue; physicians should apply this caustic substance and have liquid soap or sodium bicarbonate ready in case of accidental spillage (31). TCA is applied weekly for an average of 6 to 10 weeks (20). TCA can be used safely in pregnancy. An ablative therapy such as cryotherapy acts by thermal-induced cytolysis (19). Cryotherapy is usually applied once weekly for a maximum of 4 weeks with high clearance rates reported (about 80%) (33). It is useful for treatment of multiple small warts on the penis and vulva (31). Electrosurgery is an effective destructive approach but use of appropriate ventilation is required as smoke emanating from the treated lesion contains HPV particles similar to that generated when using carbon dioxide laser surgery (2). Carbon dioxide laser treatment is useful for treatment of warts in the urethral meatus and anal canal when lesions are extensive (19). However, clearance and recurrence rates are not encouraging (31).

Surgical treatment is considered a last resort nowadays but is useful if an extensive area is involved or they are large thereby causing obstruction and requiring immediate removal (19, 31). Clearance rates as high as 93% with recurrence rates of 29% at 1-year post-treatment have been reported (19, 29).

What are the treatment options for internal warts at the following sites:

Vaginal – Cryotherapy or TCA or electrosurgery

Cervical – Cryotherapy or TCA or electrosurgery or laser ablation or excision

Urethral meatus – Cryotherapy or electrosurgery or laser ablation or surgery

Intra-anal warts – TCA or electrosurgery or laser ablation

All of these options are recommended in a European guideline (20).

Which options are available if warts are refractory to treatment?

If there is no response to more than one treatment modality, review the differential diagnoses and consider referral for a biopsy (19, 33).

What approach is needed for management of a pregnant woman with anogenital warts?

While anogenital warts may become extensive in pregnancy, routine treatment is not obligatory and does not necessarily prevent transmission to the neonate (2). Maternal history of anogenital warts is a risk factor for juvenile-onset recurrent respiratory papillomatosis but the overall risk is low and is not reduced by caesarean section (34). However, if there is risk of pelvic obstruction during labour or bleeding from friable warts, prophylactic caesarean section or treatment with cryotherapy or surgical excision should be considered (2, 19).

How are immunosuppressed individuals with anogenital warts managed?

Increased number, large size of warts, high frequency of recurrence and refractoriness to treatments are features of this condition in immunosuppressed hosts. While the approach to treatment of warts should be similar to that for immunocompetent individuals, there should be a strong index of suspicion for malignancy and a low threshold for referral of suspicious cases for biopsy, particularly those which proliferate rapidly and/or ulcerate *(2, 19)*.

Do sexual contacts of those diagnosed with anogenital warts need follow-up?

Partners should be informed but testing them for HPV is of no value as it is likely they already have been subclinically infected with HPV. A partner in a relationship may develop condylomata acuminata following transmission of HPV from the other person who is already infected subclinically and, therefore, does not indicate sexual contact outside of the relationship *(2, 21)*.

REFERENCES (*useful reviews)

1 J.G. Baseman, L.A. Koutsky. *J. Clin. Virol.* **32** (S1), S16 (2005)

2 K.A. Workowski, G.A. Bolan. *MMWR Recomm. Rep.* **64**, 84 (2015)*

3 R.L. Winer *et al.*, *J. Infect. Dis.* **191**, 731 (2005)

4 I.U. Park, C. Introcaso, E.F. Dunne. *Clin. Infect. Dis.* **61** (S8), S849 (2015)

5 L.S. Massad *et al.*, *Obstet. Gynecol.* **118**, 831 (2011)

6 G.A. Maglennon, P.B. McIntosh, J. Doorbar. *J. Virol.* **88**, 710 (2014)

7 D.R. Brown *et al.*, *J. Clin. Microbiol.* **37**, 3316 (1999)

8 K. Sonawane *et al.*, *Ann. Intern. Med.* **167**, 714 (2017)

9 S.M. Garland *et al.*, *J. Infect. Dis.* **199**, 805 (2009)

10 H. Schofer *et al.*, *Int. J. STD AIDS.* **28**, 1433 (2017)

11 M. Blomberg *et al.*, *J. Infect. Dis.* **205**, 1544 (2012)

12 C.C. de Camargo *et al.*, *Open AIDS J.* **8**, 25 (2014)

13 H. Trottier, E.L. Franco. *Vaccine.* **24**(S1), 4 (2006)

14 M. Drolet *et al.*, *Lancet.* doi.org/10.1016/S0140-6736(19)30298-3 Published June 26 (2019)*

15 L.E. Markowitz *et al.*, *Pediatrics.* **137**, e20151968 (2016)

16 M. Checchi et al., *Sex. Transm. Infect.* doi: 10.1136/sextrans-2018-053751 (2019)

17 S.N. Tabrizi *et al.*, *Lancet Infect. Dis.* **14**, 958 (2014)

18 D. Novakovic *et al.*, *J. Infect. Dis.* **217**, 208 (2018)

19 J.B. Karnes, R.P. Usatine. *Am. Fam. Physician.* **90**, 312 (2014)*

20 C.J.N. Lacey *et al.*, *J. Eur. Acad. Dermatol. Venereol.* **27**, e263 (2013)*

21 C.M. Kodner, S. Nasraty. *Am. Fam. Physician.* **70**, 2335 (2004)

22 C. Sonnex *et al.*, *BMJ.* **303**, 1243 (1991)

23 D.A. Larson, C.S. Derkay. *APMIS.* **118**, 450 (2010)

24 N.N. Venkatesan, H.S. Pine, M.P. Underbrink. *Otolaryngol. Clin. North Am*. **45**, 671 (2012)

25 P. Ramdass, S. Mullick, H.F. Farber. *Prim. Care Clin. Office Pract*. **42**, 517 (2015)

26 R. Lee, R.A. Schwartz. *Cutis*. **86**, 230 (2010)

27 J.M. Teichman, M. Mannas, D.M. Elston. *Am. Fam. Physician*. **97**, 102 (2018)*

28 V. Madan, M. Gangopadhyay, G. Dawn. *Clin. Exp. Dermatol*. **34**, 433 (2009)

29 H.W. Buck. *Clin. Evid*. **15**, 2149 (2006)

30 D.J. Wiley. *Clin. Evid*. **9**, 1741 (2003)

31 V.R. Yanofsky *et al*., *Expert Rev. Dermatol*. **8**, 321 (2013)*

32 S.M. Meltzer, B.J. Monk, K.S. Tewari. *Am. J. Obstet. Gynecol*. **200**, 233.e1 (2009)

33 N. Scheinfeld, D.S. Lehman. *Dermatol. Online J*. **12**, 5 (2006)

34 M.J. Silverberg *et al*., *Obstet. Gynecol*. **101**, 645 (2003)

GENITAL HERPES

What is the meaning of the term genital herpes?

The most common cause of genital ulcers worldwide is herpes simplex virus (HSV) infection of anogenital skin and mucous membranes.

Outline the virology of herpes simplex viruses known to cause genital ulcers.

There are two strains of herpes simplex virus, type 1 (HSV-1) and type 2 (HSV-2), within the family *Herpesviridae*. These DNA viruses are genetically quite similar but have sufficient differences to allow distinction between them serologically *(1)*.

PATHOGENESIS

How does herpes simplex virus generally cause infection?

Herpes simplex virus (HSV) is usually acquired following direct contact with an individual who has HSV lesions (which may or may not be recognised) or is shedding the virus asymptomatically. HSV infects epithelial cells in the skin or mucous membranes following entry via micro abrasions at the sites. It replicates within these cells and may manifest as vesicles with an erythematous base *(2)*. These vesicles are filled with inflammatory cells and exudate containing large amounts of viral particles. The virus is neurotropic and invades sensory nerve endings innervating the infected area. In the sensory nerve, the virus travels in a retrograde manner along the axon to the sensory ganglion in which it may establish latency. HSV may also spread to local and regional lymph nodes on primary infection *(3)*. Resolution of HSV infection occurs with the development of a cellular immune response. HSV-specific T cell response is important as shown by the potential for cutaneous and visceral dissemination of HSV in persons with deficiency of the cellular immune system *(4)*.

What is meant by the term HSV reactivation? Does it matter in clinical practice?

HSV reactivation matters in terms of clinical disease and viral transmission to others. HSV establishes a persistent infection for life in the sensory ganglia following resolution of infection. HSV-1 infection usually involves the orofacial region with the trigeminal ganglion being the common site of latency, while for HSV-2, the sacral nerve ganglia (S2 – S5) are typically involved *(5)*. Cellular immunity maintains the virus in a state of dormancy. However, throughout life HSV may reactivate with shedding of virus from the areas of skin and mucosa innervated by nerves from latently-infected ganglia *(6)*. As a general rule, HSV-1 is the cause of recurrent infections above the waist line, whereas HSV-2 causes recurrences below the waist (e.g. genital area and buttocks) *(5)*.

EPIDEMIOLOGY OF GENITAL HERPES

Why is HSV-1 a frequent cause of genital herpes?

Both HSV-1 and HSV-2 are now common causes of genital herpes. HSV-1 is usually acquired in childhood via nonsexual contact and is the main cause of orofacial herpes. In contrast, HSV-2 is mainly acquired by sexual transmission and, historically, has chiefly caused genital herpes. However, primary HSV-1 infection is increasingly recognised as contributing significantly to the aetiology of genital herpes [7]. In 2016, 1,369 cases of genital herpes were notified to public health authorities in Ireland of which 61% and 36% were laboratory-confirmed as HSV-1 and HSV-2, respectively [8]. The explanation for this trend towards HSV-1-related genital herpes has been attributed to the large cohort of adolescents who lack antibodies to HSV-1 and acquire the virus at the time of sexual debut [9]. Furthermore, oral-genital sexual practices are likely contributory factors by transmitting HSV-1 from the mouth to genital sites of uninfected partners [2, 9].

TYPES OF GENITAL HERPES INFECTION

Primary: initial infection of an individual with either HSV-1 or HSV-2 when that person has no preexisting antibodies to HSV-1 and HSV-2.

Nonprimary: initial infection with HSV-1 in an individual who already has antibody to HSV-2 or initial infection with HSV-2 in a person with preexisting antibodies to HSV-1.

Recurrent: reactivation of latent HSV-1 in a person with preexisting antibodies to HSV-1 or reactivation of latent HSV-2 in a person who is already HSV-2-seropositive.

Does knowledge of the type of genital HSV infection matter in clinical practice?

Yes, severity of infection and frequency of recurrence can vary with the type of genital HSV infection. Many individuals probably acquire genital herpes subclinically followed by episodes of symptomatic reactivation [10]. In those who are symptomatic, primary genital HSV infection is more severe than nonprimary infection: in other words, the clinical course of a first-time HSV-2 infection is attenuated to some extent in the presence of preexisting antibody to HSV-1 [11]. The rate of recurrent HSV-2 genital infection (about four recurrences per year) is about four-fold higher than that of HSV-1 [12]. However, the frequency of clinical reactivation of HSV-2 (70% to 90%) within the first year after primary infection decreases thereafter in most patients, although some may continue to have multiple symptomatic recurrences for ≥ 10 years [11]. Between clinical episodes of recurrent infection, HSV-2 can be shed subclinically and intermittently in the anogenital area with transmission to sexual contacts [13].

CASE VIGNETTE

A female teenager attended her GP with a crop of fluid-filled blisters on her vulva and perineum. Two days before onset of the lesions, she developed a burning sensation around the genital area. Seven days before her presentation to the clinic she had unprotected sexual intercourse with a male. The GP suspected genital herpes. What are the important learning points for GPs?

LABORATORY DIAGNOSIS

Was it necessary in this case to confirm genital herpes by laboratory testing?

Yes, laboratory confirmation is advised for all suspected cases of genital herpes *(7, 14)*. Differentiation between HSV-1 and HSV-2 is important because appropriate counselling is needed for patients with HSV-2 infection in whom a higher frequency of recurrent genital herpes occurs and the risk of recurrences is more protracted over time *(11)*. Furthermore, clinical manifestations of primary genital herpes caused by HSV-1 and HSV-2 are indistinguishable. Clinical diagnosis of genital herpes by experienced physicians may be unreliable in patients with lesions suggestive of genital herpes disease *(7, 10)*. Other infections such as syphilis and, albeit rarely, chancroid, cause diseases with similar symptoms and signs as genital herpes *(2)*. A unilateral vesicular, painful and pruritic rash in the perineal area would suggest genital herpes zoster *(15)*.
Lymphogranuloma venereum is another potential mimicker of genital herpes, albeit very uncommon except in men who have sex with men (MSM).

Which laboratory test was performed by the GP to diagnose genital herpes in this case?

HSV-2 infection was confirmed. A viral swab collected from genital lesions was tested for HSV-1 and HSV-2 DNA by real-time polymerase chain reaction (PCR) which is the optimal assay for diagnosis of genital herpes because its sensitivity and specificity approach 100% *(16, 17)*.

Is there a serology test available for detection of antibody specific to HSV-1 and HSV-2?

Yes, HSV IgG type-specific (TS) serological assays are available but are not indicated for routine diagnostics: a viral swab for PCR is the current gold-standard. Advice should be sought from the genitourinary medicine (GUM) clinic before requesting HSV IgG TS serology.

Was HSV IgG TS serological testing done in this case?

Yes, a serum sample was collected when she attended the GUM clinic 10 days after presenting to the GP. The TS serology test was used to identify if it was a primary, nonprimary or recurrent HSV-2 infection. The serum sample was HSV-1 /-2 IgG negative, confirming primary HSV-2 infection (remember HSV-2 DNA was detected in the viral swab). It takes a minimum of two weeks and possibly as long as 12 weeks for type-specific IgG antibody to be reliably detected following primary infection with HSV-1 or HSV-2, therefore a viral swab for PCR is the diagnostic test of choice *(18, 19)*.

Is testing for IgM antibody to HSV-1 or HSV-2 of diagnostic value for primary genital herpes?

No because IgM antibody to HSV cannot distinguish between HSV types and may be detected coincidentally during recurrent genital or orofacial herpes infection *(20)*.

What other tests were done by the GP in this case?

The GP collected serum for hepatitis B surface antigen, syphilis screen, human immunodeficiency virus 1 & 2 antigen/antibody testing. A vaginal swab was collected and sent for *Chlamydia trachomatis* and *Neisseria gonorrhoeae* molecular testing.

When might the GP be asked by the GUM clinic to test patients for HSV IgG TS antibody?

It is helpful for asymptomatic persons who report having a sexual partner with genital herpes. A serum sample negative for HSV-1 IgG and HSV-2 IgG indicates susceptibility to genital infection with HSV-1 and HSV-2. Asymptomatic sexual contacts of individuals with a history of HSV-2 genital herpes are at risk of infection if they are found to be negative for HSV-2 IgG. Referral to a genitourinary medicine (GUM) clinic for counselling regarding transmission risk should be considered.

For women who present with a genital ulcer at any stage in pregnancy which is confirmed by PCR as HSV-1 or HSV-2 (see chapter on HSV in pregnancy). HSV IgG TS serology is done to determine whether it is a primary HSV-1 or HSV-2 infection because of its implications for management of delivery of the baby.

CLINICAL FEATURES OF GENITAL HERPES

Is the clinical presentation in the case vignette typical of genital herpes?

Yes, although almost 90% of individuals with genital HSV infection are asymptomatic, the 'typical' clinical manifestations in those with primary HSV-1 or HSV-2 infection include the appearance of crops of papules and vesicles, mostly bilateral, on the genitalia, perineum, perianal region and upper thighs which usually ulcerate before healing within 14 to 21 days *(21, 22)*. The incubation period is typically 4 to 7 days following sexual exposure *(23)*. Patients may complain of pain, burning sensation and pruritus while proctitis may be a feature in MSM *(24)*. Furthermore, those with primary genital herpes may have accompanying systemic illness with complaints of headache, malaise, fever or localised lymphadenopathy *(2, 21)*.

What other clinical manifestations of genital herpes may be seen by the GP?

Recurrent genital disease

Recurrent genital disease may be associated with a prodrome of pruritus and paraesthesia hours to days before appearance of papules and vesicles but clinical manifestations are milder and usually resolve within 5 to 10 days *(11)*. Genital herpes should be suspected in cases of recurrent, unexplained symptoms that patients often report as 'itching', 'allergy' or 'tingling'. Recurrences may occur frequently in any area innervated by sacral nerve ganglia, including buttocks and thighs, and may present as areas of excoriation or fissures similar to candidalintertrigo *(25)*.

Herpetic whitlow

This can be an extragenital manifestation of genital herpes which occurs most commonly on fingers following self-inoculation from herpetic lesions. It is important to advise patients with primary herpes to be cautious about hand hygiene.

Benign recurrent lymphocytic meningitis (BRLM)

The eponymous term for BRLM is Mollaret's meningitis. This is a rare, self-limiting condition characterised by recurrent (3 to 10) short episodes of fever and meningism that resolve spontaneously *(26)*. Episodes of BRLM vary in their frequency occurring weeks to months and, sometimes, even years apart *(27)*. Although HSV-2 is the commonest identified viral cause, genital herpetic lesions may not be present at the time of presentation with meningitis *(28)*. Because of the self-limiting nature of the illness, treatment of acute episodes with aciclovir is of questionable value. While long-term suppressive antiviral treatment for HSV-2-related BRLM is not recommended, the opinion of an infectious disease physician should be sought *(28)*.

ANTIVIRAL TREATMENT

Was treatment of the teenager in the vignette with an antiviral commenced?

Yes, valaciclovir 500 mg twice daily for five days was prescribed for the patient. In the meantime, she was referred to a GUM clinic for follow-up. Antiviral treatment should always be considered for treatment of initial symptomatic episodes of suspected genital herpes *(2)*. A proportion of immunocompetent persons with mild disease initially may still progress to severe genital ulceration *(20)*. Treatment with oral antivirals was shown to reduce significantly the duration of lesions, viral shedding and severity of clinical illness with the maximum benefit achieved when started within 72 hours of onset of lesions *(11)*.

What are the antiviral treatment options for first clinical episodes of genital herpes?

Oral treatment options for initial genital herpes include the following nucleoside analogues which inhibit viral replication: aciclovir; valaciclovir which is a valine ester prodrug of aciclovir with the advantage of higher bioavailability, and famciclovir which is a highly bioavailable prodrug of penciclovir *(29)*. Antiviral regimens of potential value include one of the following *(30)*:

Aciclovir 400 mg three times daily for 5 days

Aciclovir 200 mg five times daily for 5 days

Valaciclovir 500 mg twice daily for 5 days

Famciclovir 250 mg three times daily for 5 days

If clinical response is poor then the duration of antiviral treatment may be extended (30).

Was treatment with a topical antiviral considered in this case?

No, topical application of aciclovir is not recommended for first or recurrent episodes of genital herpes and confers no advantage when combined with oral acyclovir *(20, 30)*.

How would you manage the teenager if she developed recurrent genital herpes?

Refer her to a GUM clinic. In general, for persons with clinical episodes of recurrent genital herpes, mainly due to HSV-2, treatment can be approached in one of two ways: episodic treatment or suppressive treatment, each of which is associated with improvements in health-related quality of life *(20, 30, 31)*.

Explain the term 'episodic treatment' of recurrent genital herpes?

The episodic approach to recurrent genital herpes involves patient-initiated antiviral treatment within 24 hours of recognition of prodromal symptoms and preferably prior to development of papules. Its purpose is to attenuate the clinical course of recurrent genital herpes and is considered an option for those with mild or infrequent recurrences *(20, 30)*.

Which regimens are recommended for episodic antiviral treatment of recurrent genital herpes?

Several regimens are available including the following *(30)*:

Aciclovir 800 mg three times daily for 2 days

Valaciclovir 500 mg twice daily for 3 days

Famciclovir 1 g twice daily for one day which is the most convenient *(32)*.

Other regimens are also available *(20)*.

Explain the term 'suppressive treatment' of recurrent genital herpes?

Suppressive treatment in this clinical scenario involves long-term daily oral administration of an antiviral to prevent symptomatic genital recurrences and to reduce viral transmission rates *(30)*. Among those with frequent recurrences of genital herpes, suppressive antiviral treatment can reduce recurrent episodes by 70-80% *(33)*.

What did the GP advise her when she began a relationship with a new partner 12 months later?

The GP advised her to inform her new partner that she had a history of genital herpes before starting a sexual relationship. The male partner did not have a history of genital HSV. He was referred to the GUM clinic and tested for type-specific HSV IgG. He was HSV-2 IgG negative whereas she was HSV-2 IgG positive, known as serological discordance. To reduce HSV-2 transmission the following measures were advised: antiviral suppressive treatment of the infected partner, sexual abstinence when prodromal symptoms are present and during active infection until lesions have healed, and consistent condom use.

What suppressive antiviral treatment was recommended in this case?

Long-term use of valaciclovir 500 mg once daily was recommended for the female in this case when it was shown that her new partner was susceptible to HSV-2. The duration of suppressive treatment is unknown but should be reassessed annually *(20)*.

What other points should be highlighted when discussing genital herpes with patients in general practice?

Genital herpes is generally a mild condition, however, the GP should be aware of the potential for adverse psychological impact on the patient. A referral to GUM services should always be considered to provide advice and reassurance, and diminish the psychological burden of being told that the infection is for life. Antiviral suppression is a way of making a newly diagnosed patient feel in control of their condition while they come to terms with it. Genital herpes is of significant concern for women who acquire primary infection in the third trimester of pregnancy due to the risk of transmission to the neonate, and for immunocompromised individuals due to the risk of disseminated disease.

Useful information for patients at info@herpes.org.uk

https://www.hse.ie/eng/services/list/2/gp/antibiotic-prescribing/conditions-and-treatments/genital/genital-conditions.html.

REFERENCES (*USEFUL REVIEWS)

1 A. Dolan *et al.*, *J. Virol*. **72**, 2010 (1998)

2 R. Gupta, T. Warren, A. Wald. *Lancet*.**370**, 2127 (2007)*

3 D.W. Kimberlin, D.J. Rouse. *N. Engl. J. Med.* **350**, 1970 (2004)*

4 S. Kusne*et al.*, *J. Infect. Dis*. **163**, 1001 (1991)

5 A. Wald *et al.*, *N. Engl. J. Med.* **342**, 844 (2000)

6 K.E. Mark *et al.*, *J. Infect. Dis*. **198**, 1141 (2008)

7 D.I. Bernstein *et al.*, *Clin. Infect. Dis*. **56**, 344 (2013)

8 Health Protection Surveillance Centre. Genital herpes report. HPSC 2016

9 H. Bradley *et al.*, *J. Infect. Dis*. **209**, 325 (2014)

10 A. Langenberg *et al.*, *N. Engl. J. Med.* **341**, 1432 (1999)

11 J.W. Gnann Jr, R.J. Whitley.*N. Engl. J. Med.* **375**, 666 (2016)*

12 J. Benedetti, L. Corey, R. Ashley. *Ann. Intern. Med.* **121**, 847 (1994)

13 G.J. Mertz. *J. Infect. Dis*. **198**, 1098 (2008)

14 A. Wald, R. Ashley-Morrow. *Clin. Infect. Dis*. **35**Suppl 2, S173 (2002)

15 C.J. Birch *et al.*, *Sex. Transm. Infect*. **79**, 298 (2003)

16 M. Ramaswamy *et al.*, *Sex. Transm. Infect*. **80**, 406 (2004)

17 J. Kuypers *et al.*, *J. Clin. Virol*.**62**, 103 (2015)

18 R. Ashley-Morrow, E. Krantz, A. Wald.*Sex.Transm. Dis*. **30**, 310 (2003)

19 R. Ashley-Morrow *et al.*, *J. Clin. Virol*.**36**, 141 (2006)

20 K.A. Workowski, G.A. Bolan. *MMWR Recomm. Rep*. **64**, 1 (2015)*

21 J.G. Beauman. *Am. Fam. Physician*. **72**, 1527 (2005)

22 J.A. Schillinger *et al.*, *Sex. Transm. Dis*. **35**, 599 (2008)

23 L. Corey *et al.*, *Ann. Intern. Med.* **98**, 958 (1983)

24 M. Bissessor *et al.*, *Sex. Transm. Dis*. **40**, 768 (2013)

25 C. Johnston, L. Corey. *Clin.Microbiol. Rev*. **29**, 149 (2016)*

26 M. Shalabi, R.J. Whitley. *Clin. Infect. Dis*. **43**, 1194 (2006)

27 P.J. Poulikakos *et al.*, *J. Infect. Public Health*.**3**, 192 (2010)

28 Y. Schlesinger *et al.*, *Clin. Infect. Dis*. **20**, 842 (1995)

29 C.M. Perry, D. Faulds. *Drugs*.**52**, 754 (1996)

30 R. Patel *et al.*, *Int. J. STD AIDS*. **26**, 763 (2015)*

31 K.H. Fife, J. Almekinder, S. Ofner. *Sex.Transm. Dis*. **34**, 297 (2007)

32 F.Y. Aoki *et al.*, *Clin. Infect. Dis*. **42**, 8 (2006)

33 L. Corey *et al.*, *N. Engl. J. Med.* **350**, 11 (2004)

34 C. Celum *et al.*, *N. Engl. J. Med.* **362**, 427 (2010)

HEPATITIS (VIRAL)

- Hepatitis A

- Hepatitis B (understanding Hepatitis B virus serology)

- Hepatitis C (understanding Hepatitis C virus serology)

- Hepatitis E

HEPATITIS A

What is hepatitis A?

Hepatitis A is an acute self-limiting infection of the liver caused by the hepatitis A virus (HAV). In general, the disease is mild and self-limiting and in young children often asymptomatic, but morbidity increases with age. In older adults, hepatitis A can be debilitating and the illness can last several months. Case fatality from fulminant hepatitis is 0.1 – 0.3% overall, but reaches 2% in older individuals and those already with chronic liver disease. A safe and effective vaccine is available, and both pre and post exposure strategies can be used to prevent infection. A chronic hepatitis A carrier state does not occur in otherwise healthy persons who acquire HAV. HAV infection has become uncommon in Ireland, but is still often imported from abroad, as below.

CASE VIGNETTE

An otherwise healthy 32-year-old male presented to his GP with a 24-hour history of fever, nausea, vomiting and mild epigastric pain. Only 4 days before visiting his GP he had returned from a 5-week holiday to Brazil. On physical examination, his temperature was 38.8°C and otherwise unremarkable. The GP sent blood samples for biochemical profile, including liver function tests, and full blood count with differential. Alanine aminotransferase (ALT) and aspartate aminotransferase (AST) levels were elevated at 2,178 IU/L (* < 41 IU/L) and 1,298 IU/L (* < 40 IU/L), respectively. Total bilirubin was 20 µM (* < 21 µM). FBC parameters were normal. The GP suspected acute viral hepatitis. The patient, who worked as a nurse, was immunised successfully in the past against hepatitis B virus (HBV) and yellow fever virus when he worked in Uganda. He was homosexual and had unprotected sexual intercourse once while in Brazil and once since his return to Ireland. He denied any illicit drug use. (*Reference range)

What lessons can be learned by GPs from this case?

LABORATORY DIAGNOSIS

What further laboratory tests were collected by the GP for investigation of acute liver injury?

Serum was sent for IgM and IgG antibody to hepatitis A virus (anti-HAV IgM / IgG), hepatitis B surface antigen (HBsAg), antibody to hepatitis C virus (HCV), HCV core antigen, IgM antibody to hepatitis E virus (anti-HEV IgM), IgG antibody to Epstein Barr virus nuclear antigen (EBNA IgG), IgM and IgG antibody to cytomegalovirus (anti-CMV IgM / IgG) and human immunodeficiency virus 1&2 antigen / antibody (HIV 1&2 Ag / Ab). A sample was sent for prothrombin time (PT) and international normalised ratio

(INR). Tests for autoimmune hepatitis (anti-nuclear, anti-smooth-muscle and anti-liver-kidney antibodies) and drug toxicology screen were not regarded as relevant.

What did the initial laboratory tests reveal?

No viral aetiology was identified initially. However, a repeat serum sample collected 96 hours after onset of symptoms confirmed acute HAV infection – anti-HAV IgM / IgG were positive. Although anti-HAV IgM was negative in the initial sample collected at presentation, it had a serology index which was a 'high-negative' i.e. the reactivity value in the sample was 0.91 just below the cutoff value of 1.00, at or above which anti-HAV IgM is defined as positive.

If acute HAV infection is suspected but anti-HAV IgM / IgG are negative, should repeat testing be considered?

Yes, among those presenting clinically with HAV infection, anti-HAV IgM is usually detectable in serum, however, occasionally it may be negative (1). Therefore, negative anti-HAV IgM / IgG in a sample collected within 5 days of illness onset does not exclude current HAV infection (2, 3). However, when anti-HAV IgM is negative in serum collected ≥5 days after onset of illness, current HAV infection is unlikely.

Why should anti-HAV IgM results be interpreted cautiously?

The prevalence of HAV disease in the developed world is low and a positive anti-HAV IgM result alone has a low positive predictive value (PPV). Furthermore, over testing for anti-HAV IgM in those who do not have acute hepatitis also lowers its PPV (4).

Do false-positive anti-HAV IgM results occur?

Yes, anti-HAV IgM may be detected in the absence of clinical and biochemical hepatitis due to many reasons. False-positive anti-HAV IgM results, which typically have low positive values, are likely due to persistence of anti-HAV IgM for many months after resolution of HAV infection or following HAV vaccination (5, 6, 7). Furthermore, false-positive IgM responses may occur during active infection with completely different infectious agents. For example, detection of false-positive anti-CMV IgM and anti-EBV VCA IgM have been reported in as many as 30% of those with true acute HAV infection while false-positive anti-HAV IgM has been reported in non-HAV illnesses (4, 8, 9). Polyclonal memory B cell stimulation occurs early in any infection, with production of antibodies against conserved regions of proteins found in many unrelated pathogens, thereby leading to false-positive antibody responses (10).

When should the GP consider testing for anti-HAV IgM / IgG?

Anti-HAV IgM /IgG testing should be restricted to situations when there is acute onset of symptoms and either jaundice or elevated ALT levels or, alternatively, in instances when there is epidemiological evidence of significant exposure of a contact to a proven index case of acute HAV (5, 11). Managing contacts of confirmed hepatitis A cases should be discussed with public health authorities who may also wish to act to prevent further spread as discussed later.

EPIDEMIOLOGY

What was the most likely route by which HAV was acquired in this case?

HAV is transmitted via the faecal-oral route, most commonly from person-to-person or from ingestion of contaminated food or water. While the incubation period ranges from 15 to 50 days, the mean incubation period is 28 days. In this case, infection was likely to be the result of one of two factors: first, travel to a country with moderate-to-high endemicity of HAV, where there is a risk of infection through ingestion of contaminated food or water; second, faecal-oral transmission through sexual activity, which is well documented, particularly among men who have sex with men (MSM)*(1, 12)*. Other risk factors for HAV infection, although unlikely in this case, include living in the same household as a case, sharing needles when using drugs and homelessness or other living conditions where adequate hygiene cannot be maintained *(13)*.

For how long was the patient infectious?

HAV cases are infectious from two weeks before to one week after the onset of symptoms. If the case had presented with jaundice, then the day of onset of icterus or dark urine or pale stools would have been the time-point from which infectivity was determined. For those who are asymptomatic but have serological evidence of recent HAV infection, the period of infectivity is estimated using the date of likely exposure and 28 days as the mean incubation period.

Should the patient have been vaccinated against HAV pre-exposure?

Yes, HAV vaccination is recommended for those travelling to areas of intermediate to high HAV endemicity such as Brazil. It is most effective if given 14 days before departure to allow immunity to develop but may be given even on the day of departure. Pre-exposure HAV vaccination is also recommended for MSM, individuals with chronic liver disease, those with clotting-factor disorders and injecting drug users *(14)*. Immunisation against HAV may be considered for staff at occupational risk for HAV such as those working in facilities caring for those with mental handicap and sewage workers.

Who gets HAV-related hepatitis in Ireland?

In Ireland, the incidence of HAV-related hepatitis is low in recent years with notification rates of about 0.8/100,000 population, similar to those in other European countries *(15)*. Most cases appear to be linked to travel to areas with intermediate-to-high incidence of HAV infection, probably acquired through ingestion of contaminated food and water. Household clusters, sometimes related to a case who returned from travel abroad, occur also. These clusters occasionally extend beyond the household, in particular when one family member attends early years education, or is a food handler. Sometimes contaminated food items also enter the domestic food chain resulting in cases. Faecal-oral transmission through sexual activity among MSM is another documented route of HAV transmission. A large HAV outbreak affected more than 4,000 persons, predominantly MSM, across Europe in 2016-18 *(16)*. In many instances, however, the source of HAV is not always identified. This is mainly because young children infected with HAV are generally asymptomatic and more likely to transmit disease, because of their inability to maintain good personal hygiene. Therefore, there may be asymptomatic individuals in a transmission chain before a clinical case occurs, and it is difficult to identify the source of infection in those situations. There could also be activities which are still unrecognised as risk factors for HAV.

PUBLIC HEALTH MANAGEMENT OF THIS CASE

Why should public health authorities be notified about HAV-related hepatitis?

HAV infection is a notifiable disease in Ireland. Rates of transmission of HAV to susceptible contacts (termed secondary transmission rates) can be as high as 50% *(17)*. However, HAV transmission to contacts of cases can be prevented by administration of post-exposure prophylaxis (PEP) with a dose of inactivated HAV vaccine, combined with human normal immune globulin (HNIG) in some cases (mainly for older adults or those with chronic liver disease) *(18)*. PEP should be given within 14 days to prevent transmission. Public health authorities will issue advice on what action to take following the notification of a HAV case.

What public health advice was given to the patient?

Person-to-person transmission of HAV occurs mainly via the faecal-oral route. Therefore, until 7 days after symptom onset, the index case was advised to adhere to scrupulous hand washing after using the toilet and to avoid preparing food for others. He was also asked to abstain from sexual activity, particularly involving anal and oral contact. Furthermore, he was excluded from attending the nursing home where he worked for 7 days after illness onset.

Who did public health identify as contacts of the index case?

On returning from Brazil, the index case lived with his elderly parents, sister and niece during the infectious period of the HAV illness. They were household contacts with whom he shared toilet and kitchen facilities. The MSM with whom he had anal and oral sex on his return to Ireland was also a contact.

The index case worked in a long-term care facility for the elderly. Was this of public health concern?

Yes because of potential transmission to residents and other staff in the facility. The index case worked as a nurse in the institution for 4 hours during the infectious phase. His duty was mainly administrative but he assisted one resident with feeding and toiletry, two activities during which HAV could be transmitted. However, a serum collected from the elderly resident showed she was immune to HAV (anti-HAV IgG positive). He did not prepare food for residents, an activity which would have placed many of them at risk. The risk of HAV transmission to his colleagues was regarded as negligible: he used the toilet only once on the premises, had no diarrhoea and washed his hands thoroughly.

What post-exposure prophylactic measures were taken by public health authorities in this case?

Hepatitis A vaccine and HNIG are each known to provide good protection against HAV infection following exposure *(19)*. Immunisation with a dose of mononvalent HAV vaccine with or without HNIG was considered for all contacts:

No PEP was given to the mother (65 years of age) of the index case because she had previous laboratory evidence of HAV immunity (anti-HAV IgG positive). If she had been HAV nonimmune, both HAV vaccine and HNIG would be given as PEP because of severity of acute HAV infection in the elderly and reduced immunogenicity of HAV vaccine in this cohort *(17, 20)*.

Younger contacts very recently exposed solely need to be offered HAV vaccine. His 26-year-old sister worked as an attendant in a home for mentally handicapped children. She was given a dose of HAV vaccine as PEP within 14 days of exposure to the index case. HAV vaccine alone is an effective PEP measure in immunocompetent persons aged 1 to 59 years, although the upper age limit for use of HAV vaccine as PEP varies, with some national guidelines not stating any age restriction *(21, 22, 23)*. In addition, as a precautionary measure, she was advised regarding hand hygiene after using the toilet and before preparing food or feeding others.

His niece, who was 18 months of age, attended a crèche. She was also immunised with HAV vaccine as PEP. In addition, as a precautionary measure, management of the crèche was advised to use enhanced hygienic practices when changing her diapers for 28 days.

The 67-year-old father of the index case, who was undergoing chemotherapy for multiple myeloma, was already known to be susceptible to HAV (anti-HAV IgG negative). However, the effectiveness of HAV vaccination alone as PEP against HAV in older age groups and immunocompromised hosts is likely to be diminished. Therefore, both HAV vaccine and HNIG were given within 14 days of exposure.

The sexual contact of the index case in the infectious period had a recent diagnosis of chronic hepatitis C (HCV). He was known to be HAV seronegative. However, HAV super infection of chronic HBV or HCV carriers or those with underlying liver disease can lead to acute liver failure. The protective value of HAV vaccine as PEP in those with underlying liver disease is unknown. Therefore, both HAV vaccine and HNIG were given to this contact. All persons who were given a dose of HAV vaccine as PEP received a second dose between 6 and 12 months later. None developed HAV-related hepatitis. Post vaccination testing for HAV IgG is not indicated because of the high rate of immunity following full vaccination which, according to mathematical models, persists for as long as 40 years in ≥ 90% of vaccinees (24).

Would PEP be considered if one of the above contacts was identified > 14 days after exposure?

Yes, although secondary transmission may have occurred already, HAV vaccination can be considered for household contacts up to 8 weeks after exposure to prevent tertiary cases of HAV. Furthermore, for those at risk of severe HAV disease, it is hypothesised that PEP with HAV vaccine and HNIG may attenuate clinical disease if given as long as 28 days after exposure (21). Public health authorities will advise how to manage contacts of cases not vaccinated within 14 days of exposure.

What about serological screening of contacts for immunity to HAV?

Serological screening of contacts for HAV immunity is generally not recommended as it can delay administration of PEP. However, it may be considered for contacts for whom HNIG would be recommended as PEP (21). Therefore, the elderly contact in the long-term facility was tested for immunity to HAV in this case. However, PEP should not be delayed beyond 14 days in order to screen.

ADDITIONAL POINTS OF INTEREST

CLINICAL FEATURES AND PATHOGENESIS

Does jaundice always develop in those with acute HAV infection?

No but severity of clinical disease tends to correlate with age. Young children (< 6 years of age) are usually asymptomatic (about 90% of cases) but they may still transmit HAV to others. When young children are symptomatic, illness is usually anicteric (1). In contrast, older children and adults usually present with abrupt onset of non-specific symptoms like fever, malaise, anorexia and vomiting after an incubation period of 15 to 50 days (mean, 28 days). Jaundice occurs in > 70% of these cases but resolves typically within 4 to 8 weeks of onset.

Does HAV clinical disease cause chronic hepatitis?

No but in a proportion (about 10%) of those in whom HAV-related hepatitis seems to have resolved, episodes of clinical and biochemical hepatitis may recur for up to a year later (25). HAV can be excreted faecally during these relapses with potential viral transmission (26). In addition, a prolonged clinical course of severe cholestatic hepatitis A infection is seen occasionally (27).

Do severe complications and extra hepatic clinical features occur with HAV infection?

Although HAV infection is rarely associated with fulminant hepatitis, those in older age groups, individuals of any age with underlying liver disease and those chronically infected with HBV and HCV, are at increased risk of liver failure with acute HAV infection *(28)*. Extrahepatitic manifestations are rarely seen in clinical practice *(29)*. Immune complex deposition is the likely pathogenesis of rare manifestations such as cutaneous vasculitis, arthritis, cryoglobulinaemia and interstitial nephritis *(1)*. Other rare complications include autoimmune haemolysis, acute cholecystitis and acute pancreatitis *(29)*.

What is the pathogenesis of HAV-related hepatitis?

It appears to be immune-mediated with hepatitis caused by a HAV-specific cellular immune response induced to control viral replication in liver cells *(30)*. Ironically, HAV-related liver failure is associated with a robust cellular immune response to the virus by the host *(31)*.

REFERENCES (*useful reviews)

1 J.A. Cuthbert. *Clin.Microbiol. Rev.* **14**, 38 (2001)

2 R. Hirata *et al.*, *Am. J. Gastroenterol.* **90**, 1168 (1995)

3 L. Thomas and the Hepatitis A Guidelines Group. Health Protection Agency UK (2009)*

4 M.L. Landry. *Clin.VaccineImmunol.* **23**, 540 (2016)

5 A. Alatoom, M.Q. Ansari, J.A. Cuthbert. *Arch. Pathol. Lab. Med.* **137**, 90 (2013)

6 E. Vidor *et al.*, *Biologicals.* **24**, 235 (1996)

7 Z. Dembek *et al.*, *MMWR Morb. Mortal. Wkly. Rep.* **54**, 453 (2005)

8 C.R. Woods .*J. Pediatric Infect. Dis. Soc.* **2**, 87 (2013)

9 A.M. Roque-Afonso, D. Desbois, E. Dussaix. *Future Virol.* **5**, 233 (2010)

10 C.L. Montes *et al.*, *J.Leukoc. Biol.* **82**, 1027 (2007)

11 L. Castrodale, A. Fiore, T. Schmidt. *Clin. Infect. Dis.* **41**, e86 (2005)

12 O. Sfetcu *et al.*, *Euro. Surveill.* **16**, pii = 19808 (2011)

13 M. Kushel. *N. Engl. J. Med.* **378**, 211 (2018)

14 http://www.hpsc.ie/hpsc/A-Z/VaccinePreventable/Vaccination/*

15 P. Carrillo-Santisteve *et al.*, *Lancet Infect. Dis.* **17**, e306 (2017)*

16 D. Werber *et al.*, *Euro.Surveill.* **22**, pii = 30457 (2017)

17 J. Whelan *et al.*, *PLOS One.* **8**, e78914 (2013)

18 I. Parron *et al.*, *Hum. VaccineImmunother.* **13**, 423 (2017)

19 J.C. Victor *et al.*, *N. Engl. J. Med.* **357**, 1685 (2007)

20 R. Link-Gelles, M.G. Hofmeister, N.P. Nelson. *Vaccine.* **36**, 2745 (2018)

21 R. Mearkle *et al* on behalf of the Hepatitis A Guidelines Working Group. PHE (2017)*

22 E. Freeman *et al.*, *Vaccine.* **32**, 5509 (2014)

23 Canadian NACI. Public Health Agency of Canada. (2016)

24 H. Theeten *et al.*, *Vaccine*. **33**, 5723 (2015)

25 O.V. Nainan *et al.*, *Clin. Microbiol. Rev.* **19**, 63 (2006)

26 M.H. Sjogren *et al.*, *Ann. Intern. Med.* **106**, 221 (1987)

27 N. Coppola *et al.*, *Clin. Infect. Dis.* **44**, e73 (2007)

28 M. Ciocca. *Vaccine.***18**, S71 (2000)

29 S.C. Matheny, J.E. Kingery. *Am. Fam. Physician*. **86**, 1027 (2012)*

30 B. Fleischer *et al.*, *Immunology*. **69**, 14 (1990)

31 G. Rezende *et al.*, *Hepatology*. **38**, 613 (2003)

HEPATITIS B VIRUS SEROLOGICAL PATTERNS SEEN COMMONLY BY THE GENERAL PRACTITIONER

BACKGROUND

What is hepatitis B?

Hepatitis B is an inflammation of the liver caused by infection with hepatitis B virus (HBV). HBV may be transmitted sexually, perinatally or percutaneously. Chronic HBV infection causes significant morbidity and mortality due to cirrhosis, liver failure and hepatocellular carcinoma (HCC). About 257 million people worldwide are chronically infected by HBV (also referred to as HBV carriers). The extent of HBV endemicity differs regionally, and may be classified as: low (< 2%), intermediate (2-7%) and high (> 8%) *(1)*.

In Ireland, most notifications of HBV infection concern migrants from countries with intermediate or high HBV endemicity. Universal infant vaccination against HBV was introduced in 2008. Vaccination is also recommended for groups at high risk of HBV infection.

VIROLOGY

What is HBV?

HBV belongs to *Hepadnaviridae*. An infectious HBV virus is enveloped and has a small, partially double-stranded, relaxed circular (rc) DNA genome. When HBV infects hepatocytes, the rc DNA is transported to the cell nucleus where it is converted to a fully double-stranded DNA molecule known as covalently closed circular DNA (cccDNA). This molecule acts as a transcriptional template for viral protein expression and HBV replication. The persistence of cccDNA in nuclei of hepatocytes and the integration of HBV DNA into host chromosomes make it difficult to eradicate HBV through treatment *(2)*. There are currently 10 genotypes of HBV (designated A – I) with distinct geographic distributions, although migration to developed countries is now changing the molecular epidemiology of HBV *(3)*.

Which HBV proteins and antibodies are of clinical significance?

Hepatitis B surface antigen (HBsAg) is a viral envelope protein and a marker of current HBV infection.

Antibody to HBsAg (anti-HBs) usually indicates past, resolved infection.

Hepatitis B core antigen is the nucleocapsid protein surrounding the HBV genome; the antigen is not yet part of routine testing and detection of serum antibody to this antigen may indicate current or past HBV infection.

Hepatitis B e antigen (HBeAg) is a nucleocapsid protein secreted from infected hepatocytes and its detection in serum is a marker of high-level viral replication. It should be noted that absence of HBeAg, with or without antibody to HBeAg (anti-HBe), is often but not always an indication of low-level viral replication.

NATURAL HISTORY

What is the course of acute HBV infection?

In Western countries, most acute HBV infections occur among young adults and are acquired sexually or through injecting drug use. Acute infections are mostly self-limited and antiviral treatment is only indicated if illness is prolonged or severe *(4)*. The incubation period of 50 – 180 days, and about 30% of adult cases develop icterus. Others remain asymptomatic or anicteric but with non-specific symptoms such as anorexia and nausea. Acute infection in infants and young children is mostly subclinical. Recovery from acute infection is mediated by a robust antiviral cellular immune response directed against viral proteins *(5)*. Hepatocellular injury, indicated by high serum ALT activities, is a manifestation of this immune response *(5)*.

Why does chronic HBV develop?

Progression from acute to chronic HBV infection is related to the age of HBV acquisition. Approximately 95% of infants (aged < 1 year), 20 – 30% of children (aged 1 – 5 years), but <5% of adults develop lifelong HBV infection *(6)*. Maturation of the immune response to HBV infection is age-dependent: young children generate weak anti-HBV immune responses in contrast to adults *(7)*. Furthermore, maternally-derived HBeAg may induce tolerance of the developing fetal immune system to HBV allowing viral persistence in perinatally infected neonates. Among adults with chronic HBV infection, there is an anti-HBV immune response but it is weaker than in those who have cleared infection, and this abrogated immune response may still be followed by hepatocellular damage *(8)*.

What are the important phases in chronic HBV infection?

Chronic infection can be classified into five phases, each reflecting the extent of interaction between HBV replication and the host's immune response.

First phase: <u>HBeAg-positive chronic infection</u>: very high HBV replication as indicated by high serum HBV DNA concentration (> 10^7 IU/mL), with normal serum ALT levels. There is no liver disease owing to immune tolerance *(4)*.

Second phase: <u>HBeAg-positive chronic hepatitis</u>: indicated by moderately high HBV DNA concentration ($10^4 - 10^7$ IU/mL) with fluctuating serum ALT levels. Active liver disease is ascribable to attempts at immune clearance of HBeAg. There is an increased risk of cirrhosis and HCC *(4)*. The appearance of anti-HBe indicates clearance of HBeAg.

Third phase: <u>HBeAg-negative chronic infection</u>: indicated by low serum HBV DNA concentration (< 2 x 10^3 IU/mL), anti-HBeseropositivity, normal serum ALT activity and inactive liver disease. Loss of HBsAg in serum can then occur spontaneously, at a rate of about 1% annually *(2)*.

Fourth phase: some patients in phase three develop <u>HBeAg-negative chronic hepatitis</u>: serum HBV DNA concentration can rise to > 2 x 10^3 IU/mL with fluctuation in serum ALT levels and reactivated liver disease. There is an increased risk of cirrhosis and HCC. Loss of HBsAg is rare.

Fifth phase: <u>resolved HBV infection</u>: there is loss of HBsAg with or without the appearance of anti-HBs. Despite clinical and serological recovery from acute or chronic infection, HBV replication persists at a very low level for decades but the host remains asymptomatic and non-infectious due to control by the primed immune system *(9)*. However, immunosuppression can induce HBV reactivation.

SUMMARY

CHRONOLOGY OF APPEARANCE OF HBV SEROLOGICAL MARKERS IN ACUTE HBV INFECTION:

HBsAg (earliest**)** then **HBeAg** (pre-clinical phase with normal ALT activity)

HBsAg, **HBeAg** & then **HBV core IgM antibody/HBV core total antibody** (symptomatic acute phase with raised ALT activity)

anti-HBe(HBeAg Negative) and later **anti-HBs** (**HBsAg Negative**) (resolved acute HBV infection).

CHRONOLOGY OF APPEARANCE OF HBV SEROLOGICAL MARKERS IN CHRONIC HBV INFECTION:

Phase 1 **HBsAg** (persists ≥ 6 months in serum) and **HBeAg** with normal ALT activity.

Phase 2 **HBsAg** and **HBeAg** with increased ALT activity. (Immune response to clear HBeAg).

Phase 3 **HBsAg** and **anti-HBe** (HBeAg negative) with normal ALT activity.

Phase 4 **HBsAg** and **anti-HBe** with increased ALT activity (reactivated liver disease).

Phase 5 **HBsAg Negative** and **anti-HBe Positive** with normal ALT activity, resolved chronic HBV infection.

IMPORTANT POINTS ABOUT MANAGEMENT OF CHRONIC HBV CARRIERS

All those with a diagnosis of chronic HBV infection should be tested for HIV, HCV and HAV. Those non-immune to HAV should be vaccinated. Testing for concomitant hepatitis delta virus (HDV) infection is important in chronic HBV carriers with low HBV DNA levels because HBV replication is suppressed by co infection with HDV. All patients with HBV infection should be seen at least initially in specialist services so that an appropriate assessment can be made.

EXAMPLES OF COMMON HBV SEROLOGICAL PROFILES IN ACUTE AND CHRONIC HBV INFECTION

A 20-year-old pre-medical student had a serum sample tested for HBsAg.

HBsAg – Positive (weak) (confirmed by neutralisation)

HBV core total antibody – Negative

HBeAg – Negative

Anti-HBe – Negative

HBV core IgM antibody – Negative

Suggestive of recent immunisation with HBV vaccine. The person was vaccinated against HBV four days before the serum sample was collected. HBsAg derived from HBV vaccine is absorbed into blood and is usually detectable in serum for up to 14 days *(10)*. The GP collected a repeat serum 10 days after the first sample: HBsAg was negative, confirming transient HBsAg positivity due to recent HBV vaccination. No public health implications.

A 24-year-old male asked the GP for a screen for HIV, HBV and syphilis following a recent holiday in Thailand. HIV and syphilis screen were negative. HBV serology was as follows:

HBsAg – Positive

HBV core total antibody – Negative

HBeAg- Negative

Anti-HBe – Negative

HBV core IgM antibody – Negative

Both recent immunisation with HBV vaccine and early (incubation-phase) HBV infection must be considered. HBsAg is the first serological marker detected in acute HBV infection. Further enquiry revealed that the patient was not vaccinated recently against HBV, and had unprotected sexual intercourse with a female sex worker seven weeks earlier. The GP collected a repeat serum one week later – HBsAg was more strongly positive and HBeAg was also detected while other HBV markers were negative. He was asymptomatic and the ALT activity was 25 IU/L (normal range < 40 IU/L). The picture is consistent with early acute HBV infection in the preclinical phase. Public health authorities were notified and appropriate measures were advised for preventing infection in exposed household and sexual contacts with a view to immunise non-immune contacts with hepatitis B immune globulin and HBV vaccine. The patient was referred to a hepatology clinic for followup.

A 23-year-old male presented to the GP complaining of abdominal pain. As part of laboratory investigations, the GP requested ALT testing, which was 400 IU/L, and hepatitis screening including HBV markers:

HBsAg- Positive

HBV core total antibody – Positive

HBeAg – Positive

Anti-HBe – Negative

HBV core IgM antibody – Positive

Suggestive of acute HBV infection. A serum sample collected 16 weeks earlier was HBsAg-negative. The current result confirms acute HBV infection, since there is HBsAg and HBeAg seroconversion and appearance of HBV core IgM antibody. The patient is homosexual and had unprotected sexual intercourse on several occasions recently. Public health authorities were notified and appropriate measures were advised for preventing infection in exposed household and sexual contacts with a view to immunise non-immune contacts, with hepatitis B immune globulin and HBV vaccine. He was referred to a hepatology clinic.

A 25-year-old male sex worker was diagnosed with HBV infection. A previous serum collected 12 months earlier was also HBsAg positive. Laboratory tests showed serum ALT of 22 IU/L and the following HBV serological profile:

HBsAg- Positive

HBV core total antibody – Positive

HBeAg – Positive

Anti-HBe – Negative

HBV core IgM antibody – Negative

Persistence of HBsAg in serum for ≥ 6 months indicates chronic HBV infection. He was referred to hepatology. Serum HBV DNA was very high (10^9 IU/mL), serum ALT activity was normal and transient elastography excluded cirrhosis, consistent with HBeAg-

<u>positive chronic infection</u>. Public health was notified. Biannual review was arranged: antiviral treatment was not recommended.

Five years later, HBV markers in samples collected from the above patient were as follows:

HBsAg- Positive

HBV core total antibody – Positive

HBeAg – Positive

Anti-HBe – Negative

HBV core IgM antibody – Positive (weak).

ALT – 230 IU/L (normal < 40 IU/L) and HBV DNA concentration - 10^5 IU/mL.

He has now developed <u>HBeAg-positive chronic hepatitis</u>. Transient elastography indicated moderate liver fibrosis. The hepatology clinic commenced antiviral treatment with entecavir in accordance with international guidelines *(11)*. Tenofovir is an alternative to entecavir. HBV core IgM positivity can occur in this phase of chronic HBV infection, reflecting immune activation against HBV.

A 40-year-old female from an African country with the following HBV serology wants to work as a nursing aide:

HBsAg – Positive

HBV core total antibody - Positive

HBeAg – Negative

Anti-HBe – Positive

HBV Core IgM – Negative

Serum ALT – 12 IU/L (normal < 40 IU/L)

She was referred to a hepatology clinic. Several tests over 4 months of follow-up indicated normal ALT levels. HBV DNA was not detected in serum. Testing for concomitant antibody to hepatitis delta virus (anti-HDV) was negative (HDV suppresses HBV replication). She had an <u>HBeAg-negative chronic infection</u>. Regardless of her serum HBV DNA and HBsAg results, she was allowed to work as a nurse's aide since her work did not involve participation in exposure-prone procedures. She was monitored annually.

A 50-year-old female with the following HBV serology:

HBsAg – Positive

HBV core total antibody - Positive

HBeAg – Negative

Anti-HBe – Positive

HBV core IgM antibody – Negative

Serum ALT - 140 IU/L (normal < 40 IU/L).

She was referred to a hepatology clinic. Serum HBV DNA concentration was 3×10^3 IU/mL. Transient elastography showed moderate fibrosis. She was diagnosed with HBeAg-negative chronic hepatitis. She was started on antiviral treatment with entecavir *(11)*.

OTHER HBV SEROLOGICAL PROFILES SEEN BY GPs

Is an immunocompetent patient with the following HBV profile infectious?

HBsAg – Negative

HBV core total antibody – Positive

No. Serology indicates a past, resolved HBV infection. However, there is a risk of HBV reactivation if the patient starts immunosuppression for an underlying illness or uses direct-acting antiviral agents for hepatitis C treatment. The GP should refer such patients to the attending physician for advice on the need for antiviral prophylaxis to prevent HBV reactivation *(11)*.

A foreign national was given a 3-dose course of HBV vaccination pre-employment and anti-HBs measured 8 weeks post vaccination:

Anti-HBs – 0 IU/L

To exclude current or past infection, the GP requested testing for HBsAg and HBV core total antibody. Both serology markers were positive, consistent with current HBV infection. HBV vaccination was inappropriate. Public health authorities were notified to follow-up contacts.

A female sex worker, known to be seronegative for HBsAg and HBV core total antibody, was given a 3-dose course of HBV vaccination:

Anti-HBs – 75 IU/L

An anti-HBs level ≥ 10 IU/L in serum collected 6-8 weeks following completion of a course of HBV vaccine signifies vaccine-induced immunity to HBV infection.

Anti-HBs level (0 mIU/mL) was found in the above individual 5 years later. Would you revaccinate her?

No need for booster doses of HBV vaccine since, in most vaccine recipients, protection lasts for at least 30 years.

A nurse, known to be seronegative for HBsAg and HBV core total antibody, was given two courses of HBV vaccine:

Anti-HBs – 0 IU/L

Patient is a non-responder to HBV vaccination. She was referred to occupational health regarding protective measures to be taken after potential exposure to HBV.

REFERENCES (*useful reviews)

1 A. Schweitzer *et al., Lancet.* **386**, 1546 (2015)

2 W.K.Seto *et al., Lancet.* **392**, 2313 (2018)*

3 S. Tong, P. Revill. *J. Hepatol.* **64** Suppl 1, S4 (2016)

4 C. Trépo, H. Chan, A. Lok. *Lancet.* **384**, 2053 (2014)*

5 A. Bertoletti, C. Ferrari. *J. Hepatol.* **64** Suppl 1, S71 (2016)

6 Y.F. Liaw, C.M. Chu. *Lancet.* **373**, 582 (2009)

7 K.N. Tsai, C.F. Kuo, J.J.Ou. *Trends Microbiol.* **26**, 33 (2018)

8 C. Seeger, W.S. Mason. *J. Hepatol.* **64** Suppl 1, S1 (2016)

9 M.P. Curry, M. Koziel. *Hepatology.* **32**, 1177 (2000)

10 C.D. Rysgaard *et al., BMC Clin. Pathol.* **12**, 15 (2012)

11 EASL 2017 Clinical Practice Guidelines on the management of hepatitis B virus infection. *J. Hepatol.* **67**, 370 (2017)*

COMMON QUESTIONS ABOUT HEPATITIS C VIRUS SEROLOGY FOR THE GENERAL PRACTITIONER

BACKGROUND

What is hepatitis C virus infection?

Hepatitis C virus (HCV) is an important cause of liver disease. Globally, 71 million people are estimated to be chronically infected, most of whom are unaware of their infection *(1)*. Liver cirrhosis, end-stage liver disease and hepatocellular carcinoma (HCC) are consequences of chronic HCV infection. Although an effective vaccine is not currently available, chronic HCV infection can be cured with direct-acting antivirals (DAAs) in the vast majority of cases *(2)*. Increased accessibility to DAAs will enhance the prospect of eliminating HCV infection worldwide *(3)*.

VIROLOGY

What is hepatitis C virus (HCV)?

HCV is an enveloped virus belonging to the family *Flaviviridae*. It has a single-stranded RNA genome encoding seven non-structural proteins and three structural proteins including one core and two envelope proteins (E1, E2). There are seven known genotypes (GTs) of HCV (designated GT 1 to 7) circulating globally. Each genotype has a number of subgenotypes suffixed by a letter, for example, HCV GT 3a and GT 3b *(4)*. The distribution of genotypes varies worldwide. GT1 and subgenotypes GT 1a and 1b predominate in Europe, Asia and the Americas *(5)*. Identification of HCV genotype is important in selection of antiviral treatment, although with availability of DAAs active against all genotypes (pangenotypic), this consideration is becoming less applicable *(4)*. In people infected with a particular HCV genotype the genetic diversity of the virus is high. This diversity contributes to evasion of the host's antiviral immune response and to development of antiviral resistance *(6)*. Due to ease of the virus escaping drug pressure, curative DAA regimens must comprise combinations of agents targeting different steps of the viral life cycle, typically two agents.

EPIDEMIOLOGY

What is the prevalence of HCV in Ireland?

In Europe, the prevalence of chronic HCV infection ranges from 0.4% to 5.2% with lower rates in western and northern countries than in Eastern Europe *(7)*. In Ireland, like the United Kingdom, the prevalence of chronic HCV infection among adults in the general population is relatively low (0.57%) *(8)*.

How is HCV transmitted?

HCV transmission occurs via the parenteral route with risk factors such as previous or current injecting drug use (IVDU), receipt of blood products or blood transfusion before 1992, haemodialysis and vertical transmission from mother-to-child. HIV and HCV co-infection is common in many settings due to shared routes of transmission *(9)*. HCV is not often transmitted sexually between monogamous heterosexual couples *(10)*. Among HIV-infected men who have sex with men, the risk of HCV transmission is increased and is associated with sexual practices that damage the rectal mucosa *(11)*.

NATURAL HISTORY AND CLINICAL FEATURES

What happens in acute HCV infection?

Acute HCV (AHCV) is characterised by detection of HCV RNAemia (HCV RNA in blood) and abnormal alanine aminotransferase (ALT) activities. Appearance of HCV-specific (anti-HCV) antibody is slow and can be delayed to 12 weeks after exposure *(12)*. Most cases (~75%) of AHCV infection remain asymptomatic. Among the minority who develop clinical disease, symptoms manifest 5-12 weeks after exposure and are typically mild and non-specific, including malaise, fatigue, lethargy, anorexia, nausea and abdominal pain. The differential diagnosis includes other infection like hepatitis A, B and E, primary EBV and CMV infections and non-infectious causes like autoimmune hepatitis *(13)*. HCV RNAemia begins within 14 days of infection and the level plateaus between days 45 and 68.

How does chronic HCV infection develop?

Approximately 12 weeks after exposure, the HCV RNA level decreases and either clears spontaneously (~ 25% of cases) or persists (~ 75% of cases) leading to chronic HCV infection *(14)*. Following spontaneous resolution of HCV, reinfection with a strain of HCV different to that causing the initial HCV infection can occur particularly in IVDUs and can also occur after cure with DAAs *(2, 15)*. Among those who progress to chronic HCV infection, cirrhosis develops in 10-20% of carriers over the next 20-30 years and HCC occurs at a rate of 1-5% annually among those with cirrhosis (15). Rare extrahepatic manifestations of HCV may occur such as HCV-associated splenic lymphoma, mixed essential cryoglobulinaemia and membranous or membranoproliferative glomerulonephritis *(9)*.

LABORATORY DIAGNOSIS

What virological markers in blood are used currently for diagnosis of HCV infection?

Anti-HCV antibody: testing for anti-HCV antibody in blood using an enzyme immunoassay (EIA) is the initial approach to diagnosis of HCV infection. Detection of anti-HCV antibody indicates either current HCV infection or past exposure to HCV which has since resolved, or a false-positive result. To confirm positivity, a second EIA, containing antigens from a different manufacturer, is used to test for anti-HCV antibody in the same sample *(16)*. Alternatively, confirmation is obtained by direct virus detection (HCV RNA or HCV core antigen).

HCV RNA: detection of HCV RNA in blood confirms current HCV infection. Commercial molecular assays for HCV RNA are highly sensitive and specific. HCV RNA is detectable in blood within 14 days after infection and is invariably present at onset of symptomatic acute illness and in chronic HCV infection. In general, for those who are anti-HCV antibody positive, absence of HCV RNA in blood indicates either spontaneous resolution of HCV infection or successful antiviral treatment. For patients who are anti-HCV antibody negative but in whom recent exposure is suspected, testing for HCV RNA or HCV cAg should be considered *(2)*. For immunocompromised persons with risk factors for HCV infection, HCV RNA testing of blood should be considered regardless of an anti-HCV antibody negative result *(17)*.

HCV core antigen (HCV cAg): detection of HCV cAg in blood confirms current HCV infection. Assays for HCV cAg detect viral nucleocapsid peptide 22 (p22) which is released from infected hepatocytes into plasma during HCV replication *(18)*. HCV cAg is detected earlier than anti-HCV antibody. However, HCV cAg is a less sensitive marker of active HCV infection than HCV RNA: depending on HCV genotype, if HCV RNA levels are < 500-3,000 IU/mL, HCV cAg may yield a false-negative result, although this is rare *(19)*. HCV cAg testing has been used favourably instead of HCV RNA levels to monitor treatment responses to DAAs *(20)*.

CHRONOLOGY OF APPEARANCE OF HCV VIROLOGICAL MARKERS IN ACUTE HCV INFECTION:

HCV RNA is detected in serum followed a few days later by HCV core antigen and later by anti-HCV antibody.

TYPICAL HCV VIROLOGICAL MARKERS SEEN IN CHRONIC HCV INFECTION:

HCV RNA detected and/or HCV core antigen positive in serum for 6 months and (typically) anti-HCV antibody positive.

EXAMPLES OF COMMON HCV VIROLOGY PROFILES FOR THE GENERAL PRACTITIONER

A serum sample was sent from an injecting drug user (IVDU):

Anti-HCV – Positive (assay 1)

Anti-HCV – Positive (assay 2)

Confirmed anti-HCV antibody positive is consistent either with current HCV infection or resolved HCV infection in the past. The laboratory tested reflexedly for **HCV cAg which was positive**, confirming current infection. The patient was referred to hepatology for further management. If HCV cAg had been negative, a repeat serum for HCV RNA would have been requested to confirm either resolved HCV infection or current infection with low-level HCV RNAemia.

A serum sample from a person with chronic HBV-related cirrhosis who presented with acute jaundice:

Anti-HCV antibody – Negative

The patient admitted recent injecting drug use. The GP requested HCV cAg using the anti-HCV antibody-negative sample: **HCV cAg was positive**, confirming current HCV infection, likely acute HCV infection. Anti-HCV antibody may be negative on presentation with symptomatic acute HCV infection. The patient was referred to a hepatology clinic.

A 72-year-old retired engineer presented to the GP with a urinary tract infection. He had a transrectal ultrasound guided (TRUS) biopsy of the prostate performed 15 weeks previously. The GP collected a serum sample coincidentally for biochemistry: of note was raised ALT activity (752 IU/L, normal < 40 IU/L) and elevated total bilirubin (38 µM, normal < 20 µM). He sent an urgent serum for hepatitis B surface antigen, anti-HCV antibody and IgM antibody to hepatitis A virus. Because anti-HCV antibody was positive, the laboratory tested the sample for HCV cAg:

Anti-HCV antibody – Positive (by two EIAs)

HCV cAg - Positive

Consistent with current HCV infection. The patient was referred to hepatology. Astored serum sample, collected around the time of the TRUS biopsy, was tested for anti-HCV antibody and HCV cAg, both of which were negative. HCV RNA was detected in the current serum sample (1.9×10^6 IU/mL), genotype 1b. To prevent progression to chronic HCV infection, he was immediately treated with a combination of DAAs, sofosbuvir and ledipasvir for 8 weeks. Absence of HCV RNA in serum using a highly sensitive molecular assay at 12 weeks and 24 weeks after the end of treatment confirmed a sustained virological response to antiviral treatment. Public health authorities concluded that this was likely to be a health-care associated infection. No breaches in infection control policy such as re-use of syringes or use of multidose vials were identified. However, one study showed that hospital admission was the only documented risk factor associated with acute HCV infection, stressing the importance of strict adherence to infection control policies *(21)*.

REFERENCES (*useful reviews)

1 Polaris Observatory HCV Collaborators. *Lancet Gastroeneterol. Hepatol.* **2**, 161 (2017)

2 EASL Recommendations on Treatment of Hepatitis C 2018. *J. Hepatol.* **69**, 461 (2018)*

3 WHO: Progress report on access to hepatitis C treatment 2018: WHO/CDS/HIV/18.4

4 E.M. Wilson *et al.*, *Clin. Microbiol. Rev.* **30**, 23 (2017)*

5 J.P. Messina *et al.*, *Hepatology.* **61**, 77 (2015)

6 R.R. Gray *et al.*, *PLOS Pathogens.* **8**, e1002656 (2012)

7 ECDC.Technical Report. Hepatitis B and C in the EU neighbourhood: prevalence, burden of disease and screening policies. Stockholm: ECDC; 2010

8 P. Garvey *et al.*, *Euro. Surveill.***22**, pii=30579 (2017)

9 D.P. Webster, P. Klenerman, G.M. Dusheiko. *Lancet.***385**, 1124 (2015)*

10 C. Vandelli *et al.*, *Am. J. Gastroenterol.* **99**, 855 (2004)

11 R.A. Tohme, S.D. Holmberg. *Hepatology.***52**, 1497 (2010)

12 A. Maheshwari, S. Ray, P.J. Thuluvath. *Lancet.***372**, 321 (2008)

13 T. Wong, S.S. Lee. *CMAJ.***174**, 649 (2006)

14 B. Hajarizadeh, J. Grebely, G.J. Dore. *Nat. Rev. Gastroenterol. Hepatol.***10**, 553 (2013)*

15 R.H. Westbrook, G. Dusheiko. *J. Hepatol.* **61** Suppl 1, S58 (2014)

16https://www.cdc.gov/mmwr/pdf/wk/mm62e0507a2.pdf

17 V. Mallett *et al.*, *Lancet Infect. Dis.* **5**, 606 (2016)*

18 J.J. Feld.*Clin. Liver Dis.* **12**, 125 (2018)

19 J.M. Freiman *et al.*, *Ann. Intern. Med.* **165**, 345 (2016)

20 M. van Tilborg *et al.*, *Lancet Gastroenterol. Hepatol.***3**, 856 (2018)

21 E. Martinez-Bauer *et al.*, *J. Hepatol.* **48**, 20 (2008)

HEPATITIS E

What is hepatitis E?

Hepatitis E is a disease caused by hepatitis E virus (HEV) and is a frequent cause of hepatitis in developing and industrialised nations (1). Although most infections in humans are asymptomatic, HEV can present as a self-limiting acute hepatitis in immunocompetent individuals for which antiviral treatment is not usually required. However, HEV infection in immunocompromised hosts may result in development of chronic hepatitis for which reduction in immunosuppression and/or antiviral treatment are therapeutic options. Furthermore, in both immunocompetent and immunocompromised persons, HEV infection is associated with extrahepatic manifestations, especially neurological syndromes.

CASE VIGNETTE

A 57-year-old man presented to his GP with a 10-day history of myalgia, fatigue and malaise. He had a past history of hypertension for which his current medication included enalapril and aspirin. He had returned from a 14-day trip to India4 months previously. Physical examination was normal. The GP sent samples for full blood count (FBC) with differential and a biochemical profile which revealed abnormal liver function tests (LFTs): alanine aminotransferase (ALT) 435 IU/L (* < 41 IU/L), aspartate aminotransferase (AST) 220 IU/L (* < 40 IU/L) with normal total bilirubin 19 µM (* < 21 µM) and normal synthetic function. The GP suspected drug-induced liver injury (DILI) rather than acute viral hepatitis because previous serology reports showed the patient to be immune to hepatitis A virus and hepatitis B virus with evidence of past infection to Epstein Barr virus and cytomegalovirus (CMV). Hepatitis C virus (HCV) infection was felt to be unlikely since he had no history of injection drug use. (* Reference range)

LABORATORY DIAGNOSIS

What further virological test(s) did the GP request in this patient with suspected DILI?

The GP sent serum for IgM antibody to hepatitis E virus (anti-HEV IgM) which was strongly positive. To confirm acute HEV infection, the serum sample was also tested for HEV RNA which was detected. HEV RNA testing of a stool sample also confirmed HEV. Testing for anti-HCV and HCV core antigen were performed and shown to be negative.

Why test for HEV in this case?

A diagnosis of DILI should not be made without excluding acute HEV infection particularly when aminotransferase levels are elevated (2). Laboratory testing of samples from cases with suspected DILI found that a small but significant proportion (3% to 13%) had acute HEV infection (3, 4).

In what other circumstances should the GP request testing for markers of HEV infection?

Some national guidelines recommend that all immunocompetent persons with suspected acute viral hepatitis should be tested for HEV infection, particularly if ALT levels are ≥ 300 IU/L *(5)*. In fact, in many European countries HEV acquired locally is the commonest cause of acute viral hepatitis *(6)*. Testing for HEV is also indicated among those with chronic liver disease who develop a hepatitis flare, or especially acute-on-chronic liver failure. Furthermore, hospital physicians may consider HEV testing in those with suspected HEV-related neurological findings (discussed below) even when ALT levels are < 300 IU/L *(5)*.

Was anti-HEV IgM sufficient to diagnose HEV infection in this case?

No, confirmatory molecular testing for HEV RNA in serum was necessary. Testing of stool samples for HEV RNA is another confirmatory option. Current serological assays for anti-HEV IgM / IgG show significant variations in sensitivity and specificity, in particular high-level cross-reactivity with CMV and EBV *(7, 8)*. Furthermore, false-negative and false-positive anti-HEV IgM results may have adverse effects on clinical management due to delayed diagnosis and inappropriate therapeutic interventions, respectively *(9)*.

For how long are virological markers of acute HEV infection detectable?

Anti-HEV IgM is usually detectable at the time of illness onset and persists for about 3 months but occasionally may be detected for as long as 12 months *(10)*. In contrast, anti-HEV IgG persists for up to 20 years *(11)*. In immunocompetent individuals HEV RNA is detectable in serum for only about 3 to 4 weeks after onset of symptoms while in faeces it is detectable usually for about 6 weeks *(2)*. The short-lived circulation of HEV RNA in serum means that recent HEV infection cannot be excluded if serum is collected late in the course of infection.

Was follow-up virological testing for HEV markers needed in this patient?

No, detection of anti-HEV IgM and HEV RNA in serum confirmed acute HEV infection in this immunocompetent person.

EPIDEMIOLOGY

Why is knowledge of HEV genotypes relevant to understanding its epidemiology?

Four major genotypes of HEV (designated GT 1 – GT 4) are currently known to cause infection in humans and can be divided into two main groups: anthropotropic (GT 1/2) and enzootic (GT 3/4) *(12)*. In developing countries, GT 1 and GT 2 circulate in humans only, not animals, and are spread by contaminated drinking water with large water-borne outbreaks of hepatitis occurring sometimes due to poor sanitation *(2)*. High attack rates of HEV GT 1/2 occur mainly among adults aged between 15 and 45 years. In developed countries, HEV is a zoonosis in which GT 3 and GT 4 circulate in animals, in particular pigs, with humans infected as accidental hosts (enzootic) mainly by consumption of contaminated food. The pattern of spread of HEV GT 3/4 is mostly sporadic and locally acquired ('autochthonous'), with older age groups and immunocompromised hosts at high risk for clinical disease (10).

Are there other routes of HEV transmission?

Vertical and parenteral routes of HEV transmission occur infrequently. In developing countries, HEV GT 1 infection in pregnancy has been associated with acute liver failure in the mother (mortality rate as high as 20%) and with an increased risk of spontaneous abortion, fetal death in utero and premature delivery (13, 14). In Europe, iatrogenic transmission of HEV GT 3 between humans has been reported via blood and blood products (15, 16). In Ireland and the United Kingdom (UK), screening of blood donations for HEV RNA was implemented to reduce the risk of transfusion-transmitted HEV, particularly to immunosuppressed individuals who are at risk of developing chronic HEV infection. Furthermore, HEV transmission to humans has been demonstrated in single cases with dromedaries (GT 7/8) and rats (completely different GT) but the significance of these routes is ill-understood.

What was the likely route of acquisition of HEV in the current case?

He probably acquired HEV in Ireland: HEV GT 3 (subtype i) caused his infection, a GT associated with food consumption. Although he consumed cooked pork products in the two months before diagnosis of HEV, he also ate mussels that may have been undercooked about four weeks before diagnosis of HEV. High loads of HEV are shed by infected pigs into the environment, including waterways, which can lead to contamination of shellfish which are a possible source of infection (17, 18). However, the source of HEV is not always identified (19). It was unlikely to be travel-associated HEV since he was last abroad four months before presentation and the incubation period of HEV ranges from about 15 days to a maximum of 63 days.

Why do locally acquired HEV cases in Europe exceed travel-associated cases?

Sporadic autochthonous cases of HEV are increasingly notified in some European countries as shown recently among young adults in Scotland and also observed in England and the Netherlands (20, 21, 22). Strains of HEV GT 3 associated with recent human infections in the UK were shown to originate mainly from pigs in Continental Europe, suggesting importation of HEV-contaminated food from abroad (20, 22). It has been speculated that changes in the way food is cooked may predispose to HEV acquisition due to consumption of undercooked HEV-contaminated food (23).

CLINICAL FEATURES

What was the clinical course of acute HEV infection in this case?

Within four weeks of presentation, the patient's symptoms resolved spontaneously and biochemical recovery was complete, similar to that seen in the majority of symptomatic HEV infections among immunocompetent individuals (2). Autochthonous HEV GT 3 infections are mostly asymptomatic, particularly in young adults and females, while clinical disease is mainly a feature of infection in older males (10). While the clinical presentation in this case was non-specific, this is not unusual with almost 50% of those with acute HEV in one study presenting with features such as influenza-like illness, arthralgia with myalgia and abdominal pain with diarrhea (24).

Which patients groups are at risk of severe autochthonous HEV genotype 3 infection?

Acute HEV infection in those with underlying chronic liver disease, which may have pre-existed subclinically, can progress to acute liver failure which has a poor prognosis (10). HEV infection in immunocompromised individuals can become chronic, defined as persistence of HEV RNA in blood for > 3 months (25). Persons who are lymphopenic and those on immunosuppression are at risk of chronic HEV including solid organ and haematopoietic stem cell transplant recipients, those on chemotherapy and HIV-infected persons (2). Patients are typically asymptomatic with persistently high ALT levels. Because anti-HEV IgM / IgG may be negative in those with chronic HEV, HEV RNA testing of blood or stool is best.

What is the relationship between HEV infection and pregnancy?

Autochthonous HEV GT 3 or 4 infection in developed countries occurs rarely during pregnancy and, in general, the clinical outcome is favourable probably because of better medical care or possibly because of lower virulence of GT 3 (26). By contrast, in developing countries acute HEV infection with GT1 or 2 in pregnancy, especially in the third trimester, may lead to fulminant hepatitis with high maternal and fetal morbidity and mortality (13, 14). Host immune response, hormonal factors, nutritional status and viral load and genotype are believed to interact in a complex way during pregnancy potentially leading to severe HEV infection (26).

What are the common extrahepatic manifestations of HEV infection?

HEV infection is commonly associated with neuralgic amyotrophy (NA), Guillain-Barré syndrome and encephalitis/myelitis (27). The relationship between HEV and NA appears to be causal (28). Testing for HEV should be done for persons presenting with these conditions irrespective of ALT levels (29). Other manifestations for which there is anecdotal evidence include glomerular disease, aplastic anaemia, thrombocytopenia and pancreatitis (2).

TREATMENT

How was the patient managed in this case in terms of treatment and infection control?

Treatment was supportive with frequent clinical monitoring and assessment of ALT levels. Although the duration of infectivity of HEV in infected persons is unknown and person-to-person transmission is uncommon, strict adherence to hand hygiene was advised for 14 days after illness onset and he was advised not to cook for others *(30)*.

When should the GP consider referral of patients with acute HEV for antiviral treatment?

Antiviral treatment is not indicated in otherwise immunocompetent individuals with acute HEV. However, anecdotal evidence implies that those with severe acute HEV infection can be considered for treatment with oral ribavirin which has been shown to be effective in shortening the symptomatic period of infection and lowering the severity of the course *(31)*. In the setting of HEV-related acute-on-chronic liver failure, oral ribavirin treatment may be beneficial although properly designed controlled trials are needed *(32)*.

What should the GP know about management of chronic HEV infection in immunocompromised individuals?

Management of HEV infection in immunocompromised persons involves, if feasible, reducing the immunosuppressive drug regimen thereby allowing development of an immune response to control viral replication. However, if HEV RNA in serum persists for> 3 months, treatment with oral ribavirin for at least 3 months is the next step *(33)*. Oral ribavirin is currently the antiviral treatment of choice for those with chronic HEV *(34)*. However, this has not yet been approved for use in HEV-infected patients (off-label).

PREVENTION

What advice should the GP give a pregnant woman who plans to travel to Pakistan and wants to avoid HEV infection?

Any person travelling to a HEV-endemic area should follow precautions used to avoid travellers' diarrhea: drink only bottled water, do not add ice cubes to drinks, avoid raw or undercooked pork products or other meats, including seafood, and do not eat unpeeled fruits or raw vegetables. Hand washing should be performed after handling raw meat and good hygienic practice observed to avoid cross-contamination with cooked food.

Does cooking food easily inactivate HEV?

The current opinion in Ireland recommends cooking pork products to a minimum temperature of 75°C in the thickest part of the meat to inactivate HEV *(35)*. Cooking sausages until they are brown is likely to achieve inactivation of HEV and other microorganisms.

Is there a vaccine available currently in Ireland for prevention of HEV infection?

No, a HEV vaccine has been available commercially only in China since 2011. The vaccine was shown to be efficacious (vaccine efficacy 86.8%) with sustained protection for up to 4.5 years after first vaccination *(36)*. However, its protective efficacy against HEV GT 3, the main genotype circulating in Europe, is still unclear *(37)*. There is no role currently for prophylaxis against HEV with immune globulin although this needs to be studied further *(38)*.

REFERENCES (*useful reviews)

1 N. Kamar *et al.*, *Lancet*. **379**, 2477 (2012)

2 N. Kamar *et al.*, *Clin.Microbiol. Rev.* **27**, 116 (2014)*

3 T.J. Davern *et al.*, *Gastroenterology*. **141**, 1665 (2011)

4 H.R. Dalton *et al.*, *Aliment. Pharmacol.Ther.***26**, 1429 (2007)

5 S.J. Wallace *et al.*, *Eur. J. Gastroenterol. Hepatol.***29**, 215 (2017)*

6 C. Adlhoch *et al.*, *J. Clin. Virol.***82**, 9 (2016)

7 Q. Huang *et al.*, *Antivir. Ther.***21**, 171 (2016)

8 L.S. Friedman *et al.*, *N. Engl. J. Med.***375**, 2082 (2016)

9 P.K. Sue *et al.*, *Transpl. Infect. Dis.***17**, 284(2015)

10 J.H. Hoofnagle, K.E. Nelson, R.H. Purcell. *N. Engl. J. Med.* **367**, 1237 (2012)

11 M.S. Khuroo, M Khuroo.*Hepatol. Int.***4**, 494 (2010)

12 M.A. Purdy, Y.E. Khudyakov. *PLOS One.***5**, e14376 (2010)

13 N. Jilani *et al.*, *J. Gastroenterol.Hepatol.***22**, 676 (2007)

14 S. Sharma *et al.*, *J. Viral Hepat.***24**, 1067 (2017)

15 P.E. Hewitt *et al.*, *Lancet*. **384**, 1766 (2014)

16 D. Domanovic *et al.*, *EuroSurveill.***22**, pii=30514 (2017)

17 B. Said *et al.*, *Emerg. Infect. Dis*. **15**, 1738 (2009)

18 Z. O'Hara *et al.*, *Food Environ. Virol.***10**, 217 (2018)

19 H.R. Dalton *et al.*, *Lancet Infect. Dis*. **8**, 698 (2008)

20 K. Thom *et al.*, *Euro. Surveill.***23**, pii=17-00174 (2018)

21 E. Slot *et al.*, *Euro. Surveill.***18**, pii=20550 (2013)

22 S. Ijaz *et al.*, *J. Infect. Dis*. **209**, 1212 (2014)

23 D.B. Smith *et al.*, *J. Gen. Virol*. **96**, 3255 (2015)

24 C. Renou *et al.*, *Aliment. Pharmacol.Ther.***27**, 1086 (2008)

25 N. Kamar *et al.*, *Am. J. Transplant.***13**, 1935 (2013)

26 M. Perez-Garcia, B. Suay-Garcia, M. Mateos-Lindemann. *Rev. Med. Virol.* **27**, e1929 (2017)

27 H.R. Dalton *et al.*, *Nat. Rev. Neurol.* **12**, 77 (2016)*

28 H.R. Dalton *et al.*, *J. Hepatol.* **68**, 1256 (2018)*

29 J.J.J. van Eijk *et al.*, *Neurology.* **89**, 909 (2017)

30 E.T. Clayson *et al.*, *J. Infect. Dis.* **172**, 927 (1995)

31 J.M. Peron *et al.*, *Liver Int.***36**, 328 (2016)

32 G.Y. Lee *et al.*, *World J. Virol.* **4**, 343 (2015)

33 N. Kamar *et al.*, *Nat. Rev. Dis. Primers.* **3**, 17086 (2017)*

34 N. Kamar *et al.*, *N. Engl. J. Med.* **370**, 1111 (2014)

35 Food Safety Authority of Ireland: https://www.fsai.ie/faq/hepatitis_E.html

36 J. Zhang *et al.*, *N. Engl. J. Med.* **372**, 914 (2015)

37 J. Hartl, M.H. Wehmeyer, S. Pischke. *Viruses.* **8**, 299 (2016)

38 M. Ankcorn *et al.*, *J. Infect. Dis.* **219**, 245 (2019)

INFECTIOUS MONONUCLEOSIS-LIKE ILLNESS

- EBV & CMV
- Acute HIV-1
- Toxoplasmosis

INFECTIOUS MONONUCLEOSIS

What is infectious mononucleosis?

Infectious mononucleosis (IM), otherwise known as 'glandular fever', is an acute clinical syndrome with the classical triad of fever, pharyngitis and lymphadenopathy, usually with an atypical lymphocytosis and mainly due to primary infection with Epstein-Barr virus (EBV). EBV (human herpes virus type 4), is a DNA virus which is ubiquitous with 90% seropositivity in adults worldwide. It establishes latency following the resolution of primary infection.

CASE VIGNETTE

A 17-year-old male rugby player, who was otherwise healthy, presented to the GP with a 72-hour history of fever, sore throat and fatigue. His temperature was 38.5°C at presentation and clinical examination revealed pharyngeal inflammation, enlarged tonsils with a whitewash exudate and prominent cervical lymphadenopathy in the anterior and posterior triangles of the neck. A rapid antigen test for Group A Streptococcus was negative. The GP suspected acute infectious mononucleosis (IM) on clinical grounds.

What are the learning points in this case?

LABORATORY DIAGNOSIS

What laboratory tests did the GP request to confirm EBV-related IM?

A sample of whole blood was sent for white blood cell count with differential and heterophile antibody. These tests should be requested from any young adult, who is otherwise immunocompetent, presenting with fever and pharyngitis, especially when accompanied by fatigue and posterior cervical, pre-auricular or occipital lymphadenopathy. A positive rapid agglutination (monospot) test for heterophile antibody supports the diagnosis of acute IM in those with the above clinical features and lymphocytosis as well as ≥ 10% atypical lymphocytes on blood film *(1)*. In this case, heterophile antibody was positive and typical haematological features were present (see later).

Does a negative result for heterophile antibody exclude the diagnosis of acute EBV-related IM?

No, false negative rates of the rapid agglutination (monospot) assay for heterophile antibody are as high as 25% in patients for the first week of illness, 5% to 10% in the second week and 5% in the third week *(2)*. Furthermore, heterophile antibody production occurs in only 25% to 50% of children with acute IM aged <12 years *(3)*.

Therefore, ordering the white blood cell count with differential is particularly important when IM is suspected early in the course of the illness, or in younger children.

Does detection of heterophile antibody always support a diagnosis of acute EBV-related IM?

No, a positive monospot result for heterophile antibody does not always indicate IM, particularly if the clinical presentation is not typical. Monospot results must always be interpreted in the light of clinical findings. It is known that heterophile antibody may persist in blood for as long as a year after primary EBV infection and thereby confound diagnosis of a patient's current illness *(4)*. Furthermore, false-positive monospot test results may occur in several conditions such as acute viral hepatitis, human immunodeficiency virus (HIV) infection, autoimmune disease and malignancy *(5)*.

What should be done if the monospot test for heterophile antibody is negative in a suspected IM case?

A serum sample should be sent for EBV-specific antibody testing to confirm or exclude EBV-related IM when the heterophile antibody screen is negative or when it is positive but the clinical picture is atypical. In general, detection of IgM antibody to viral capsid antigen (anti-VCA IgM) confirms definitively recent EBV infection. If anti-VCA IgM is negative, it excludes current EBV infection.

What are the EBV-specific serology reports seen typically in serum samples from those with acute IM?

Scenario 1: anti-VCA IgM – Positive: anti-VCA IgG – Positive: [a]anti-EBNA IgG – Negative

Scenario 2: anti-[b]VCA IgM – Positive: [c]anti-VCA IgG – Negative: anti-EBNA IgG – Negative

[a]anti-EBNA IgG becomes positive in the convalescent phase between 4 and 8 weeks after illness onset.

[b]Suggestive of primary EBV but send follow-up serum within 1 week to confirm by showing anti-VCA IgG seroconversion.

[c]anti-VCA IgG becomes detectable at or shortly after presentation and persists for life.

Does a negative heterophile antibody and negative anti-VCA IgM exclude a diagnosis of acute IM?

No, these results exclude primary EBV infection but there are several other causes of mononucleosis with the typical clinical syndrome of IM, known as 'mononucleosis-like illness' (MLI), including primary infection with cytomegalovirus (CMV), *Toxoplasma gondii* and human immunodeficiency virus (HIV).

What tests should be done for other common causes of mononucleosis-like illness (MLI)?

The serum sample used for VCA IgM can be tested for anti-CMV IgM / IgG and anti-*T gondii* IgM / IgG. Primary CMV (5% to 7%) and toxoplasmosis (3%) are two frequent causes of non-EBV-related IM seen in clinical practice *(3, 6)*. Testing for HIV 1&2 Ag/Ab (antigen/antibody) should always be requested in adults with MLI (see chapter on acute HIV-1 infection).

Were haematological and biochemical findings of value in diagnosis of acute IM in this case?

Yes, in this case a peripheral blood film showed atypical lymphocytes and the absolute lymphocyte count was raised at 5.5×10^3 mm^{-3} (total white cell count 8.8×10^3 mm^{-3}). About 80% of patients with acute IM have raised liver function tests, particularly alanine aminotransferase (101 IU/L in this case; normal value < 35 IU/L). Identification of $\geq$ 10% atypical lymphocytosis in a peripheral blood film increases the likelihood of IM in those with relevant clinical findings *(1)*. Similarly, an absolute lymphocyte count > 4,000 mm^{-3} also suggests IM while a value $\leq$ 4,000 mm^{-3} makes it unlikely (predictive value of 99% for a negative heterophile antibody test) (7). However, in children and the elderly with acute IM, atypical lymphocytosis may be absent *(8)*.

What does the term 'mononucleosis' mean?

The haematological picture reflects the response of the cellular arm of the immune system to acute viral infection. Atypical lymphocytes, also known as Downey cells, indicate proliferation of virus-specific CD8+ T cells and natural killer (NK) cells during the acute phase of the infection.

EPIDEMIOLOGY

Does the patient in this case belong to a cohort at risk of IM?

Yes, primary EBV infection with development of IM is most commonly diagnosed in adolescents and young adults aged 15-24 years living in developed countries like the United Kingdom and Ireland *(9)*. Primary EBV infection among adolescents and young adults results in development of the clinical syndrome of IM in 30% to 70% and may rarely require hospitalization *(10, 11)*. Unsurprisingly, IM is frequent in situations where many young adults are in close proximity such as in universities and military barracks *(12, 13)*. In contrast, among lower socioeconomic groups and in populations in developing countries, primary EBV infection is common in childhood (< 10 years of age) when it is usually asymptomatic or only a mild nonspecific illness *(14)*. In recent decades, improvements in living conditions have probably led to a decline in EBV infection during childhood with increased susceptibility among adolescents and young adults in the United Kingdom *(15)*.

By which route is the patient likely to have acquired EBV?

Transmission of EBV between people occurs mainly via infected saliva: between young children by sharing contaminated fomites like toys and bottles, while among young adults by kissing, although transmission via infected genital secretions is also a possibility *(16, 17)*.

CLINICAL PRESENTATION

What other key clinical features may be seen in young adults with acute IM?

Young adults with IM present most frequently with sore throat, fatigue, cervical lymphadenopathy, fever and tonsillar enlargement *(2)*. Four physical signs strongly associated with acute IM include palatine petechiae, posterior cervical lymphadenopathy and axillary or inguinal lymph nodes *(1)*. Furthermore, a thin, grey exudate on the tonsils may sometimes be seen and aids in differentiating IM from Group A streptococcal infection which is associated with a more speckled exudate. A diffuse maculopapular rash may develop in those with IM who have been prescribed amoxicillin or ampicillin, for presumed streptococcal pharyngitis *(3)*. These antibiotics should be avoided when IM is suspected.

Is the clinical presentation of acute IM in those at the extremes of age different to that in young adults?

Young children (< 5 years of age) rarely develop the typical clinical syndrome of acute IM, primary EBV infections being asymptomatic or nonspecific and not recognised clinically as IM *(1, 14)*. However, older adults (> 60 years of age) with symptomatic primary EBV infection tend to have a severe illness with prolonged fever and hepatitis leading to jaundice, and presenting less frequently with pharyngitis, lymphadenopathy and splenomegaly *(10)*.

CLINICAL MANAGEMENT

What was the clinical course of acute IM in this young man?

Most clinical features of IM resolved within four weeks of illness onset, although fatigue persisted for several weeks. This is typical of the natural history of IM seen in otherwise healthy young adults *(18)*. Biochemical and haematological laboratory abnormalities returned to normal values within a month of onset of illness.

What treatment was recommended?

The approach used was symptomatic management, including acetaminophen and non-steroidal anti-inflammatory drugs as antipyretics and for analgesia. He was advised to maintain adequate hydration and nutrition.

Would you prescribe an antiviral agent such as aciclovir for EBV-related acute IM?

No, current data do not support the use of oral aciclovir for treatment of acute IM as no clinical benefit in terms of duration or severity of symptoms has been shown *(3, 19)*. Even use of both oral aciclovir and prednisolone did not reduce duration of clinical illness *(20)*. Further studies are needed to determine if use of antiviral agents might confer clinical benefit in severe EBV infections *(21)*. Although oral aciclovir and valganciclovir were shown to reduce the rate and quantity of EBV shed from the oropharynx, this was a transient effect of no clinical benefit, with resumption of viral shedding once the antiviral was stopped *(22, 23)*.

Is the use of corticosteroids recommended in management of acute IM?

No, there is a lack of evidence to support the use of corticosteroids for symptom control in uncomplicated IM *(24, 25)*. However, steroid treatment is usually given in those with life-threatening complications such as airway obstruction and those with severe thrombocytopenia or haemolyticanaemia *(4, 26)*.

If he had MLI due to acute CMV or *T. gondii* infection, would you offer an antiviral or antiparasitic agent?

No, primary CMV and acute toxoplasmosis are mostly self-limiting illnesses in immunocompetent individuals with MLI. However, if there is evidence of end-organ disease, such as pneumonitis, colitis, chorioretinitis or encephalitis, which develops rarely in otherwise healthy persons including pregnant women, referral to hospital for assessment is advised.

RETURN TO NORMAL ACTIVITIES

When might the patient return to playing rugby?

Caution is advised because splenic rupture due to trauma is a potential consequence of acute IM. The general advice is that patients may return to non-contact sports as early as three weeks after onset of IM and at four weeks for those participating in contact sports or activities known to increase intraabdominal pressure, provided that splenomegaly is not identified on physical examination and patients are a febrile, well-hydrated and have sufficient energy to exercise *(27)*. Although splenic rupture is rare (< 0.5%) in IM, it can occur spontaneously or with modest trauma. However, most cases of splenic injury in IM occur within the first 21 days of illness onset and are rare after 28 days *(28)*. Ultrasonographic examination of the spleen at one month in athletes with acute IM has been suggested before return to contact activities but it is argued that this is of limited value due to lack of knowledge of splenic size before onset of illness *(27, 29)*.

Should an IM patient be allowed to return to school? Should they be separated from other pupils in the classroom on return?

They can return to school when feeling well enough, and need not be quarantined from other students. Even though they will shed EBV in saliva immediately post-infection and intermittently throughout their lives, other students of their age are likely to be EBV seropositive and therefore immune to primary infection.

ADDITIONAL POINTS ABOUT EBV-RELATED INFECTIOUS MONONUCLEOSIS PATHOGENESIS

How does EBV cause IM?

The incubation period between infection and clinical manifestation of IM is about 30 to 50 days. EBV infection begins with virus replication in tonsillar B cells probably followed by early switching of the site of replication to tonsillar epithelium leading to high-level shedding of virus in the oropharynx *(30)*. EBV-infected B cells proliferate and differentiate into memory B cells while simultaneously inducing development of EBV-specific cytotoxic T cells which eliminate rapidly EBV-infected B cells from blood *(30)*. However, shedding of infectious EBV from the oropharynx continues after clinical resolution of infection suggesting differences in the timing of immune control of EBV-infected B cells and infected tonsillar epithelium *(31)*. The high proportion of atypical 'Downey' lymphocytes usually seen in blood films of patients in the acute phase of IM are activated CD8+ T cells and CD16+ natural killer cells reflecting the exaggerated cellular immune response to EBV-infected B cells *(32)*. Production of high levels of proinflammatory cytokines from the activated immune cells is thought to be responsible for the clinical manifestation of acute IM *(4)*. Following resolution of primary EBV infection, it is proposed that about 1 in 10^6 B cells carries the EBV genome in a latent state i.e. there is persistent infection but no active viral replication *(4)*. This reservoir of EBV genomes is probably maintained in latency by EBV-specific cellular immunity. However, EBV reactivation from infected B cells may occur with intermittent shedding of infectious virus into saliva throughout the lifetime of the host and subsequent transmission to EBV-susceptible individuals *(3, 30)*.

Is the clinical severity of acute IM related to the individual's immune response to EBV infection?

Recent data support the notion of immunopathogenesis as the cause of symptoms in acute IM, specifically related to an excessive CD8+ T cell response by the individual to viral infection resulting in elevated levels of proinflammatory cytokines and chemokines in plasma. A hyperactive, adaptive cellular immune response to EBV contributes significantly to the clinical course of IM as has been proposed by many investigators *(4, 14, 31, 33, 34, 35)*.

COMPLICATIONS

What complications of acute IM may be seen in clinical practice?

Complications are uncommon rarely progressing to fulminant disease. Although fatigue may be present in 9% to 12% of persons 6 months after acute IM, it resolves in the majority of cases within a year *(36)*. IM may be a risk factor for chronic fatigue syndrome (CFS), but this is unproven and the cause of CFS is likely to be multifactorial *(36, 37)*. Extreme tonsillar enlargement and pharyngeal oedema may lead to airway obstruction and dehydration requiring hospitalization *(4)*. Children under six years of age with IM are at highest risk for airway obstruction due to oropharyngeal swelling. Haematological complications, which are usually mild and transient, occur in 25% to 50% of acute IM cases and include haemolyticanaemia and thrombocytopenia, both thought to be immune-mediated conditions *(3, 4)*. In addition, thrombotic thrombocytopenia purpura, disseminated intravascular coagulation and aplastic anaemia may develop. Meningoencephalitis is the most common neurological complication while others such as Guillain-Barré syndrome and optic neuritis are rare *(38)*. Peritonsillar abscess formation may also occur due to localised secondary bacterial infection in those with acute IM. Splenic rupture is often highlighted as a complication in acute IM but occurs rarely (0.1% to 0.5%) *(3)*.

Can primary EBV infection develop into fulminant IM and lead to death in otherwise healthy individuals?

Yes, although fulminant acute IM is rare, any individual with persistent IM-like illness, other than symptoms of fatigue or malaise alone, should be referred to hospital. Primary EBV infection may rarely develop into fulminant disease in the following three circumstances: haemophagocytic lymphohistiocytosis (HLH), in those with X-linked lymphoproliferative (XLP) disorder and chronic active EBV (CAEBV) infection.

Although primary EBV infection is rarely fatal, it is known to be a common trigger for haemophagocytic lymphohistiocytosis (HLH), a syndrome of persistent hyperactivation of immune cells with massive production of cytokines leading to multiorgan failure *(39)*. There is evidence of a genetic defect in some children while other cases appear to be sporadic. HLH is characterised clinically by prolonged fever, hepatosplenomegaly, lymphadenopathy, hepatitis and cytopenia *(40)*. Typical changes on examination of bone marrow shows activated macrophages with ingested red blood cells.

A rare inherited disorder in males, X-linked lymphoproliferative (XLP) disease, predisposes to development of potentially fatal IM and malignancy. XLP is a rare inherited immunodeficiency state caused by mutations in a gene (*SH2D1A*) which is needed to activate certain immune cells (T cells and natural killer (NK) cells). Carriers of XLP are otherwise healthy until they acquire primary EBV infection. Normally T cells and NK cells control proliferation of EBV-infected B cells thereby resolving the infection. T /

NK cells are activated against EBV when they are presented with viral antigen by EBV-infected B cells *(41)*. In XLP carriers, EBV-specific CD8+ T-cells cannot be activated by antigen-presenting B cells due to mutations in the *SH2D1A* gene.

Chronic active EBV (CAEBV) infection is a rare, life-threatening condition occurring in otherwise healthy individuals following primary EBV infection. Most patients with CAEBV present with fever, hepatitis, hepatosplenomegaly, lymphadenopathy and pancytopenia which persist for > 6 months, although more acute onset may occur also *(42)*. Although EBV infects B cells, it is detected in T cells and natural killer (NK) cells in most CAEBV cases reported in Asian and South/Central American populations *(43)*. Furthermore, CAEBV cases tend to progress to lymphoproliferative diseases of B, T or NK cell origin. Defective cellular immune control of EBV-infected cells appears to lead to CAEBV and lymphomagenesis *(44)*.

REFERENCES (*useful reviews)

1 M.H. Ebell *et al.*, *JAMA*. **315**, 1502 (2016)*

2 M.H. Ebell. *Am. Fam. Physician*. **70**, 1279 (2004)

3 K. Luzuriaga, J.L. Sullivan. *N. Engl. J. Med*. **362**, 1993 (2010)*

4 O.A. Odumade, K.A. Hogquist, H.H. Balfour Jr. *Clin. Microbiol. Rev*. **24**, 193 (2011)*

5 B.A.C. Fisher, S. Bhalara. *J. Clin. Microbiol*.**42**, 4411 (2004)

6 C. Hurt, D. Tammaro. *Am. J. Med*. **120**, 911 (2007)

7 T.C. Biggs *et al.*, *Laryngoscope*. **123**, 2401 (2013)

8 M. Papesch, R. Watkins. *Clin.Otolaryngol*.**26**, 3 (2001)

9 B. Candy *et al.*, *Br. J. Gen. Pract*. **52**, 844 (2002)

10 P.G. Auwaerter. *JAMA*.**281**, 454 (1999)

11 P. Tattevin *et al.*, *J. Clin. Microbiol*.**44**, 1873 (2006)

12 D.H. Crawford *et al.*, *Clin. Infect. Dis*. **43**, 276 (2006)

13 H. Levine *et al.*, *Eur. J. Clin. Microbiol. Infect. Dis*. **31**, 757 (2012)

14 S. Jayasooriya *et al.*, *PLoSPathog*.**11**, e1004746 (2015)

15 M.C. Morris, W.J. Edmunds. *J. Infect*. **45**, 107 (2002)

16 C.D. Higgins *et al.*, *J. Infect. Dis*. **195**, 474 (2007)

17 R. Thomas *et al.*, *J. Med. Virol*. **78**, 1204 (2006)

18 T.D. Rea *et al.*, *J. Am. Board Fam. Pract*. **14**, 234 (2001)

19 M. De Paor *et al.*, *Cochrane Database Syst. Rev*. **12**, CD011487 (2016)

20 E. Tynell *et al.*, *J. Infect. Dis*. **174**, 324 (1996)

21 P.I. Rafalidis *et al.*, *J. Clin. Virol*.**49**, 151 (2010)

22 H.H. Balfour Jr *et al.*, *J. Clin. Virol*.**39**, 16 (2007)

23 J.E. Yager *et al.*, *J. Infect. Dis*. **216**, 198 (2017)

24 B. Candy, M. Hotopf. *Cochrane Database Syst. Rev*. **3**, CD004402 (2006)

25 E.K. Vouloumanou, P.I. Rafailidis, M.E. Falagas. *Curr.Opin.Hematol*. **19**, 14 (2012)*

26 Y. Kagoya *et al.*, *Int. J. Hematol.* **91**, 326 (2010)

27 J.A. Becker, J.A. Smith. *Sports Health.* **6**, 232 (2014)

28 J. Turner, M. Garg. *Curr.Sports Med. Rep.* **7**, 113 (2008)

29 T.E. O'Connor *et al.*, *Ear Nose Throat J.* **90**, E21 (2011)

30 H.H. Balfour Jr *et al.*, *J. Infect. Dis.* **192**, 1505 (2005)

31 A.B. Rickinson, C.P. Fox. *J. Infect Dis.* **207**, 6 (2013)

32 A.D. Hislop *et al.*, *Ann. Rev. Immunol.* **25**, 587 (2007)

33 S.L. Silins *et al.*, *Blood.* **98**, 3739 (2001)

34 V. Hadinoto *et al.*, *Blood.* **111**, 1420 (2008)

35 R.J. Abbott *et al.*, *J. Virol.* **91**, e00382-17 (2017)

36 B.Z. Katz *et al.*, *Pediatrics.* **124**, 189 (2009)

37 J.M. Harvey *et al.*, *BMC Pediatr.* **16**, 54 (2016)

38 H.B. Jenson. *Curr.Opin.Pediatr.* **12**, 263 (2000)

39 H.R. Freeman, A.V. Ramanan. *Arch. Dis. Child.* **96**, 688 (2011)

40 N.R. Maakaroun *et al.*, *Rev. Med. Virol.* **20**, 93 (2010)

41 U. Palendira *et al.*, *PLoS Biol.* **9**, e1001187 (2011)

42 J.I. Cohen *et al.*, *Blood.* **117**, 5835 (2011)

43 H. Kimura *et al.*, *Blood.* **98**, 280 (2001)

44 N. Sugaya *et al.*, *J. Infect. Dis.* **190**, 985 (2004)

ACUTE HIV-1 INFECTION

What is acute human immunodeficiency virus type 1 (HIV-1) infection?

Acute HIV-1 infection (AHI) (also termed primary HIV-1 infection or acute retroviral syndrome) is a transient clinical syndrome that may occur in a substantial proportion (as high as 90%) of individuals during HIV-1 seroconversion. Onset of illness is usually one week to four weeks after acquiring infection when there is high-level HIV-1 viraemia and a strong host inflammatory response *(1)*. A mononucleosis-like illness (MLI) is a common presentation of AHI. Illness resolves usually within 14 to 21 days, coinciding with the beginning of a decline in HIV-1 viraemia to a semi-steady state level (termed viral load set point) due to development of a host immune response. However, there is large variation in duration and severity of symptoms in the various case series. Acute HIV-2 infections may occur also but are rare in Ireland so far. This review focuses on acute HIV-1 infection.

EPIDEMIOLOGY OF ACUTE HIV IN THOSE WITH MLI

Unlinked anonymous HIV testing of samples collected in primary care from patients with MLI in London found an overall HIV prevalence of 1.3% *(2)*. A similar finding was identified in a Spanish study *(3)*. Furthermore, in HIV cases identified in the UK study, 75% were missed at initial presentation because HIV testing was not requested. While there are no data on HIV incidence among those persons with MLI in Ireland, the national prevalence of HIV is about 0.2% in adults, such that offering HIV testing to those with MLI should be considered *(4, 5)*. This is particularly relevant for adults in traditional high-risk groups such as men who have sex with men, those engaging in unprotected intercourse with new partners and intravenous drug users.

CASE VIGNETTE

An otherwise healthy 33-year-old male presented to his GP with a 48 hour history of fever, fatigue, myalgia, sore throat and headache. He had not travelled abroad recently. Physical examination revealed a temperature of 38.8°C, pharyngeal erythema without exudate and palpable posterior cervical lymphadenopathy. A diagnosis of mononucleosis-like illness (MLI) was suspected by the general practitioner.

What lessons can the GP learn from management of this case?

LABORATORY DIAGNOSIS

What samples were sent for laboratory testing?

A whole blood sample was sent for white blood cell count with differential and heterophile antibody (monospot agglutination assay). In addition, serum was sent for anti-EBV VCA IgM / IgG, anti-CMV IgM / IgG and anti-*T. gondii* IgM / IgG. A rapid antigen test for Group A *Streptococcus* was negative.

What were the findings of the above tests?

Although heterophile antibody was weakly positive, this was a false-reactive monospot result since EBV anti-VCA IgM was negative and anti-VCA IgG positive, indicating a past, resolved EBV infection. Furthermore, there was no serological evidence of recent primary CMV and *T.gondii* infections. White blood cell differential showed lymphopenia (0.8 mm^{-3}) and thrombocytopenia (140 mm^{-3}); there was no evidence of the relative lymphocytosis usually seen in acute MLI.

Two days after his initial presentation, he reattended because of appearance of a rash. Physical examination showed an erythematous, non-pruritic, maculopapular rash involving his trunk, neck, arms and legs.

What did the GP consider as the most likely diagnosis at this point?

The GP suspected secondary syphilis which can present with constitutional symptoms and a rash. On questioning, the patient revealed that he had unprotected sexual intercourse with multiple female sex workers, with the last encounter 14 days before his initial presentation. The GP sent samples for syphilis serology and testing for HIV-1&2 Ag / Ab (antigen / antibody) using a fourth-generation enzyme immunoassay (EIA). The syphilis screen was negative. HIV-1 p24 antigen was positive (confirmed by neutralisation) while HIV-1&2 antibody results were negative using an assay which detected antigen and antibody separately. The result was consistent with recent acute HIV-1 infection (AHI). The patient was then referred to an Infectious Disease clinic.

What further tests relating to AHI were done on referral of the patient to the Infectious Disease clinic?

A plasma sample collected 24 hours after onset of the rash was tested for HIV-1 RNA quantitation and indicated high-level viraemia (HIV-1 RNA 3.3 x 10^5 copies/mL). Antibody to HIV-1 was still negative. HIV-1 seroconversion (detection of antibody to HIV-1) was confirmed in a serum sample collected 26 days after his initial presentation to the GP. In addition, the patient was screened for other sexually transmitted infections including chlamydia, gonorrhoea and hepatitis B and C, and had a chest X-ray and skin testing for tuberculosis. A test to detect any transmitted HIV drug resistance was also performed. Two sets of CD4+ T-cell counts performed at the time of diagnosis and two weeks later, showed CD4+ T-cell counts of 423 cells mm^{-3} and 451 cells mm^{-3}, respectively.

What is the laboratory definition of AHI?

Acute HIV-1 infection (AHI) can only be diagnosed by detection of HIV-1 p24 antigen, which can be detected around day 14 after acquiring the virus, or by demonstrating HIV-1 RNA in plasma, which becomes detectable around day 10 post-infection *(6)*. Antibody to HIV-1 is negative in AHI. There is a delay of approximately three weeks after initial infection (or one week to 10 days after HIV-1 p24 antigen or HIV-1 RNA first appear) before antibody to HIV-1 is detectable using current fourth-generation EIAs. Seroconversion signals the start of the next phase which is commonly defined as recent HIV infection.

What would you do as a GP if you suspected AHI clinically but the HIV 1&2 Ag / Ab test was negative?

Given that HIV-1 RNA is the first marker to become detectable, send an EDTA blood for HIV-1 RNA quantification, although the patient should be referred to an Infectious Disease physician for this test.

If an asymptomatic individual presents to the GP following a potential exposure for HIV 'a few weeks ago', should the GP send serum for HIV testing at this time?

Yes, the patient should be tested immediately using a fourth-generation EIA for HIV Ag / Ab. Provided a 4th generation laboratory-based test is being used, the test can be expected to become reactive within 4-6 weeks of exposure. Depending on time of last exposure, if the result is negative, recent acquisition of HIV infection is not fully excluded and a repeat serum sample should be sent at least four weeks after the date of the last exposure. A further negative serology result at this point has a high likelihood of excluding recent HIV infection *(7)*. However, referral to Infectious Diseases clinic should be considered if the exposure was high-risk and within 72 hours in which case post exposure prophylaxis could be given *(8)*.

CLINICAL PRESENTATION

AHI was not obvious on the initial presentation in this case. Is the syndrome difficult to diagnose clinically?

Yes, many of those with AHI have nonspecific symptoms and signs. Individuals with the clinical syndrome of AHI may present with MLI or may have clinical features suggestive of conditions as diverse as secondary syphilis, measles, influenza, streptococcal pharyngitis, acute toxoplasmosis or even brucellosis *(1)*.

Should the GP have considered AHI initially?

Yes, all adults presenting with MLI should be tested for HIV *(4, 5)*. AHI should also be considered by GPs in persons who present with a febrile viral-like syndrome and engage in high-risk behaviour such as unprotected sexual intercourse and injection drug misuse. Clinical presentation with a febrile illness and oral, genital or anal mucocutaneous lesions is highly suggestive of AHI while a maculopapular rash is recognised as its most common skin manifestation *(9, 10)*. Those presenting with anorexia, weight loss and diarrhea should also be thoroughly assessed regarding high-risk behaviours for acquiring HIV *(1)*.

In what other circumstances should GPs consider testing for HIV?

HIV testing should be considered for any adult presenting to primary care or other healthcare settings with one of the following 'indicator' conditions, so-called because of their strong association with current HIV infection: sexually transmitted infection, lymphoma, cervical or anal cancer/dysplasia, shingles, hepatitis B or C, mononucleosis-like illness, leukocytopenia/thrombocytopenia lasting at least 28 days, seborrheic dermatitis/exanthema *(11)*.

ACQUISITION OF HIV-1

What was the most likely route of HIV transmission in this case?

Exposure of mucosal surfaces in the genital tract to HIV during sexual activity, as in this case, is the most common (80%) route of transmission globally *(12)*.

What factors increase and decrease the risk of sexual transmission of HIV-1?

HIV-1 viral load in semen and endocervical fluid are significant factors which heighten the risk of viral transmission *(13)*. Other contributory factors include unprotected receptive anal intercourse, local infection at site of exposure, in particular genital ulceration, HSV-2 coinfection, trauma to the genital tract and the presence of foreskin *(8, 14)*. Factors that reduce the risk include pre-exposure prophylaxis (PrEP) which prevents acquisition of HIV by the HIV-negative partner who engages in high risk sexual activities *(15)*. Suppression of plasma HIV-1 RNA load in a HIV-infected man leads to virtual elimination of the risk of HIV transmission *(16)*.

SIGNIFICANCE OF DIAGNOSIS OF AHI

Why is diagnosis of AHI so important?

The public health implications of AHI are significant: a sizeable proportion (almost 50%) of all new HIV-1 infections are likely to be acquired from individuals with AHI who are yet to be diagnosed and have a very high viral load *(17, 18)*. Therefore, diagnosing AHI is critical to controlling the HIV epidemic allowing rapid initiation of antiretroviral therapy (ART) which reduces significantly the risk of transmission. Furthermore, early administration of ART has significant benefits for the individual patient *(19, 20)*.

MANAGEMENT OF AHI IN GENERAL PRACTICE, INCLUDING PREVENTION

Was the patient treated with antiretroviral agents in this case?

Yes, the HIV specialist prescribed a combination of antiretroviral agents including elvitegravir, cobicistat, emtricitabine and tenofovirdisoproxil. The patient's illness resolved within 10 days of starting antiretroviral treatment and he did not complain of side-effects due to medication. HIV-1 RNA level had declined markedly within 4 weeks of commencing ART and became fully suppressed within 4 months. In addition, CD4+ T-cell count was 832 cells mm^{-3} indicating immune recovery. Treatment is generally recommended in AHI, regardless of timing and CD4+ T-cell count because of the established benefits of preventing progression of disease in the individual and reducing viral transmission to sexual contacts (16, 22). Starting ART very early after infection may also translate into smaller viral reservoirs, better preservation of immunity and less damage to organs and tissues (e.g. GI tract, CNS). Adherence to lifelong treatment is essential in preventing development of antiretroviral drug resistance.

What are the other aspects of management of AHI about which the GP should be aware?

Patients with AHI should be educated and counselled about their potential infectivity to sexual contacts. Strategies to reduce the risk of HIV-1 transmission need to be addressed with the patient such as safe sexual practices that do not involve exchange of body fluids and including effective use of condoms (23). The protective effects of ART on the risk of transmission to sexual contacts should be regarded as starting about 6 months after the viral load is suppressed in plasma, to allow sufficient time for suppression to extend to other compartments. Tracing of sexual contacts needs to be performed by Public Health.

Was post exposure prophylaxis (PEP) against HIV-1 recommended to sexual contacts in this case?

No, he had no sexual contacts since the last exposure with commercial sex workers which was outside the window of effectiveness of PEP. Antiretroviral agents for PEP should be given to contacts as soon as possible but not more than 72 hours after potential exposure for maximum effectiveness. PEP is given for four weeks. Where available, the ART and viral load status of the source case can be used to judge the need for PEP in contacts (no need when stably suppressed viral load). For contacts with ongoing at-risk behaviours, pre-exposure prophylaxis (PrEP) should be considered (15, 24).

REFERENCES (*useful reviews)

1 J.O. Kahn, B.D. Walker. *N. Engl. J. Med.* **339**, 33 (1998)

2 D.T. Hsu *et al.*, *HIV Med.* **14**, 60 (2013)

3 I. Menacho *et al.*, *HIV Med.* **14**Suppl 3, 33 (2013)

4 European Centre for Disease Control;

https://ecdc.europa.eu/en/publications-data/public-health-guidance-hiv-hepatitis-b-and-c-testing-euea

5 National Institute for Health and Care Excellence;
https://www.nice.org.uk/guidance/ng60/chapter/Recommendations*

6 J.K. Cornett, T.J. Kim. *Clin. Infect. Dis.* **57**, 712 (2013)*

7 BASHH.BASHH/EAGA.Statement on HIV window period.www.bashh.org November 2014

8 https://www.bhiva.org/PEPSE-guidelines

9 F.M. Hecht *et al.*, *AIDS.* **16**, 1119 (2002)

10 E.N. Vergis, J.W. Mellors. *Infect. Dis. Clin. North Am.* **14**, 809 (2000)

11 A.K. Sullivan *et al.*, *PLoS One.* **8**, e52845 (2013)

12 M.S. Cohen *et al.*, *N. Engl. J. Med.* **364**, 1943 (2011)*

13 J.M. Baeten *et al.*, *Sci. Trans. Med.* **3**, 77ra29 (2011)

14 R A. Royce *et al.*, *N. Engl. J. Med.* **336**, 1072 (1997)

15. Centers for Disease Control. https://wwwcdc.gov/hiv/pdf/risk/prep/dcd-hiv-prep-guidelines.2017.

16. A.J. Rodger *et al.*, *Lancet.* **393**, 2428 (2019)

17 M.J. Wawer *et al.*, *J. Infect. Dis.* **191**, 1403 (2005)

18 B.G. Brenner *et al.*, *J. Infect. Dis.* **195**, 951 (2007)

19 INSIGHT START Study Group. J.D. Lundgren *et al.*, *N. Engl. J. Med.* **373**, 795 (2015)

20 L. Gras *et al.*, *AIDS.* **25**, 813 (2011)

21 S. Fidler, J. Fox.*Clin. Med.* **16**, 180 (2016)*

22www.bhiva.org/documents/Guidelines/Treatment/2015/2015-treatment-guidelines.pdf

23 The Healthy Living Project Team. *J. Acquir. Immune Defic.Syndr.***44**, 213 (2007)

24. R.H. Goldschmidt. *Clin. Infect. Dis.* **64**, 150 (2017)

TOXOPLASMOSIS

What is toxoplasmosis?

Toxoplasmosis is caused by the protozoan parasite *Toxoplasma gondii* (*T.gondii*). Almost a third of the world's population may become infected. Although primary infection with *T.gondii* is mainly asymptomatic, some individuals present with a mild and self-limiting influenza-like illness, or infectious mononucleosis-like illness. Furthermore, in those who acquire toxoplasmosis postnatally, a small proportion (< 2%) may develop ocular disease, most commonly posterior uveitis. In certain vulnerable groups toxoplasmosis has potentially serious consequences. Primary infection in pregnancy may result in transmission to the fetus with devastating neurological or ocular sequelae.

Following primary infection, *T.gondii* becomes latent (encystment in tissues) and persists in this state due to the individual's cellular immune system. Consequently, if the cellular arm of the immune system is impaired, for example, with iatrogenic immunosuppression following transplantation or with human immunodeficiency virus (HIV) infection, the encysted latent form of *T.gondii* may reactivate causing life-threatening visceral diseases such as encephalitis, pneumonitis or disseminated disease. The latter manifestations occur rarely in otherwise immunocompetent persons.

CASE VIGNETTE

A 26-year-old previously healthy woman presented with a 2-week history of fatigue and malaise. She had recently returned from a 6-week holiday to South America. On physical examination, the patient was afebrile with normal vital signs but she had enlarged, non-tender cervical and occipital lymphadenopathy. How would you approach this case?

LABORATORY DIAGNOSIS

What infections would you suspect? What laboratory tests would you request?

A 'mononucleosis-like illness' was considered likely. Serum was sent for heterophile antibody, anti-CMV IgM / IgG, anti-*T.gondii* IgM / IgG and HIV Ag/Ab (antigen / antibody) testing. Because she had travelled to Brazil, anti-Zika virus IgM / IgG and Zika virus RNA were included in the testing panel. A full blood count (FBC) and biochemical profile were also requested.

What did the above laboratory tests reveal?

The FBC showed a slight lymphocytosis (lymphocytes 4,000 mm^{-3}) without atypical lymphocytes on peripheral film and anti-*T.gondii* IgM / IgG results were positive, suggestive of primary toxoplasmosis. Biochemical findings were within the normal range.

Does anti-*T.gondii* IgM result confirm recent primary toxoplasmosis?

No, anti-*T.gondii* IgM can persist for up to 6 months after onset of primary infection and, furthermore, false-positive IgM results are known to occur with commercial assays for toxoplasmosis *(1)*. Therefore, anti-*T.gondii* IgM results alone must be interpreted with caution.

What other test is of value in the laboratory diagnosis of recent primary toxoplasmosis?

Anti-*T.gondii* IgG avidity testing is helpful in distinguishing recent versus past infections by testing the strength with which antibody binds to antigen (strength of binding increases over the months following exposure to the pathogen as the immune response matures). With the toxoplasma avidity test used in this laboratory, low avidity (< 30%) suggests infection within the last 3 months while high avidity (> 40%) indicates infection > 6 months ago. The woman's serology revealed that anti-*T.gondii* IgM was strongly positive and anti-*T.gondii* IgG avidity was low (15%), which together with the clinical presentation, was consistent with primary *Toxoplasma* infection. A repeat sample four weeks later showed a significant increase in the avidity result (30%) and a rise in anti-*T.gondii* IgG titre (determined by Dye test in a reference laboratory), confirming primary toxoplasmosis.

Does low anti-*T.gondii* IgG avidity always indicate recent primary infection?

No, low-avidity results are not necessarily diagnostic of recent primary toxoplasmosis *(1)*. Caution is needed because IgG avidity may remain stable at low level for ≥ 3 months *(2)*. Therefore, referral of samples to a Toxoplasma reference laboratory is advised to confirm any suspected primary infection, particularly in pregnancy. An alternative way of confirming primary toxoplasmosis is to show either a significant rise in anti-*T.gondii* IgG levels, or seroconversion (from IgG negative to IgG positive) if earlier samples are available from before the onset of symptoms, e.g. an antenatal booking blood.

Does high anti-*T.gondii* IgG avidity reliably exclude recent infection?

Yes, even in the presence of positive anti-*T.gondii* IgM, high-avidity IgG values indicate evolution from acute to chronic latent toxoplasmosis since there is a minimum time for this process to take place *(1)*.

TREATMENT OF TOXOPLASMOSIS IN IMMUNOCOMPETENT INDIVIDUALS

Would you treat the patient in this case with antiparasitic drugs for acute toxoplasmosis?

No, treatment with pyrimethamine, sulfadiazine (and folinic acid) is rarely warranted unless there is evidence of visceral disease or prolonged and severe symptoms. In the latter circumstances, referral to hospital for clinical review is advised.

What would you do if the patient had visual problems and fundoscopy suggested ocular toxoplasmosis?

The woman should be referred to an ophthalmologist. Ocular toxoplasmosis in immunocompetent persons is usually a self-limiting condition lasting about 4 to 8 weeks *(3)*. While some ophthalmologists monitor individuals with small peripheral lesions, treatment with antiparasitic agents should be considered for those presenting with ocular toxoplasmosis if lesions are sight-threatening such as when they are within the vascular arcades, proximal to the optic disc or larger than two optic disc diameters *(4)*. Corticosteroids are added if there is severe vitreous inflammation, lesions are large or near the fovea or optic disc *(5)*. The classic combination for treatment of ocular disease is oral pyrimethamine (folinic acid supplement), oral sulfadiazine (or oral clindamycin) and topical corticosteroids.

TRANSMISSION OF TOXOPLASMOSIS TO HUMANS

What are the infectious forms of *T.gondii*?

There are three forms of the parasite which are potentially infectious: sporozoites, tachyzoites and bradyzoites. Large numbers of oocysts (containing sporozoites) are shed infaeces of infected cats into the environment. If infectious oocysts are ingested by humans or mammals like cows, goats and pigs, sporozoites are released in the intestine and develop into tachyzoites which then disseminate to many organs, including the fetus in pregnancy, and multiply causing tissue damage. The immune system responds and clears most tachyzoites, although a tiny number persist in muscle, myocardium, brain and eye, as tissue cysts containing bradyzoites, the dormant form of the parasite. Ingestion of inadequately cooked meat containing tissue cysts (bradyzoites) can cause toxoplasmosis in non-immune humans *(6)*. Cats, a source of human infection, acquire the parasite by eating rodents and birds that are already encysted with *T.gondii*.

How does toxoplasmosis develop in immunocompromised individuals infected in the past?

If the human immune system is severely impaired due to iatrogenic immunosuppression or HIV infection, bradyzoites in tissue cysts of those infected with *T.gondii* in the past may revert to actively replicating tachyzoites. This reactivation of the parasite may cause end-organ diseases such as toxoplasmic encephalitis, retinitis and/or pneumonitis.

How did the woman in this case acquire toxoplasmosis?

Often exposure is due to under processed meat. She ate undercooked meat on several occasions, including steak tartare and barbequed lamb, while in Argentina. Humans often acquire *T.gondii* through eating undercooked, raw or improperly cured meat containing viable tissue cysts of the parasite. Alternatively, ingesting untreated water, raw fruits or vegetables covered with soil that is contaminated with oocysts of *T.gondii* shed by cats, can act as a source *(7)*. Travel outside Europe, the United States and Canada is associated with acquisition of toxoplasmosis in pregnant women *(7)*.

PREVENTION OF HUMAN TOXOPLASMOSIS

What advice should be given to women of childbearing age and immunocompromised persons to avoid toxoplasmosis?

Ensure meat is cooked all the way through and to a safe temperature (71.1°C) to kill tissue cysts of *T.gondii*.

Freezing meat for 2-3 days prior to use will kill bradyzoites in tissue cysts.

Wash hands thoroughly after contact with raw meats or unwashed fruits and vegetables to prevent ingestion of oocysts via hands.

All kitchen utensils used to prepare raw meat should be cleaned thoroughly.

Individuals should wear gloves when handling soil and wash hands thoroughly to eliminate contamination with oocysts in soil.

Ideally, a nonpregnant and immunocompetent household member should clean cat litter boxes. Otherwise, pregnant or immunocompromised individuals should wear gloves when handling cat litter and wash hands thoroughly. Cats should be fed only commercial diets or well-cooked table food. Cat litter should be disposed of daily because oocysts in excrement need at least 24 hours to become infectious.

If the woman in this case was planning to conceive, for how long should she wait?

It seems prudent to avoid conception until six months after diagnosis of primary toxoplasmosis in women *(8)*.

Should a domestic cat owned by a pregnant woman or immunocompromised person be rehomed?

No, ownership of a cat or contact with one does not pose a risk for *Toxoplasma*. When cats acquire *T.gondii*, they can shed up to 100 million oocysts daily in faeces for about 21 days, but such large numbers are usually only shed once in their lifetime. Oocysts require 1 to 5 days in the environment to become infectious and then persist for as long as 18 months in soil *(6)*. Interestingly, cats usually groom faeces, which potentially carries oocysts of *T.gondii*, from their fur before the oocysts have time to become infectious *(9)*. Therefore, humans do not usually acquire *Toxoplasma* from direct contact with cats. However, caution is needed when handling and changing cat litter trays *(10)*.

REFERENCES (*useful reviews)

1 R. Dhakal *et al.*, *J. Clin.Microbiol.***53**, 3601 (2015)

2 G. Findal *et al.*, *PLoS ONE.***10**, e0145519 (2015)

3 N.J. Butler *et al.*, *Clin. Exp. Ophthalmol.* **41**, 95 (2013)

4 G.N. Holland, K.G. Lewis. *Am. J. Ophthalmol.* **134**, 102 (2002)

5 C. Ozgonul, C.G. Besirli. *Ophthalmic Res.* **57**, 1 (2017)

6 A.M. Tenter, A.R. Heckeroth, L.M. Weiss. *Int. J. Parasitol.* **30**, 1217 (2000)

7 A.J.C. Cook *et al.*, *BMJ.* **321**, 142 (2000)*

8 C. Paquet, M.H. Yudin. *J. Obstet. Gynaecol. Can.* **40**, e687 (2018)*

9 J.P. Dubey. *J. Parasitol.***81**, 410 (1995)

10 S.A. Elmore *et al.*, *Trends Parasitol.***26**, 190 (2010)

MUMPS

CLINICAL VIROLOGY

What is mumps virus?

Mumps is a single-stranded RNA virus of the genus *Rubulavirus* in the family *Paramyxoviridae (1)*. There are currently 12 known genotypes (designated A to N) of mumps virus based on molecular analysis of the small hydrophobic gene (SH), the most diverse area in its genome *(2)*. However, since there is only one serotype, immunity to one genotype would be expected to provide protection against all others.

What is the clinical definition of mumps?

Mumps is a viral illness characterised by acute onset of painful swelling of the jaw or parotid gland, less commonly involving other salivary glands, and persisting for ≥ 2 days in the absence of another obvious cause.

Are there other clinical presentations compatible with mumps virus infection?

Common complications of mumps virus infection include orchitis in post-pubertal males and aseptic meningitis. Less common complications are mastitis, transient hearing loss, Bell's palsy, oophoritis and pancreatitis *(3)*.

Can mumps infection be asymptomatic or cause very mild infections?

Yes, estimates suggest that about 30% of unvaccinated individuals have subclinical infection or minimally symptomatic infections *(4)*. The younger the patient at the time of infection, the higher is the probability of asymptomatic or mild infection.

Are complications more severe in immunocompromised individuals with mumps?

Despite deficiency in humoral and cellular immunity, mumps virus rarely causes severe infections in immunosuppressed individuals *(5)*. However, there are anecdotal reports of mumps-related encephalomyelitis and nephritis in this cohort, reflecting the neurotropism of the virus and its preference for infection of epithelium in renal distal tubules *(6, 7)*. With persistent circulation of mumps in the community, immunocompromised patients are potentially at risk of mumps and therefore it should be considered when a viral cause of central nervous system or renal complications is suspected.

PATHOGENESIS

How does mumps virus cause disease?

The virus probably replicates in the upper respiratory tract of the host and later disseminates systemically most likely via blood mononuclear cells. Furthermore, it has tropism for cells in parotid glands, central nervous system and gonads where it replicates rapidly thereby causing its characteristic clinical features and complications *(1)*.

EPIDEMIOLOGY

Almost half of all notified cases of mumps in 2018 were in those aged 15 to 24 years, of whom 43% reported having had≥ 1 dose of MMR vaccine *(8)*. Outbreaks of mumps are also reported among vaccinated young adults attending educational institutions, including secondary schools and third-level colleges / universities; however, the number of cases is much lower than in the pre-vaccine era and spread beyond these settings into the community is limited *(9)*.

Why do outbreaks of mumps still occur?

Uptake of two-dose MMR vaccination is suboptimal in young Irish adults *(10)*. MMR vaccination uptake among children at 24 months of age in Ireland is currently 92% which is below the World Health Organisation target of 95% *(11)*. One study in 2004 suggested that the seroprevalence of antibodies to mumps virus in Irish 15–24 year olds was only 80%-85%, which is below the herd immunity threshold of 88% to 92% proposed as necessary to prevent onward transmission of mumps in the community *(11)*. This inadequate immunity may reflect reduced natural boosting due to lower natural disease incidence.

Why do outbreaks of mumps occur in populations with high rates of two-dose vaccination coverage?

It is likely that those living in congregated settings that allow exposure to infectious saliva are at risk of mumps because a high virus inoculum may overwhelm vaccine-induced immunity *(3, 12)*. In these circumstances, waning of immunity and a two-dose vaccine effectiveness against mumps of 66% to 95% may also be contributory *(13)*. Waning of vaccine-induced immunity probably contributed significantly to a recent mumps outbreak among a highly vaccinated population of university students *(12)*. There is currently no evidence of emergence of a viral strain capable of wholly evading vaccine-induced humoral immunity *(14, 15)*.

CASE VIGNETTE

An 18-year-old female student presented to her GP with a 36-hour history of left-sided facial swelling with fever and malaise. Twelve hours before attending the GP she also developed right-sided facial swelling. She had no dental problems. On examination, both parotid glands were swollen and tender with swelling extending to the retromandibular area. The GP had documented evidence of the student's previous immunisation with two doses of MMR vaccine. There was an ongoing outbreak of mumps in the girl's school. What can GPs learn from this case?

LABORATORY DIAGNOSIS

Was laboratory testing necessary for confirmation of mumps in this patient with mumps-like illness?

No, laboratory confirmation is generally not required for notification of patients with an illness compatible with mumps. However, as in this case, it should be considered in MMR-vaccinated individuals with suspected infection since there are other infectious causes of mumps-like illness. Diagnostic testing is important in defining the epidemiology of clinical mumps and evaluating limitations of the current MMR vaccine.

What laboratory tests are most frequently used to diagnose mumps?

Laboratory diagnosis of mumps is based on detection of either mumps virus RNA by a real-time reverse transcription PCR (rRT-PCR) that targets the small hydrophobic protein (SH) gene, or mumps virus-specific IgM antibody in clinical samples using capture IgM enzyme immunoassays.

Which clinical samples were collected for laboratory diagnosis of mumps in this case?

Oral fluid (using saliva collection swab) was tested for mumps RNA and mumps-specific IgM. Mumps RNA was detected and mumps-specific IgM was negative. Serum was tested for mumps-specific IgM which was negative and mumps-specific IgG which was positive.

If serum was unavailable, would oral fluid have sufficed for diagnosis of recent mumps infection?

Yes, detection of mumps virus RNA confirmed current infection. In addition, oral fluid collected in acute- and convalescent-phases could have been tested for mumps virus-specific IgM *(16)*.

If molecular and serological findings for mumps virus were negative in a case with mumps-like illness, what other tests would you request?

Consider testing for other viruses which may present clinically as parotitis *(17, 18)*. If influenza virus is circulating in the community, test oral fluid for influenza A / B RNA. Otherwise, test for parainfluenza virus RNA and send serum for EBV serology. Sporadic cases of parotitis have also been associated with human herpes virus 6, adenoviruses and enteroviruses.

FACTORS AFFECTING VIROLOGY TEST RESULTS

Did the patient's MMR vaccination status impact on performance of virology tests for mumps?

Yes, mumps virus-specific IgM production is commonly diminished or delayed or may even be absent in individuals with recent mumps infection who previously received ≥ 1 dose of MMR vaccine (18, 19). In contrast, mumps virus-specific IgM is usually present in unvaccinated individuals who acquired recent infection. Therefore, in vaccinated persons with clinical mumps, as in this case, an acute-phase sample may be negative for mumps IgM. However, a repeat serum should be collected ≥ 10 days after illness onset in vaccinated persons with clinical mumps as it may improve detection rates (19). While mumps virus RNA was detected in this case, there is evidence that viral shedding in oral fluid may be short-lived and low-level in previously vaccinated individuals with clinical mumps because of rapid clearance of virus due to residual immunity (20, 21). Therefore, detection rates of mumps RNA can be lower in those exhibiting a secondary immune response.

Is timing of collection of clinical samples relevant to serological confirmation of mumps?

The rate of detection of mumps-specific IgM is also influenced by the timing of sample collection. Mumps-specific IgM can be negative in the acute phase of infection (≤ 3 days) in persons with mumps (22). In vaccinated individuals with clinical mumps, detection rates for mumps-specific IgM using capture EIAs improved significantly when samples were collected ≥ 5 days after symptom onset (20). Another study recommended testing serum collected ≥ 10 days after onset of symptoms for mumps-specific IgM if negative in the acute-phase samples (19).

What factors may affect molecular confirmation of mumps?

In contrast to serology, as the time interval from onset of illness to collection of oral fluid was increased to ≥ 5 days, the proportion of swabs positive for mumps virus RNA by rRT-PCR decreased significantly, limiting the diagnostic value of molecular testing in samples collected later in the course of mumps, although it may still be detected until day 9 after onset (22). Furthermore, the quality of a clinical specimen, specifically its concentration of RNA, can be adversely affected by improper storage conditions thereby influencing diagnostic yield (21). Therefore, a negative result on molecular testing does not necessarily exclude mumps.

OPTIMAL DIAGNOSTIC APPROACH

What would be a reasonable approach to laboratory confirmation of mumps?

If ≤ 7 days since onset of illness, oral fluid should be collected (using saliva collection swab) for mumps virus RNA and mumps virus-specific IgM.

INTERPRETATION OF MUMPS VIRUS (MuV) TEST RESULTS IN ORAL FLUID

The following virological results are encountered frequently in samples collected ≤ 7 days after onset of mumps-like illness. Interpret them.

MuV-specific IgM NEGATIVE: MuV RNA DETECTED:

Current mumps virus infection. Notify public health authorities.

MuV-specific IgM NEGATIVE: MuV RNA NOT detected:

Does not exclude current mumps infection in persons vaccinated previously with MMR or with past history of mumps. Notify public health authorities if illness is clinically compatible with mumps. Collect a <u>serum</u> sample ≥ 10 days after onset of illness for MuV-specific IgM/IgG. MuV-specific IgM may be detected.

MuV-specific IgM POSITIVE: MuV RNA DETECTED:

Consistent with current mumps virus infection. Notify public health authorities.

MuV-specific IgM POSITIVE (weak): MuV RNA NOT detected:

While suggestive of recent mumps virus infection when clinical findings are compatible, send a serum sample collected ≥ 10 days after illness onset and check for MuV-specific IgM. In addition, test serum for EBV VCA IgM/IgG. During primary EBV infection, polyclonal B cell stimulation can generate false-positive mumps IgM results *(3)*.

PUBLIC HEALTH CONSIDERATIONS

What was the likely route of transmission in this case?

In general, transmission occurs by exposure of mucous membranes in the nose, throat and conjunctiva of a contact to infectious saliva or respiratory droplets from an index case or to contaminated fomites *(5)*. Close and prolonged contact with an infectious case is required for transmission. Therefore, communal living conditions as in dormitories of boarding schools as well as enclosed settings such as third-level institutions (as in this case) and barracks facilitate transmission, potentially leading to outbreaks *(1, 5)*.

What was the period of infectivity in this case?

An index case is infectious from two days before to five days after onset of symptoms *(5)*. Therefore, she was advised not to attend college or work for five days after onset of illness. She recovered with supportive and symptomatic care.

Was post exposure prophylaxis advised for contacts of this newly diagnosed case of mumps?

No, neither active immunisation with MMR vaccine nor passive immunisation with immune globulin is recommended as immediate postexposure prophylaxis. However, MMR vaccination would be beneficial in reducing the risk of transmission to nonimmune individuals who are subsequently exposed to mumps *(23)*.

Should the GP be concerned if a pregnant woman had contact with this index case with mumps?

No, there is no consistent evidence that mumps acquired during pregnancy is associated with increased rates of spontaneous abortion or teratogenicity *(24)*. However, pregnant women should try to avoid exposure to mumps cases if possible.

Why does mumps-specific IgG positivity not guarantee protection against mumps?

Because there is no known immune marker which defines immunity to mumps *(14)*. Therefore, mumps-specific antibody may be ineffective in protecting against infection particularly with a large inoculum of virus. Seropositivity for mumps indicates past infection or vaccination and, while it undoubtedly reduces the risk of mumps, it does not guarantee complete protection as shown in this case and by outbreaks in populations with high vaccine coverage *(3, 25)*.

If a fully vaccinated person is mumps-specific IgG negative in serum, is she/he susceptible to mumps?

Not necessarily since other components of immunity such as cell-mediated responses combined with subdetectable neutralising antibody may still protect against clinical mumps *(26)*.

Is there a role for use of a third dose of MMR in control of mumps outbreaks?

A third dose of MMR vaccine is recommended for individuals who are at increased risk of infection during mumps outbreaks *(27)*. This includes those who have had two-dose MMR vaccination in the past and attend settings such as universities and colleges where there is prolonged and close contact with infected individuals during an outbreak. Recent data from an outbreak suggest that a third dose of MMR vaccine may be of value in control of mumps outbreaks in these settings even with > 90% two-dose vaccine coverage *(12)*. Waning of vaccine-induced immunity was probably a contributory factor in the outbreak: a long interval between receipt of the second dose of MMR vaccine and exposure to mumps seemed to correlate with increased susceptibility to the virus even among two-dose vaccine recipients.

For information on mumps vaccination in Ireland see
https://www.hse.ie/eng/health/immunisation/hcpinfo/guidelines/chapter14.pdf

REFERENCES (*useful reviews)

1 A. Hviid, S. Rubin, K. Mühlemann. *Lancet*.**371**, 932 (2008)*

2 World Health Organisation. *Weekly Epid. Rec.* **87**, 217 (2012)

3 A.E. Barskey *et al.*, *N. Engl. J. Med.* **367**, 1704 (2012)*

4 M.M. Cortese *et al.*, *J. Infect. Dis.* **204**, 1413 (2011)

5 P.K. Kutty *et al.*, *Clin. Infect. Dis.* **50**, 1619 (2010)

6 T.A. Eyre *et al.*, *J. Clin. Virol.***57**, 165 (2013)

7 M.C. Baas *et al.*, *Am. J. Transplant.* **9**, 2186 (2009)

8 Annual Epidemiological Report November 2018 Health Protection Surveillance Centre

9 S. Gee *et al.*, *Eurosurveill.* **13**, pii=18857 (2008)

10 Health Protection Surveillance Centre, Ireland. *Epi-Insight***16**, 8 (2015)

11 M. Di Renzi *et al.*, *Eurosurveill.* **8**, pii=2608 (2004)

12 C.V. Cardemil *et al.*, *N. Engl. J. Med.* **377**, 947 (2017)

13 C. Cohen *et al.*, *Emerg. Infect. Dis.* **13**, 12 (2007)

14 S.A. Rubin *et al.*, *J. Virol.***86**, 615 (2012)

15 M. May, C.A. Rieder, R.J. Rowe. *Int. J. Infect. Dis.* **66**, 1 (2018)

16 F. Reid *et al.*, *J. Clin. Virol.***41**, 134 (2008)

17 A.E. Barskey*et al.*, *J. Infect.. Dis.* **208**, 1979 (2013)

18C. Thompson *et al.*, *EuroSurveill.* **20**, pii=21203 (2015)

19 C.H. Krause *et al.*, *J. Clin. Virol.***38**, 153 (2007)

20 J.S. Rota *et al.*, *Clin. Vaccine.Immunol.***20**, 391 (2013)

21 R.H. Bitsko *et al.*, *J. Clin. Microbiol.***46**, 1101 (2008)

22E.J. Baron *et al.*, *Clin. Infect. Dis.* **57**, e22 (2013)*

23 Centers for Disease Control.*Morb.Mortal.Wkly. Rep.* **61**, 986 (2012)

24 M. Siegel. *JAMA.***226**, 1521 (1973)

25M. Marin *et al.*, *Vaccine.* **26**, 3601 (2008)

26S. Jokinen *et al.*, *J. Infect. Dis.* **196**, 861 (2007)

27 M. Marin *et al.*, *Morb. Mortal. Wkly. Rep.* **67**, 33 (2018)

PREGNANCY and VIRAL INFECTIONS

- CMV
- HSV
- Parvovirus B19
- Toxoplasmosis
- Varicella

CYTOMEGALOVIRUS IN PREGNANCY

CASE VIGNETTE

A 26-year-old female who works in a crèche and is pregnant, 18 weeks' gestation, presented to her GP with a 72-hour history of fever, sore throat and malaise. She already has a 2-year-old child who is clinically well. On physical examination, her temperature is 38.8°C with diffuse pharyngeal erythema and mild lymphadenopathy in anterior and posterior cervical lymph nodes. Your clinical impression is of infectious mononucleosis (IM) but her clinical notes showed that she had laboratory-confirmed EBV-related IM several years previously.

The GP requested a rapid group A streptococcal antigen test, which was negative, a full blood count which revealed lymphocytosis (5,000 mm^{-3}) and atypical lymphocytes on the peripheral blood film. Her liver function tests showed raised alanine aminotransferase (ALT) level at 111 IU/L (normal range < 35 IU/L).

How would you manage this case?

LABORATORY DIAGNOSIS

What infectious causes of mononucleosis-like illness (MLI) would you consider important in pregnancy?

Primary infections with cytomegalovirus (CMV), a member of the *Herpesviridae* family which establishes latency following acute infection, the parasite *Toxoplasma gondii*, which also becomes dormant following infection, and human immunodeficiency virus (HIV) are relevant in this case. A serum sample collected from the patient was tested for CMV IgM / IgG, *T.gondii* IgM / IgG and HIV 1&2 Ag/Ab (antigen/antibody).

While results excluded toxoplasmosis and HIV infection, she was CMV IgM and CMV IgG positive in her serum sample collected at 18 weeks' gestation. Does this confirm primary CMV in this patient?

No, CMV IgM can be positive in serum for several reasons: primary CMV infection; non-primary (or recurrent) infection either due to CMV reactivation or reinfection with a different viral serotype; persistence of CMV IgM for months after resolution of primary infection; IgM cross-reactivity between different herpes viruses; even infection with unrelated viruses like measles and parvovirus B19 may induce CMV IgM reactivity *(1, 2)*.

How was primary CMV infection confirmed in this case?

By demonstrating CMV IgG seroconversion in two serum samples collected at different times. A 'booking blood' (serum), collected from the woman when she first attended the antenatal clinic at 10 weeks' gestation, was tested for CMV IgM / IgG and both serological markers were negative. So primary CMV infection in pregnancy was confirmed by showing CMV IgM and CMV IgG seroconversion between 10 weeks' and 18 weeks' gestation.

How would you confirm primary CMV infection in this case if her 'booking blood' was unavailable?

By showing the concomitant presence of CMV IgM and low-avidity CMV IgG in serum collected at 18 weeks' gestation. The principle of avidity testing is as follows: in the initial phase of infection, virus-specific IgG antibodies are produced which are of low avidity (strength of binding of antibody to antigen). However, avidity matures over time so that in the convalescent stage of infection, virus-specific IgG is of higher avidity and, in general, remains high for life. In this case, the serum collected at 18 weeks' gestation was CMV IgM positive and CMV IgG avidity was low (< 0.20), which indicated primary CMV infection acquired by the woman sometime in the 12 weeks before the sample was collected. A subsequent sample collected several months later showed development of high avidity CMV IgG (> 0.65).

PRIMARY VERSUS NON-PRIMARY CMV INFECTION IN PREGNANCY

Why is CMV infection in pregnancy of clinical significance?

Human CMV can cause significant damage to the central nervous system of the fetus. Although most primary CMV infections in all age groups are asymptomatic, CMV is the most common viral cause of intrauterine infection, affecting 0.2-0.6% of all live births in Ireland and Europe. It is a major viral cause of birth defects (3, 4, 5). The annual rate of primary CMV infection in pregnancy is estimated to be 1%-2% and approximately 10% of infants with congenital CMV (cCMV) infection have clinical evidence of disease at birth (6, 7). Among symptomatic neonates with cCMV, there is a 40%-50% risk of mental retardation, sensorineural hearing loss (SNHL) and neurodevelopmental disorders. In fact, even among neonates with cCMV who are asymptomatic at birth, between 5% and 17% may develop neurological sequelae in the first years of life, particularly SNHL (8, 9).

Why is confirmation of primary CMV infection in pregnancy, as in this case, important?

The risk of viral transmission to the fetus is approximately 30%-40% following primary CMV infection in the mother. This fact needs to be discussed during counselling of the mother by the clinical team.

Can a mother give birth to a child with cCMV if she is CMV seropositive before pregnancy?

Yes, even with preconceptional immunity to CMV, the fetus may acquire the virus from the mother during pregnancy. Non-primary CMV infection may develop in the pregnant woman due to endogenous viral reactivation or exogenous reinfection with a different strain of CMV. There is a much lower risk of CMV transmission to the fetus, in contrast to the 40% transmission risk with primary CMV infection *(10)*. However, neurological sequelae, such as SNHL, may develop in some infants (10%-20%) who acquire infection from mothers with non-primary CMV infection in pregnancy *(9, 11)*.

OUTCOME

How was this case managed after laboratory confirmation of primary CMV infection in the mother?

The patient was referred to her obstetrician. Antiviral treatment for prevention of maternal transmission of CMV to the fetus is not recommended. To determine if the fetus was infected, an amniocentesis was performed. This procedure is optimally performed after 21 weeks' gestation and at least 6 weeks after onset of maternal infection *(12)*. Amniotic fluid collected at 24 weeks' gestation was tested by real-time PCR and CMV DNA was detected. The mother opted to continue with the pregnancy and attended hospital regularly for ultrasound monitoring of the fetus. The baby was asymptomatic at birth. Neonatal urine and saliva were tested for CMV DNA in the first 21 days of life and confirmed cCMV infection. Audiological assessment was normal at birth but a programme for clinical and audiological follow-up every six months in the first three years was recommended. SNHL and neurodevelopmental disorder were not observed.

Antiviral treatment of neonates with cCMV infection who are asymptomatic is not recommended even if there is evidence of an audiological abnormality. In contrast, in neonates who are symptomatic at birth and either have central nervous system (CNS) involvement or end-organ disease, treatment with ganciclovir intravenously or oral valganciclovir is recommended *(13)*.

PREVENTION OF MATERNAL CMV INFECTION

What advice would you give a woman with primary CMV infection who is planning to conceive?

Waiting one year following primary CMV infection in a woman planning to conceive has been suggested but there is a paucity of data available to support this time interval *(14)*. There is evidence of an increased risk of CMV transmission if primary infection occurs months before conception *(15)*. Although the risk is not as high as 30%-40% seen in primary infection during pregnancy, it appears to be greater than the background risk of viral transmission (about 1%) seen among those with preexisting CMV immunity long before conception (non-primary infection) *(14)*. Couples need to consider what they think is an acceptable risk of CMV transmission to the fetus and factor other issues such as reduced fertility with increasing maternal age.

What was the most likely source of CMV acquired by the pregnant woman in this case?

She worked in a créche and probably acquired CMV through contact with fomites, like toys, contaminated with saliva and urine from infected children in whom CMV is shed asymptomatically *(16)*. In addition, she had a child at home and it is recognised that mothers of young children who are shedding CMV are particularly at risk for CMV transmission via childrens' urine and saliva *(17)*. Furthermore, it has been shown that adolescents and adults of child-bearing age who work with children in day-care centres, especially children under two years of age, are at risk of acquiring CMV infection *(19)*. CMV may also be acquired in the community through sexual contact since infected individuals may shed the virus in semen and vaginal fluid.

Are healthcare workers in hospitals at high risk for CMV infection?

There is no evidence for an increased risk of CMV infection among healthcare workers in paediatric hospitals compared to other women in the community, presumably because staff are trained in infection control measures, including regular hand washing, and infection requires prolonged contact *(19, 20, 21)*.

How can pregnant women reduce their risk of acquiring CMV infection?

It is important to educate pregnant women working in child care centres or who have young children at home about CMV as a pathogen in pregnancy as simple hygienic measures can reduce the risk of CMV infection significantly *(20, 22)*. Effective measures to reduce the risk for CMV transmission include frequent hand washing after exposure to childrens' saliva or urine and following contact with fomites and surfaces likely to be touched by children, like toys and tables on high chairs. In addition, adults should not use the same eating utensils or drinking cups as children and should avoid kissing them on the mouth or cheek *(13)*. There is no licensed vaccine against congenital CMV infection (cCMV) currently, however, it is a priority public healthcare goal due to the toll on society of the sometimes devastating neurological sequelae of cCMV infection *(23)*.

Useful information for parents – www.cmvaction.org.uk

REFERENCES (*useful reviews)

1 D. Lang *et al.*, *Clin.Diagn. Lab. Immunol.* **8**, 747 (2001)

2 H.I. Thomas *et al.*, *J. Clin. Virol.* **14**, 107 (1999)

3 A. Waters *et al.*,*J.Clin. Virol.* **59**, 156 (2014)

4 G. Benoist *et al.*,*Gynecol. Obstet. Fertil.* **36**, 248 (2008)

5 S.C. Dollard, S.D. Grosse, D.S. Ross. *Rev. Med. Virol.* **17**, 355 (2007)

6 P. Duff. *Am. J. Obstet. Gynecol.* **196**, 196 (2007)

7 S.B. Boppana *et al.*, *Pediatr. Infect. Dis. J.* **11**, 93 (1992)

8 K.B. Fowler *et al.*, *J. Pediatr.* **130**, 624 (1997)

9 D.H. Spector.*J. Infect. Dis.* **209**, 1497 (2014)

10 K.B. Fowler, S. Stagno, R.F. Pass. *JAMA.***289**, 1008 (2003)

11 S.A. Ross *et al.*, *J. Pediatr.***148**, 332 (2006)

12 C. Liesnard *et al.*, *Obstet. Gynecol.* **95**, 881 (2000)

13 W.D. Rawlinson *et al.*, *Lancet Infect. Dis.* **17**, e177 (2017)*

14 M.G. Revello *et al.*, *J. Infect. Dis.* **193**, 783 (2006)

15 K.B. Fowler, S. Stagno, R.F. Pass. *Clin. Infect. Dis.* **38**, 1035 (2004)

16 J.F. Bale Jr *et al.*, *Arch. Pediatr. Adolesc. Med.* **153**, 75 (1999)

17 T.B. Hyde, D.S. Schmid, M.J. Cannon.*Rev. Med. Virol.***20**, 311 (2010)*

18 S.P. Adler.*N. Engl. J. Med.* **321**, 1290 (1989)

19 K.B. Balcarek *et al.*, *JAMA.* **263**, 840 (1990)

20 S.P. Adler. *EBioMedicine.***2**, 1027 (2015)

21 T.L. Chin *et al.*, *J. Hosp. Infection.* **87**, 11 (2014)

22 M.G. Revello *et al.*, *EBioMedicine.* **2**, 1205 (2015)

23 K.M. Anderholm, C.J. Bierle, M.R.Schleiss. *Drugs.***76**, 1625 (2016)

GENITAL HERPES IN PREGNANCY

CASE VIGNETTE

A 28-year-old pregnant woman at 38 weeks' gestation presented to her GP with a crop of vesicular lesions around the mons pubis. The GP sent a viral swab for HSV molecular testing which identified HSV-2 DNA. She referred the patient immediately to the genitourinary medicine (GUM) clinic. How was the case managed?

LABORATORY DIAGNOSIS

Why was laboratory confirmation of genital herpes important in the pregnant woman?

HSV-2 transmission from mother to the neonate could occur. Neonatal herpes due to HSV-1 or HSV-2 is associated with significant morbidity and mortality *(1)*. Clinical manifestations include disseminated disease, central nervous system (CNS) disease and skin, eye and/or mouth (SEM) disease, each of which presents usually around day 10 to 12 of life *(2)*. The incidence in Ireland is currently unknown but the overall pooled rate of neonatal HSV in Europe is low (8.9 cases per 100,000 live births) *(3)*.

How may the neonate acquire HSV infection?

The most common route of transmission (~85%) is direct exposure of the neonate to HSV-1 or HSV-2-infected maternal secretions in the birth canal during labour and delivery *(1)*. The mother may shed HSV asymptomatically during delivery in primary or recurrent genital herpes *(2)*. Intrauterine transmission (~5%) and post-natal acquisition (10%) of HSV infection may also occur. Neonatal HSV is a notifiable disease *(3)*.

Why did the GUM clinic send maternal serum for HSV type-specific (TS) serology testing?

To identify if this was a primary or recurrent HSV-2 maternal infection. Most neonatal HSV occurs when mothers acquire HSV-1 or HSV-2 for the first time (primary infection) during the third trimester, particularly within six weeks of delivery *(6, 7)*. The transmission rate is much higher among women who have primary HSV infection (30-50%) in late pregnancy than those with recurrent genital herpes (< 1%) *(8)*. This difference reflects the time required by the mother to develop neutralising antibodies after primary HSV infection which then cross the placenta to protect the neonate from HSV infection or attenuate its clinical course *(6)*.

What did HSV TS serology show in this case?

IgG antibody to HSV-2 (anti-HSV-2 IgG) was positive indicating that current genital disease in the mother was not due to primary HSV-2 infection. Remember, it takes a minimum of two weeks and possibly as long as 12 weeks for type-specific antibody to be reliably detected following primary infection with HSV-1 or HSV-2 (9).

CLINICAL MANAGEMENT

Was she treated with an antiviral agent?

Yes, initially she was given oral aciclovir 400 mg three times daily for five days at the GUM clinic and then the obstetrics team continued this antiviral regimen as suppressive treatment until delivery. Even though the risk of vertical transmission with recurrent genital herpes is very low, the antiviral is thought to decrease the likelihood of viral shedding and lesions in the genital tract at delivery (10). For those with primary HSV infection in the third trimester, anitiviral treatment with oral aciclovir (400 mg every 8 hours) is advised and it should be continued after resolution of lesions until delivery (11, 12). Moreover, for those with primary HSV infection in the first and second trimesters and those with recurrent HSV episodes, daily suppressive treatment with oral aciclovir (400 mg every 8 hours) is recommended from 36 weeks' gestation until delivery (11, 12).

Did the pregnant lady in this case need to have a Caesarean section?

No, for women presenting with recurrent genital herpes around the time of delivery, no study is currently available to show that delivery by Caesarean section (CS) avoids the risk of neonatal herpes (13). Even when lesions are present during labour in women with recurrent genital disease, the risk of neonatal HSV developing is low (<3%) due to the protective effect of maternal type-specific HSV neutralising antibody (11, 14). Therefore, in the UK and other parts of Europe vaginal delivery is the preferred option in these circumstances (13). In contrast, some guidelines recommend CS for recurrent genital herpes, although this approach is based on limited data and has been questioned (13,15, 16). If spontaneous rupture of membranes occurs, delivery should be expedited to reduce neonatal exposure to HSV-infected genital fluids.

When is Caesarean section recommended for prevention of neonatal herpes?

Current UK and Irish guidelines recommend CS for any pregnancy in which primary maternal HSV-1 or HSV-2 infection occurs in the third trimester, particularly infection when acquired within 6 weeks of delivery date. This reflects the lack of neutralising antibody to type-specific HSV needed to protect the neonate from infection or at least attenuate its clinical course (11, 15).

REFERENCES (*useful reviews)

1 Z.A. Brown et al., N. Engl. J. Med. 337, 509 (1997)

2 D.W. Kimberlin *et al.*, *Pediatrics.* **108**, 223 (2001)

3 K.J. Looker *et al.*, *Lancet Glob. Health.***5**, e300 (2017)

4 Z.A. Brown *et al.*, *Obstet. Gynecol.* **87**, 483 (1996)

5 http://www.hpsc.ie/notifiablediseases/notifyinginfectiousdiseases

6 Z.A. Brown *et al.*, *JAMA.* **289**, 203 (2003)

7 D.W. Kimberlin, J. Baley. *Pediatrics.***131**, 383 (2013)

8 C. Gardella, Z. Brown. *BJOG.***118**, 187 (2011)

9 R. Ashley-Morrow, E. Krantz, A. Wald.*Sex.Transm. Dis.* **30**, 310 (2003)

10 S.G. Pinninti, D.W. Kimberlin. *Clin.Perinatol.* **41**, 945 (2014)

11 E. Foley *et al.*, London; Royal College of Obstetricians&Gynaecologists. October 2014*

12 K.A. Workowski, G.A. Bolan. *MMWR Recomm. Rep.* **64**, 31 (2015)*

13 C. Akilswaran, D. Cohan. *N. Engl. J. Med.* **375**, 1906 (2016)

14 C.G. Prober *et al.*, *N. Engl. J. Med.* **316**, 240 (1987)

15 https://ssstdi.ie/laravel-filemanager/files/shares/preventing-perinatal-transmission-2015.08.pdf

16 J.W. Gnann Jr, R.J. Whitley. *N. Engl. J. Med.* **375**, 1906 (2016)

PARVOVIRUS B19 IN PREGNANCY

EPIDEMIOLOGY

What is the risk of fetal disease due to B19V?

The annual incidence of acute B19V infection in pregnancy is estimated to vary from 1.5% to 13.5% during endemic and epidemic seasons, respectively *(1)*. While 30% to 50% of pregnant women are nonimmune to B19V, in general, there is a favourable outcome for the fetus *(2)*. The rate of fetal transmission in pregnant women with B19V infection varies between 30% to 50%, while the frequency of fetal loss is around 1 in 10 pregnancies when maternal infection occurs in the first 20 weeks of gestation but thereafter the risk of fetal loss is negligible *(3, 4)*. Among those infected during weeks 9–20 of gestation, there is an overall 3% chance of development of nonimmune hydrops fetalis which usually develops 4 to 8 weeks after maternal infection and is commonly diagnosed between 17 to 24 weeks' gestation *(4)*. Furthermore, the mortality rate due to severe hydrops fetalis has been reduced significantly with timely administration of intrauterine transfusion *(2, 4)*.

PATHOGENESIS OF B19V INFECTION IN THE FETUS

Why is acute maternal B19V infection during the first 20 weeks of pregnancy potentially detrimental to the fetus?

Fetal outcome due to B19V infection in the first 20 weeks of pregnancy is worse than infection thereafter *(5)*. In the second trimester, fetal erythropoiesis occurs mainly in the liver. During this period of rapid fetal development, there is a 34-fold increase in demand for red blood cells but erythrocytes produced in the fetal liver have a short half-life of only 45 to 70 days. Consequently, the fetus needs to maintain a high rate of red blood cell production at this stage and cannot tolerate inhibition of erythropoiesis because it has a low haematological reserve. Therefore, fetal B19V infection contributes significantly to fetal loss and development of hydrops by causing anaemia through inhibition of erythropoiesis *(6, 7)*. In contrast, later in pregnancy the demand for fetal red blood cells is reduced and their life span is longer when erythropoiesis occurs in the bone marrow, thereby negating the adverse pathophysiological effects of fetal B19V infection. Furthermore, in the first 20 weeks' gestation, the fetus is highly susceptible to B19V infection because globoside (P blood antigen), which acts as a receptor for B19V, is significantly expressed on placental villous trophoblasts *(5)*. Moreover, cardiac failure due to increased venous return related to anaemia may be exacerbated by B19V-induced myocarditis. Fetal myocytes express globoside and, although these cells are not permissive for B19V replication, production of the cytotoxic viral protein NS1 within them may lead to myocarditis *(8)*.

CASE VIGNETTE

A 26-year-old primary school teacher who was pregnant (18 weeks' gestation) attended her GP with a 48-hour history of fleeting polyarthralgia. On examination, the temperature was 37.4°C and the remainder of the examination was normal. Her 4-year-old son had a transient disseminated maculopapular rash 14 days before onset of her complaint. A 5-year-old boy in her classroom was diagnosed with slapped check syndrome around that time. The GP suspected B19V-related arthropathy. How was the pregnancy managed?

LABORATORY DIAGNOSIS

What laboratory tests were performed by the GP?

The GP contacted the obstetrics team who requested testing of her 'booking' blood, collected at 10 weeks' gestation, for anti-B19V IgG. This was negative, indicating she was susceptible to acute B19V infection. A fresh serum sample was collected from the woman following her presentation and tested for anti-B19V IgM / IgG: both were positive indicating seroconversion to B19V and confirming recent acute B19V infection.

Are there limitations with laboratory diagnosis of B19V infection in pregnancy?

Yes, expert opinion should be sought with interpretation of laboratory results. Persistence of anti-B19V IgM at low levels for several months after resolution of infection may simply reflect late convalescence or nonspecificity but can result in unnecessarily high numbers of requests for fetal ultrasound *(9, 10)*. Similarly, persistence of low-level B19V DNA in serum for ≥ 1 year will not differentiate recent versus past infection and may reflect B19V infection prior to conception *(11, 12)*.

MANAGEMENT OF CASE

What was the management plan for this pregnant woman who acquired BI9V infection at ≤ 20 weeks' gestation?

The pregnant woman with acute B19V infection was referred to the obstetrics team for counselling on issues such as the risk of vertical transmission, potential risk of adverse fetal outcome, investigation of the fetus for infection and possible therapeutic intervention. She underwent weekly Doppler ultrasound examination of the fetal middle cerebral artery peak systolic velocity (MCA-PSV) beginning within 4 weeks of diagnosis and continuing until 30 weeks' gestation (monitoring until at least 12 weeks after diagnosis is advised) *(13)*. MCA-PSV is noninvasive and determines accurately fetal anaemia *(14)*. Blood viscosity is decreased in the anaemic fetus leading to increased venous return and increased cardiac output *(15)*. Therefore, high MCA-PSV readings correlate with severe fetal anaemia which can lead to hydrops fetalis *(14)*. In this case, there was no evidence of fetal anaemia. However, if MCA-PSV readings were high, percutaneous umbilical vein blood sampling would have been performed to confirm fetal B19V infection and to measure fetal haemoglobin and platelet count *(16)*. Intrauterine fetal transfusion of packed red cells is considered as a therapeutic option for severe fetal anaemia while, in contrast, mild or moderate fetal anaemia usually resolves spontaneously.

CASE VIGNETTE

An asymptomatic pregnant school teacher ≤ 20 weeks' gestation presented to your practice following exposure to a child with acute B19V infection. ('Booking blood' is unavailable)

LABORATORY TESTING

What laboratory tests should be performed?

If testing of the 'booking blood' is not feasible, the GP should collect a fresh serum sample and test it for anti-B19V IgM / IgG. Three possible serological profiles can be reported:

(a) **anti-B19V IgM NEG / IgG POS**: patient can be assured of her immunity to B19V and that she was not infected recently.

(b) **anti-B19V IgM POS / IgG POS or NEG**: suggests patient acquired infection recently and should be referred to the obstetric team.

(c) **anti-B19V IgM NEG / IgG NEG**: patient is susceptible to infection and another serum should be collected 4 weeks after exposure. If the repeat sample is anti-B19V IgM POS, irrespective of IgG result, she should be referred to the obstetric team with suspected acute B19V infection. However, if the repeat serum is anti-B19V NEG / IgG NEG, then she was not infected recently but is still susceptible to subsequent exposure.

PUBLIC HEALTH CONSIDERATIONS

Should a pregnant school teacher ≤ 20 weeks' gestation who is seronegative for B19V IgG be excluded from school if a case of erythema infectiosum is identified in the classroom?

Contact public health for advice. In general, a policy of automatic exclusion of nonimmune teachers early in pregnancy from the workplace where sporadic cases of erythema infectiosum are occurring is not recommended *(17)*. Their risk of acquiring B19V infection in the classroom is likely to be similar to that in the community or at home if the teacher has school-aged children. Transmission from children and adults who are infected asymptomatically as well as high circulating levels of B19V activity in the community imply that furloughing from school may reduce but not eliminate the risk of acquiring infection (18). Furthermore, the child with erythema infectiosum is likely to be infectious only before the rash appears so exposure may have already occurred by the time disease is recognised (19, 20). If there is an outbreak of erythema infectiosum in the school, then exclusion of the pregnant teacher until she is at > 21 weeks' gestation can be considered (21).

Should pregnant healthcare workers (HCWs) be excluded from caring for patients with acute B19V infection if they are known to be nonimmune to the virus?

Advice should be sought from occupational health. In general, pregnant HCWs in the first 20 weeks of pregnancy who are seronegative for anti-B19V IgG should avoid contact with individuals with acute B19V infection in which patients are likely to have high viral loads (20). Those with B19V-related transient aplastic crisis and immunosuppressed patients with pure red cell aplasia due to chronic B19V infection usually have high levels of B19V replication (parvovirus B19 chapter) and pregnant HCWs should not be assigned to care for them. Individuals with erythema infectiosum have negligible levels of virus in respiratory secretions once the rash appears and thus are not likely to be infectious (19).

Following significant contact with a confirmed case, should a midwife or obstetrician who is nonimmune to B19V be excluded from the workplace?

Advice should be sought from occupational health. Exclusion from work is not justified although the HCW may be incubating B19V infection and therefore could be potentially infectious. The risk of acquiring infection from patients and then transmitting it is regarded as low (21, 22). However, to reduce the risk even further the HCW could change their work practice temporarily to avoid direct contact with pregnant women or wear a surgical mask for 15 days after exposure (period of highest infectivity) or until a rash develops (21).

REFERENCES

1 A.K. Valeur-Jensen et al., JAMA. **281**, 1099 (1999)

2 E. Miller et al., BJOG. **105**, 174 (1998)

3 O. Norbeck et al., Clin. Infect. Dis. **35**, 1032 (2002)

4 M. Enders et al., Prenat. Diagn.**24**, 513 (2004)

5 J.A. Jordan, J.A. DeLoia. Placenta.**20**, 103 (1999)

6 H. Chisaka et al., Rev. Med. Virol. **13**, 347 (2003)

7 A.L .Bittencourt, A.G. Garcia.Pediatr.Pathol. Mol. Med. **21**, 353 (2002)

8 T. Marton, W.L. Martin, M.J. Whittle. Prenat.Diagn.**25**, 543 (2005)

9 M. Enders et al., J. Virol. Methods.**146**, 409 (2007)

10 M. Enders *et al.*, *J.Clin. Virol*.**35**, 400(2006)

11 J.J. Lefrére *et al.*, *Blood*. **106**, 2890 (2005)

12 A. Lindblom *et al.*, *Clin. Infect. Dis*. **41**, 1201 (2005)

13 P. Morgan-Capner, N.S. Crowcroft.*Comm. Dis. Public Health*. **5**, 59 (2002)

14 S. Borna *et al.*, *J. Clin.Ultrasound*.**37**, 385 (2009)

15 E. Hernandez-Andrade *et al.*, *Ultrasound Obstet. Gynecol*. **23**, 442 (2004)

16 C. Puccetti *et al.*, *Prenat. Diagn*.**32**, 897 (2012)

17 American Academy of Pediatrics.*Pediatrics*.**85**, 131 (1990)

18 S.P. Adler *et al.*, *J. Infect. Dis*. **168**, 361 (1993)

19 F.A. Plummer *et al.*, *N. Engl. J. Med*. **313**, 74 (1985)

20 T.L. Chin *et al.*, *J. Hosp. Infect*. **87**, 11 (2014)

21 N.S. Crowcroft *et al.*, *J. Public Health Med*. **21**, 439 (1999)

22 J.H. Harger *et al.*, *Obstet Gynecol*. **91**, 413 (1998)

PRIMARY TOXOPLASMOSIS IN PREGNANCY

CASE VIGNETTE

A 31-year-old pregnant woman, at 21 weeks' gestation, presented to your practice requesting testing for CMV and Toxoplasmagondii (T.gondii) infection. She had just returned to Ireland from a 14-day holiday in Poland. While on holiday, she had a bout of diarrhea which resolved within 72 hours. There was no specific risk factor for CMV or T.gondii infection. IgM and IgG antibody to T.gondii (anti-T.gondii IgM / IgG) were reported as positive with low IgG avidity (20%), suggestive of a recent primary infection. What are the important issues in management of this case?

LABORATORY DIAGNOSIS

How was primary *T.gondii* infection confirmed in this case?

Acute toxoplasmosis in pregnancy was confirmed by demonstrating anti-*T.gondii* IgM and IgG seroconversion. The patient had a stored serum ('booking blood') which was collected on her first antenatal visit at 9 weeks' gestation. This sample was tested and shown to be negative for anti-*T.gondii* IgM and IgG. The serum collected at 21 weeks' gestation was anti-*T.gondii* IgM / IgG positive. In addition, both serum samples were sent to a Toxoplasmosis Reference laboratory in the United Kingdom which confirmed seroconversion in pregnancy, using the gold-standard Sabin-Feldman dye test.

What laboratory tests were performed next?

The patient was referred to a fetal medicine specialist to determine if the fetus was infected. *T.gondii* DNA was detected in amniotic fluid (AF) confirming intrauterine infection. Amniocentesis should be considered in cases where there is confirmed primary maternal infection even in the absence of abnormal ultrasound findings *(1)*. The recommended timing of amniocentesis is > 4 weeks after the estimated date of infection in the mother, and the risk of false negative findings is significantly reduced after 18 weeks' gestation *(2)*.

TIMING OF MATERNAL TOXOPLASMOSIS IN PREGNANCY

Was the gestational age at which the mother acquired toxoplasmosis significant?

Yes, the risk of maternal-fetal transmission is known to increase with the gestational age at which maternal infection occurs: transmission rates vary from 2% at eight weeks, 6% at 13 weeks, 40% at 26 weeks and 72% at 36 weeks of gestation *(3)*. In contrast, the severity of congenital toxoplasmosis (CT) is inversely related to the gestational age at which maternal infection occurs i.e. the prognosis of CT appears better when maternal infection occurs late in pregnancy. Although maternal treatment with antiparasitic agents may lessen the severity of CT, it does not appear to prevent fetal infection *(1, 4)*.

CLINICAL MANAGEMENT

Was antiparasitic treatment recommended in this case?

Yes, the mother opted to continue with the pregnancy. Once primary maternal infection was diagnosed, she was started on spiramycin 1 g three times daily. This oral antibiotic is a macrolide which concentrates in the placenta and is thought to reduce transmission of the parasite from mother to fetus *(5)*. If fetal toxoplasmosis had not been confirmed by PCR, spiramycin would still be given for the duration of pregnancy since the placenta acts as a potential source of transmission of *T gondii* to the fetus throughout pregnancy *(1)*. However, when fetal infection was confirmed in this case, spiramycin was switched to oral pyrimethamine and sulfadiazine with folinic acid (to avoid bone marrow toxicity). Spiramycin levels achieved in fetal blood are not sufficient to kill the parasite effectively and therefore cannot treat fetal infection while, in contrast, the combination of pyrimethamine and sulfadiazine can clear the parasite from placenta and fetus, thereby decreasing significantly the severity of fetal toxoplasmosis *(4, 6)*.

What was the outcome of the pregnancy?

Although serial fetal ultrasonography performed in pregnancy showed intracranial calcifications, the baby boy appeared normal at birth, like most neonates with congenital toxoplasmosis (CT). However, if infected infants are not treated, including those who are asymptomatic, they are at risk of severe neurological sequelae *(7)*. The baby was commenced on treatment with pyrimethamine, sulfadiazine and folinic acid at birth for 12 months. A later ophthalmological examination revealed a chorioretinal lesion near the macula in the left eye, suggestive of chorioretinitis. Laboratory tests were performed to confirm CT: a serum sample was collected at day 10 of life (time gap needed to avoid false-positiveIgM results due to contamination from maternal blood at birth) and tested for anti-*T.gondii* IgM, IgA and Sabin-Feldman dye test. Anti-*T.gondii*-specific IgM and IgA were both positive confirming CT. Furthermore, placental tissue was tested for *T.gondii* DNA by PCR and also confirmed infection. In addition, the Sabin-Feldman dye test was positive at day 10 of life and one year later, when tested after completion of treatment. Follow-up of the child after treatment showed resolution of intracranial calcifications and chorioretinitis, with normal neurodevelopmental outcome.

The woman asked if congenital toxoplasmosis could recur in any future pregnancy?

Not unless she developed severe deficiency of her cellular immune system due to advanced HIV infection or iatrogenic immunosuppression. Depletion of *T.gondii*-specific CD4+ / CD8+ T cells can facilitate reactivation of bradyzoites in tissue cysts to actively replicating tachyzoites which could potentially infect the fetus causing CT *(7, 8)*.

PLANNING PREGNANCY

If a woman was diagnosed recently with primary toxoplasmosis, should she wait before trying to conceive?

It seems prudent to avoid conception until six months after diagnosis of primary toxoplasmosis in the woman *(1)*.

REFERENCES (*useful reviews)

1 C. Paquet, M.H. Yudin. *J. Obstet. Gynaecol. Can.* **40**, e687 (2018)*

2 J.B. Murat *et al.*, *Expert Rev. Anti Infect. Ther.***11**, 943 (2013)

3 D. Dunn *et al.*, *Lancet.***353**, 1829 (1999)

4 F. Peyron *et al.*, *Cochrane Database Syst. Rev.* CD001684 (2000)

5 J.G. Montoya, J.S. Remington. *Clin. Infect. Dis*. **47**, 554 (2008)

6 R. McLeod *et al.*, *Mem. Inst. Oswaldo Cruz.* **104**, 320 (2009)

7 P.A Moncada, J.G. Montoya. *Expert Rev. Anti Infect. Ther.***10**, 815 (2012)*

8 K.M. Azevedo *et al.*, *Braz. J. Infect. Dis.* **14**, 186 (2010)

VARICELLA IN PREGNANCY

Why is varicella of clinical significance in pregnancy?

Maternal varicella infection in the first and second trimesters of pregnancy is associated with an increased risk of teratogenicity, known as congenital varicella syndrome (CVS). VZV infection *in utero*, when not resulting in CVS, may lead to recurrent zoster early in childhood. In addition, primary varicella in the mother in the week before and the week after delivery can cause neonatal varicella with serious sequelae. Furthermore, varicella in the third trimester may lead to life-threatening viral pneumonia in the mother (1, 2).

What is congenital varicella syndrome?

Congenital varicella syndrome (CVS) is a rare condition which was first described in 1947 (3). Multiple congenital defects may occur following transplacental transmission of VZV during maternal varicella. It is characterised by scarring of skin in a dermatomal manner; limb hypoplasia; neurological defects such as microcephaly, cortical atrophy and mental retardation; ocular abnormalities including microphthalmia, chorioretinitis and cataracts, while gastrointestinal and genitourinary tract abnormalities may occur less commonly (1, 4). A mortality rate of 30% has been associated with CVS in the first few months of life while long-term neurodevelopmental disorders may occur among survivors (5).

Does herpes zoster in pregnancy cause congenital varicella syndrome?

There is no evidence of CVS developing from localised herpes zoster in pregnant women (4). HZ involving dermatomes T10-L1 could theoretically result in intrauterine shedding of VZV but no adverse clinical outcomes for the fetus have been reported (1).

What is the clinical significance of varicella pneumonia in the pregnant mother?

Morbidity and mortality rates from varicella pneumonia in pregnant women is higher than in nonpregnant subjects, particularly among those in the third trimester (6, 7). This complication is probably due to the restriction of movement of the mother's diaphragm caused by the large gravid uterus (1).

POSTEXPOSURE PROPHYLAXIS AGAINST VARICELLA IN PREGNANCY

What should the GP do if a pregnant woman at any gestational age presented following a recent VZV exposure?

A past history of varicella in a pregnant woman is a reliable marker of immunity to VZV and serology screening is not necessary (8). However, for individuals born or raised in tropical climates (sub-Saharan Africa, South East Asia, the Caribbean and Central America), a past history of varicella is unreliable, therefore the pregnant woman's booking blood should be checked or a fresh serum sample collected for VZV IgG to diagnose immunity or susceptibility to VZV. A past history of shingles is unreliable unless there was laboratory confirmation of VZV because it can be difficult to distinguish clinically from HSV.

What should the GP do if the pregnant woman is unsure about previous VZV infection?

Check the pregnant woman's booking blood or collect a serum sample for VZV IgG to confirm immunity or susceptibility to VZV.

What should the GP do if the pregnant contact is not immune to VZV?

Refer the pregnant woman to the Obstetrics team. Passive immunisation with varicella-zoster immune globulin (VZIG) within 10 days of significant exposure is recommended (9). By preventing or modifying maternal VZV viraemia with VZIG, it is assumed that the risk of transplacental transfer of virus will be decreased (10). However, passive immunisation with VZIG does not guarantee prevention of infection. Therefore, all VZV contacts given VZIG are potentially infectious until day 28 after exposure which needs to be considered when organising any follow-up for the woman e.g. clinic visits where other pregnant women or immunocompromised patients may be present.

MANAGEMENT OF VARICELLA IN PREGNANCY

What should the GP do if the pregnant contact develops a varicella-like rash?

Advice should be sought from the Obstetrics team. In general, oral aciclovir (800mg five times daily until lesions crust) may be started within 24 hours of onset of the rash at any stage of pregnancy (4, 11). Teratogenicity in neonates has not been associated with use of aciclovir (12). Those with varicella should be advised that they are highly infectious and should avoid contact with other pregnant women, neonates and immunocompromised persons.

When should the GP refer a pregnant woman with varicella to the obstetric service?

Development of complicated varicella is indicated by occurrence of respiratory or neurological symptoms or the appearance of new crops on skin and/or mucosal vesicles or haemorrhagic lesions (13). These patients need treatment with intravenous aciclovir (10-15 mg/kg three times daily) and should be isolated in hospital with airborne precautions. Pregnant women at high risk of severe varicella should also be referred for clinical review including those who are smokers or have underlying chronic obstructive pulmonary disease or received systemic steroids in the previous three months or when varicella occurs in the third trimester (2, 9, 11).

Should the GP be concerned if an expectant mother developed varicella near delivery?

Yes, because neonatal varicella can be severe when the mother's rash appears seven days before to seven days after delivery *(1, 13)*. Furthermore, the mortality rate in the neonate is particularly high (31%) if onset of the maternal rash occurs five or fewer days before to two days after delivery without prophylaxis and/or antiviral treatment for the neonate *(14, 15)*. The severity of neonatal disease appears to be related to the high inoculum of VZV from the mother combined with the absence of passively-acquired protective maternal VZV-specific antibody *(14)*. Infants born more than seven days after onset of the maternal rash are not regarded as being at risk of severe varicella because they have probably acquired protective maternal antibody *(10)*. Advice should be sought from a neonatologist about any neonate born to a mother who had varicella in pregnancy *(9)*.

REFERENCES (*useful reviews)

1 M.P. Tan, G. Koren. *Reprod. Toxicol.* **21**, 410 (2006)*

2 J.H. Harger *et al.*, *J. Infect. Dis.* **185**, 422 (2002)

3 E.G. LaForet, C.L. Lynch Jr. *N. Engl. J. Med.* **236**, 534 (1947)

4 R.F. Lamont *et al.*, *BJOG.* **118**, 1155 (2011)

5 A. Schulze, H.J. Dietzsh. *J. Pediatr.* **137**, 871 (2000)

6 H. Rawson, A. Crampin, N. Noah. *BMJ.* **323**, 1091 (2001);

7 T.J. Schutte, L.C. Rogers, P.R. Copas. *Infect. Dis. Obstet. Gynecol.* **4**, 338 (1996)

8 E. MacMahon *et al.*, *BMJ.* **329**, 551 (2004)

9 Royal College of Obstetricians and Gynaecologists; Green-top Guideline No. 13; 2015*

10 C.K. Smith, A.M. Arvin. *Semin. Fetal Neonatal Med.* **14**, 209 (2009)

11 A.J. Daley, S. Thorpe, S.M. Garland. *Aus. N.Z. J. Obstet. Gynaecol.* **48**, 26 (2008)

12 K.M. Stone *et al.*, *Birth Defects Res. A Clin. Mol. Teratol.* **70**, 201 (2004)

13 Department of Health UK. The Green Book; 2018*

14 D. McIntosh, D. Isaacs. *Arch. Dis. Child.* **68**, 1 (1993)

15 E. Miller. *Arch. Dis. Child.* **70**, F157 (1994)

RESPIRATORY TRACT VIRAL INFECTIONS

- Influenza A and B
- Respiratory Syncytial Virus / Parainfluenza / Human Metapneumovirus
- Adenovirus

INFLUENZA VIRUS

VIROLOGY

What are influenza viruses?

Influenza viruses are members of the *Orthomyxoviridae* family. Each one has a single-stranded RNA genome in the form of eight segments coding for at least 17 proteins.

Which influenza viruses cause infections in humans?

Three types of influenza viruses have been identified in humans and are designated as A, B and C *(1)*. Type C virus appears to be of low pathogenicity and is not regarded as clinically significant, in contrast to types A and B which cause seasonal global epidemics of influenza *(2)*. Other than humans, influenza A viruses infect a wide range of hosts including pigs, horses, seals and whales as well as the natural reservoir of type A viruses, aquatic birds *(3)*. In contrast, influenza virus types B and C are only known to infect humans *(2)*. Type A viruses are subclassified into subtypes according to variations in antigenic properties of two viral surface glycoproteins, haemagglutinin (HA) and neuraminidase (NA). There are 18known HA subtypes and 11 NA subtypes of which 16 HA subtypes and 9 NA subtypes have been identified in birds *(4)*. Subtypes of influenza A are named according to their HA and NA content: for example, H1N1, H2N2, H3N2, and so on. In contrast, influenza B viruses are more homogenous with two antigenically distinct lineages that emerged about 40 years ago and known as Victoria and Yamagata *(5, 6)*. Each of these lineages carries only one form of HA and one of NA, albeit slight variation in amino acid sequences of each protein may occur between strains of influenza B every season *(5)*.

RISK FACTORS FOR COMPLICATED INFLUENZA

Which patient groups are at high risk of complicated influenza infection?

Six at least: children aged < 2 years, the elderly (≥ 65 years), women during pregnancy and ≤ 2 weeks postpartum, those with chronic medical conditions such as chronic pulmonary diseases (including asthma), cardiac disease, diabetes, obesity, renal, hepatic and neurological disorders, residents of nursing homes or long-term care institutions and those who are immunocompromised *(7)*.

Why is the elderly population annually at risk of complicated influenza virus infection?

Impairment of the cellular arm of the immune system in the elderly (known as immunosenescence) contributes to the high morbidity and raised mortality following influenza infection, and especially with influenza vaccine failure *(8, 9, 10)*.

CASE VIGNETTE

A 75-year-old male residing in a nursing home complained to staff of nasal congestion, chills, myalgia in his legs and slight nonproductive cough. The GP attended the patient within 10 hours of the onset of illness in the patient. On physical examination, the temperature was 38.3^{0}C, oxygen saturation was 99% while breathing ambient air, and the remainder of the examination was normal. Although this elderly man had been vaccinated against influenza 10 weeks previously, the GP diagnosed a viral upper respiratory tract infection (URTI), probably influenza. How was the case managed?

LABORATORY DIAGNOSIS

What samples did the GP collect for laboratory diagnosis of viral URTI in this case?

Combined nose and throat swabs in viral transport medium were collected and sent to the laboratory. Samples were tested by real-time reverse transcription polymerase chain reaction (rRT-PCR) for the following community-acquired respiratory viruses (CARVs) - influenza A and B, respiratory syncytial virus (RSV), parainfluenza types 1-4 (PIV), human metapneumovirus (hMPV), adenovirus (ADV) and rhinovirus. Influenza A RNA was detected and later confirmed as subtype influenza A H3N2.

What other specimens could be sent by the GP for diagnosis of infection with CARVs?

For patients with a productive cough, sputum can be submitted for viral testing and for bacterial culture. For hospitalised individuals, collection of nasopharyngeal aspirates is an option.

Should the GP send follow-up samples for influenza testing from people who recently have had a laboratory-confirmed infection?

In the majority of cases there is no need to send follow-up samples for influenza testing. Among individuals who are deteriorating or not improving despite five days of antiviral treatment, repeat samples may be sent for virological testing to exclude the rare possibility of antiviral resistance. In addition, sputum should be sent for bacterial culture.

CLINICAL FEATURES

Was the clinical presentation typical of influenza infection?

Yes, uncomplicated influenza infections are characterised by an abrupt onset of fever accompanied by other constitutional symptoms including headache, myalgia, arthralgia and malaise, as well as respiratory illness such as coryza, dry nonproductive cough and sore throat *(11)*. However, the absence of these classical clinical findings of influenza-like illness does not exclude current infection in elderly cohorts who may only present with acute onset of physical and/or mental deterioration *(12, 13)*. In immunocompetent individuals, uncomplicated influenza illness usually resolves within 3-7 days *(11)*. In children, the clinical presentation of influenza may include otitis media, laryngotracheobronchitis, vomiting and diarrhea *(4)*. In children with influenza who are < 5 years of age, fever and cough may not be present *(14)*.

What clinical complications may develop following infection with seasonal influenza virus?

During the 2009 H1N1 pandemic, secondary bacterial infection with *Streptococcus pneumoniae*, *Haemophilus influenzae*, *Streptococcus pyogenes* and *Staphylococcus aureus* was associated with significant morbidity and mortality *(15)*. Furthermore, influenza infection in those with chronic lung diseases and cardiac disease can lead to increased morbidity and mortality due to exacerbation of these illnesses *(16, 17)*. There is a significant association between laboratory-confirmed influenza infection and acute myocardial infarction (MI) with a six-fold increased risk of MI in the following seven days *(18)*. Primary influenza-associated viral pneumonia, which has a high mortality, is an uncommon but potential pulmonary complication of influenza, particularly during pandemics of influenza *(4)*. Young children with asthma are also known to be at risk of primary influenza pneumonia but it has been reported among otherwise healthy young adults in non-pandemic years *(19, 20)*. Pregnant women admitted to intensive care units with severe influenza appear to be more likely to have preterm and/or low birth weight babies than pregnant women with mild or no influenza infection *(21)*. Complications infrequently associated with influenza include myocarditis, pericarditis, myositis, transverse myelitis, Reye's syndrome and encephalopathy *(22, 23)*.

PATIENT MANAGEMENT

How did the GP manage the case in the vignette?

Bed rest and fluids combined with acetaminophen were advised to maintain hydration and relieve feverishness and myalgia, respectively. Antiviral treatment with oral oseltamivir, which inhibits neuraminidase activity (NA) of influenza A and B viruses, was prescribed without delay for 5 days as the elderly man was at risk of complicated influenza infection. Antiviral therapy with oseltamivir should ideally be started within ≤ 48 hours of onset of illness in persons with laboratory-confirmed influenza, or with suspected influenza in the following situations: when individuals have risk factors for influenza-related complications or when clinical judgement favours its use even in the absence of risk factors *(7, 24)*. That said, antiviral treatment may be considered even > 48 hours after illness onset for those with a moderately complicated course of illness.

What are the current antiviral agents used for treatment of influenza in primary care?

Oseltamivir is given orally and therefore commonly selected for treatment of infection and use as a prophylactic agent. It is easy to administer and surveillance data indicate that most circulating strains are oseltamivir-susceptible. Resistance can infrequently emerge during treatment with oseltamivir although almost exclusively in severely immunocompromised individuals *(25)*. Although oral oseltamivir is not licensed for use in children ≤ 1 year, a treatment dose of 3mg/kg twice daily has been recommended if it is clinically indicated *(26, 27)*. Dose adjustment based on creatinine clearance is needed for use of oral oseltamivir in those with renal dysfunction, but not for hepatic dysfunction *(28)*. For patients with nasogastric tubes, oseltamivir may be administered via the tube (https://online.lexi.com).

Inhaled zanamivir is an alternative agent and is approved for treatment of those aged ≥ 7 years and for prophylactic use in those aged ≥ 5 years *(27)*. No dose adjustment is needed in patients with hepatic and renal dysfunction. However, use of inhaled zanamivir may cause respiratory distress in those with chronic obstructive pulmonary disease and asthma and, furthermore, elderly patients find it difficult to use *(29, 30)*. Baloxavir marboxil is a new effective single-dose oral agent for treatment of uncomplicated influenza infection but is not widely available at the time of writing *(31)*.

Is the use of oseltamivir or zanamivir contraindicated in pregnancy?

There is no evidence of an association between use of these antivirals in pregnancy and development of congenital malformations, preterm delivery or low birth weight *(32)*.

INFECTION CONTROL

What infection control measures were advised by the GP in this case?

The patient was isolated in a single room while staff attending him implemented contact and droplet precautions, wearing personal protective equipment (PPE) including a surgical mask with full-face visor, plastic apron and gloves *(33)*.

For how long were infection control precautions implemented in this case?

For five days after onset of illness. In immunocompetent adults the period of communicability of influenza is 3-5 days after illness onset while this may extend to 10 days in young children *(34, 35)*. Immunocompromised patients may shed virus for prolonged periods of weeks to months and should be regarded as infectious at least until they are asymptomatic *(36)*. Advice on further isolation of immunocompromised patients should be sought from a public health specialist.

Another three residents in the nursing home developed acute onset of malaise, somnolence and anorexia within 30 hours of onset of illness in the index case.

Although all residents had recently been vaccinated against influenza, the GP suspected an outbreak of influenza in the nursing home. Why did he suspect the outbreak and how was it managed?

Within a 48-hour period, four residents had developed either acute onset of respiratory illness including cough and rhinorrhoea, or acute physical and mental deterioration, with or without fever, during a period of high influenza activity in the community (rate of influenza-like illness > 17 / 100,000 population). Onset of two cases of laboratory-confirmed influenza within 48 hours is regarded as an outbreak *(37)*. Public health were notified and gave advice on management: in brief, all residents, regardless of vaccination history, were offered chemoprophylaxis until at least 10 days after onset of illness in the last case. In addition, staff at high risk of influenza-related complications were offered chemoprophylaxis. In the meantime, samples were collected for laboratory testing (rRT-PCR) from symptomatic residents and treatment with oral oseltamivir was initiated. As in the index case, influenza A RNA (H3N2) was also detected in samples from these three cases. Therapeutic doses of oral oseltamivir were advised for at least 5 days, though longer treatment (up to 10 days) may be given to severely ill patients or immunocompromised individuals *(7)*. The symptomatic individuals were isolated in single rooms. Cases were regarded as potentially infectious for 5 days after illness onset. Staff implemented contact and droplet precautions. Personal protective equipment (PPE) worn by staff included a surgical mask with full-face visor, plastic apron and gloves *(33)*. Symptomatic staff were excluded from work until resolution of illness. Unvaccinated staff were offered immunisation but were advised to maintain PPE when attending ill patients because it may take 14 days to elicit protective immunity following vaccination. If there was a shortage of single rooms, cohorting of cases in a ward with beds separated by at least 1 metre, and ideally partitioned to reduce cross-contamination, was recommended.

What is the likely reason for the elderly residents developing influenza in spite of recent vaccination?

In general, elderly individuals (≥ 65 years of age) show poor immune responses to standard influenza vaccines *(10)*. Use of high-dose inactivated influenza vaccines and adjuvanted formulations are among the strategies developed to overcome age-related immunosenescence by eliciting a more robust immune response *(39, 40)*. Recent results from the United Kingdom showed improved effectiveness of adjuvanted inactivated trivalent influenza vaccine among vaccine recipients aged ≥ 65 years in the 2018-2019 influenza season (41).

REFERENCES (*useful reviews)

1 L.C. Lambert, A.S. Fauci. *N. Engl. J. Med.* **363**, 2036 (2010)

2 J.C. Kash, J.K. Taubenberger. *Am. J. Pathol.* **185**, 1528 (2015)

3 R.D. Slemons *et al.*, *Avian Dis.* **18**, 119 (1974)

4 C. Paules, K. Subbarao. *Lancet.***390**, 697 (2017)*

5 P.A. Rota *et al.*, *Virology.* **175**, 59 (1990)

6 Y. Kanegae *et al.*, *J. Virol.* **64**, 2860 (1990)

7 S.A. Harper *et al.*, *Clin. Infect. Dis.* **48**, 1003 (2009)*

8 Y. Deng *et al.*, *J. Immunol.* **172**, 3437 (2004)

9 J.E. McElhaney *et al.*, *J. Immunol.* **176**, 6333 (2006)

10 J.H. Kreijtz, R.A..Fouchier, G.F. Rimmelzwaan. *Virus Res.* **162**, 19 (2011)

11 K.G. Nicholson.*Semin.Respir. Infect.* **7**, 26 (1992)

12 A.M. v.d.Hoeven *et al.*, *Infection.* **35**, 65 (2007)

13 E.E. Walsh, C. Cox, A.R. Falsey. *J. Am. Geriatr. Soc.* **50**, 1498 (2002)

14 K.A. Poehling *et al.*, *N. Engl. J. Med.* **355**, 31 (2006)

15 E. Bautista *et al.*, *N. Engl. J. Med.* **362**, 1708 (2010)

16 A. Kumar *et al.*, *JAMA.* **302**, 1872 (2009)

17 M.B. Rothberg, S.D. Haessler.*Crit. Care Med.* **38**Suppl 4, e91 (2010)

18 J.C. Kwong *et al.*, *N. Engl. J. Med.* **378**, 345 (2018)

19 F.S. Dawood *et al.*, *Pediatr. Infect. Dis. J.* **29**, 585 (2010)

20 Y.C. Ho *et al.*, *J. Infect.* **58**, 439 (2009)

21 K. Newsome *et al.*, *Birth Defects Res.* **111**, 88 (2019)

22 M.B. Rothberg, S.D. Haessler, R.B. Brown. *Am. J. Med.* **121**, 258 (2008)

23 R.D. Mistry *et al.*, *Pediatrics.***134**, e684 (2014)

24 N.J. Cooper *et al.*, *BMJ.***326**, 1235 (2003)

25 M.G. Ison *et al.*, *J. Infect. Dis.* **193**, 760 (2006)

26 D.W. Kimberlin *et al.*, *J. Infect. Dis.* **207**, 709 (2013)

27 A.E. Fiore *et al.*, *MMWR Recomm. Rep.* **60**, 1 (2011)*

28 S. Karie *et al.*, *Nephrol. Dial. Transplant.***21**, 3606 (2006)

29 J.C. Williamson, P.S. Pegram. *N. Engl. J. Med.* **342**, 661 (2000)

30 P. Diggory *et al.*, *BMJ.* **322**, 577 (2001)

31 F.G. Hayden *et al.*, *N. Engl. J. Med.* **379**, 913 (2018)

32 H.J. Dunstan *et al.*, *BJOG.* **121**, 901 (2014)

33 J.E. Coia *et al.*, *J. Hosp. Infect.* **85**, 170 (2013)*

34 F.Carrat *et al.*, *Am. J.Epidemiol.* **167**, 775(2008)

35 C.B. Hall, R.G. Douglas Jr. *Pediatrics.***55**, 673 (1975)

36 J.A. Englund *et al.*, *Clin. Infect. Dis.* **26**, 1418 (1998)

37 Public Health England (2016) https://www.gov.uk/government/publications/acute-respiratory-disease-managing-outbreaks-in-care-homes*

38 S.M. Ryoo *et al.*, *Influenza Other Respir. Viruses.***7**, 833 (2013)

39 C.A. DiazGranados *et al.*, *N. Engl. J. Med.* **371**, 635 (2014)

40 S. Mannino *et al.*, *Am. J. Epidemiol.* **176**, 527 (2012)

41. Public Health England. Surveillance of influenza & other respiratory viruses in the UK: Winter 2019 to 2019: May 2019

INFLUENZA VACCINATION

BACKGROUND

Prevention and control of transmission of influenza virus among humans, particularly in those at risk of influenza-related complications, is best achieved through vaccination. Inactivated influenza vaccine (IIV) is used more commonly in Ireland than live attenuated influenza vaccine (LAIV) and recombinant influenza vaccine (RIV), therefore this review will focus on inactivated influenza vaccines. Because influenza A viruses of the H3N2 and H1N1 subtypes and influenza B (Victoria or Yamagata lineage) are responsible for seasonal influenza, the vaccine contains antigens from these three viruses, known as an inactivated trivalent vaccine. In addition, an inactivated quadrivalent vaccine containing antigens from each lineage of influenza B and both influenza A subtypes is available (1). However, seasonal influenza vaccine requires annual review and change in its composition because vaccine-induced antibody targets mainly the viral haemagglutinin (HA) protein which, in influenza A, easily acquires mutations causing changes in its antigenicity, known as antigenic drift.

How is the composition of the influenza vaccine reformulated every season?

In brief, 142 national influenza centres in 115 WHO member states worldwide monitor circulating strains of the virus noting how efficiently they are transmitted and the protective efficacy of the corresponding vaccine strain components (2). Laboratories characterise circulating seasonal strains by genomic sequencing and antigenic characterisation and also collate epidemiological and clinical data and vaccination history on patients infected. The numbers of individuals presenting to primary care with influenza-like illness, even when not laboratory-confirmed, are also monitored. These surveillance data are given to one of five World Health Organisation (WHO) Collaborating Centres for Reference and Research on Influenza which are located in Atlanta, London, Melbourne, Tokyo and Beijing. Experts from these centres analyse global surveillance data to identify new emergent strains of influenza, to determine which strains are most likely to circulate in the forthcoming season and to assess how closely they 'match' with the proposed reference vaccine strains(3). Every February and September, these WHO experts meet to recommend which strains of virus should be included in the vaccine for the upcoming influenza season in the northern and southern hemispheres, respectively (4).

These recommendations for seasonal vaccine composition are based on global surveillance data from the preceding 5 to 8 months and occur 6 to 9 months before the influenza season begins (5).

VACCINATION IN CLINICAL PRACTICE

Who should be advised to receive the seasonal influenza vaccine?

Individuals who are at high risk of influenza-related complications should be offered the inactivated vaccine annually including children aged < 2 years, the elderly (≥ 65 years), women during pregnancy and ≤ 2 weeks postpartum, those with chronic medical conditions like chronic pulmonary diseases (including asthma), cardiac disease, diabetes, obesity, renal, hepatic and neurological disorders, residents of nursing homes or long-term care institutions and those who are immunocompromised *(6)*. Similarly, healthcare workers (HCWs) attending hospitalised patients, particularly those at risk of severe complications, or HCWs who care for patients in nursing homes and long-term care facilities should be included.

When should individuals be offered influenza vaccine?

Influenza vaccine should be offered before the influenza season begins, therefore immunisation by the end of October is ideal. It takes at least 14 days following vaccination for protective antibodies to develop. However, because it is difficult to predict accurately the beginning and duration of the influenza season in any year, the vaccine should be offered throughout the season while influenza activity persists.

Who should avoid immunisation with inactivated influenza vaccine?

Any individual who developed a severe anaphylactic reaction to influenza vaccine should not receive it *(3)*. Any person who developed Guillaine-Barré syndrome (GBS) within 6 weeks of influenza vaccination should also avoid it; there is a small but statistically significant association between influenza vaccination and GBS *(7, 8)*. If an individual is clinically unwell, vaccination should be postponed unless illness is mild.

Influenza vaccine can be given to those who are allergic to egg protein?

Yes, but referral to hospital is recommended in Irish guidelines for those with severe egg allergy *(6)*. Recent evidence states that no special precautions are needed when vaccinating individuals with influenza vaccines even if they have a history of severe allergy to eggs *(9)*. The egg protein content is too low to induce an allergic reaction in vaccines derived from influenza viruses grown in embryonated chick eggs. However, immunisation with influenza vaccine is contraindicated in individuals who had an allergic reaction linked to previous vaccination against influenza *(3)*. All vaccination providers should know how to manage anaphylaxis in vaccine recipients.

How do I explain the myth among some healthcare workers, that they 'got the flu' following injection with the vaccine?

The injectable vaccine is inactivated, not live. Furthermore, some vaccine recipients may develop a mild reaction following immunisation characterised by constitutional symptoms like fever and myalgia but no coryza, which is unrelated to viral infection. In addition, some may acquire other community-acquired respiratory viruses with clinical features similar to influenza. Moreover, because it takes around 14 days for the vaccine recipient to become immune to influenza A and B, sometimes they may become infected with a circulating influenza virus before protective immunity develops to all vaccine components.

Should a pregnant woman, who had influenza A H3N2 infection recently, be offered immunisation with inactivated influenza vaccine after her recovery?

Yes, because she is still at risk of infection with seasonal influenza A subtype H1N1 and influenza B. Inactivated influenza vaccine can be given safely in any trimester.

Should a seven-year-old child with asthma be given one or two doses of influenza vaccine?

For children under nine years of age who were never vaccinated against influenza, two doses of influenza vaccine at least four weeks apart is recommended. If the child received a total of ≥ 2 doses of influenza vaccine in previous seasons, a single dose of inactivated trivalent or quadrivalent vaccine is advised (3).

Should a patient who is undergoing chemotherapy be given inactivated influenza vaccine during the influenza season?

Yes, immunisation should ideally be started two weeks before beginning chemotherapy to allow time for induction of an antibody response, although, if this is not feasible, vaccinating between courses of chemotherapy is effective (10). However, a second dose of vaccine should be given at least four weeks after the first and, optimally at the end of chemotherapy if there is influenza activity in the community (6). Such patients should be aware that the protective effectiveness of influenza vaccination may be lowered.

Does immunisation with seasonal influenza vaccine guarantee protection against infection?

No, but it should still be promoted among at-risk groups. Vaccine effectiveness may be reduced when there is a poor match between circulating virus and those used to formulate the seasonal vaccine (1). Antigenicity of the predominant circulating viral strain may vary from that in the vaccine due to spontaneous mutations in the gene encoding haemagglutinin (termed antigenic drift), the main immunogenic determinant (11). However, even if the match is suboptimal, vaccination in high-risk groups should be encouraged (5). In addition, antigenic differences between vaccine and circulating strains can occur without antigenic drift. Most influenza vaccines are composed of viral proteins, haemagglutinin (HA) and neuraminidase (NA), derived from influenza viruses propagated in embryonated eggs, a process which introduces mutations in the immunogenic component of HA, particularly in influenza A H3N2 subtype. This process, known as egg adaptation, reduces antigenic similarity between vaccine and circulating viral strains thereby contributing to reduced vaccine effectiveness *(12)*. Furthermore, host factors such as age and coexisting morbidities may impact adversely on vaccine effectiveness *(5)*.

Can the immune response of the elderly to influenza vaccination be improved?

Yes, two approaches have been used to improve the immune response to vaccine in the elderly *(11)*. One strategy was to increase the dose of haemagglutinin (HA) antigen four-fold in inactivated influenza vaccine (HA 60 µg) which was shown to be more effective in reducing hospital admissions due to respiratory disease in elderly residents of nursing homes than standard-dose vaccine (HA 15 µg) *(13)*. Use of an adjuvant in inactivated influenza vaccine to elicit a robust immune response was shown to reduce hospitalisation rates due to influenza in the elderly compared to standard IIV *(14)*. In the UK, adjuvant influenza vaccine was offered to the elderly during the 2018-2019 season with encouraging results *(15)*.

Should prophylactic use of antiviral agents against influenza be considered in primary care?

Prophylaxis of individuals at risk for severe influenza is an option but an acceptable alternative is to monitor individuals at high risk of influenza-related complications who are either unvaccinated or who are vaccinated but there is a poor match between circulating virus and vaccine composition, and then administer an antiviral at treatment doses immediately if symptoms develop *(16)*. Otherwise, chemoprophylaxis during periods of intense influenza activity in the community, the duration of which varies from 4 to 6 weeks, can be considered *(17, 18)*.

For more information on influenza vaccination in Ireland see
https://www.hse.ie/eng/health/immunisation/hcpinfo/guidelines/chapter11.pdf

REFERENCES (*useful reviews)

1 C. Paules, K. Subbarao. *Lancet*. **390**, 697 (2017)*

2 http://www.who.int/influenza/vaccines/virus/en/

3 L.A.Grohskopf *et al.*, *MMWR Recomm Rep*.**67**, 1 (2018)*

4 http://www.who.int/gb/pip/pdf files/Fluvaccvirusselection.pdf

5 C.I. Paules *et al.*, *N. Engl. J. Med.* **378**, 7 (2018)*

6 https://www.hse.ie/eng/health/immunisation/hcpinfo/guidelines/chapter11.pdf

7 L.H. Martín Arias *et al.*, *Vaccine*. **33**, 3773 (2015)

8 J.C. Kwong *et al.*, *Lancet Infect. Dis.* **13**, 769 (2013)

9 M. Greenhawt, P.J. Turner, J.M. Kelso. *Ann. Allergy Asthma Immunol.* **120**, 49 (2018)

10 L. Melcher.*Clin.Oncol*.**17**, 12 (2005)

11 K. Houser, K. Subbarao. *Host Cell Microbe*. **17**, 295 (2015)

12 V.G. Dugan *et al.*, *MMWR Morb. Mortal. Wkly. Rep.* **66**, 1318 (2017)

13 S. Gravenstein *et al.*, *Lancet Respir. Med.* **5**, 738 (2017)

14 S. Mannino *et al.*, *Am. J. Epidemiol.* **176**, 527 (2012)

15. Public Health England. Surveillance of influenza & other respiratory viruses in the UK: Winter 2019 to 2019: May 2019

16 A.E. Fiore *et al.*, *MMWR Recomm. Rep.* **60**, 1 (2011)*

17 C. LaForce *et al.*, *Clin. Ther.* **29**, 1579 (2007)

18 F.G. Hayden *et al.*, *N. Engl. J. Med.* **341**, 1336 (1999)

COMMUNITY-ACQUIRED RESPIRATORY VIRUSES OTHER THAN INFLUENZA

Multiple viruses other than influenza viruses can cause community-acquired upper and lower respiratory tract disease. The most frequent viruses include picornaviruses (rhinoviruses, enteroviruses), coronaviruses (the commonest causes of colds), respiratory syncytial virus (RSV), human metapneumovirus (HMPV), human parainfluenza viruses (HPIV) and adenoviruses. Respiratory viruses cause clinical syndromes that are difficult to differentiate on a clinical basis and range from the common cold to exacerbations of underlying airways disease to severe pneumonia. This chapter focuses on RSV and two other common community-acquired respiratory viruses (CARVs), HPIV and HMPV.

What is the virology of RSV, HPIV and HMPV?

RSV, HPIV and HMPV, are important respiratory pathogens in children and adults and share similar virological features. They are single-stranded, enveloped RNA viruses belonging to the *Paramyxoviridae* family. For more information on taxonomy read references *(1, 2)*.

VIRAL TRANSMISSION

How are CARVs transmitted in the community?

RSV and other CARVs likely share the same modes of transmission from patient-to-patient, although formal studies on transmission of HMPV are unavailable so far *(3)*. The main route of transmission is by respiratory droplet (> 5 μm diameter) from an infectious source causing direct inoculation of mucous membranes of the nose, mouth and conjunctiva *(4, 5)*. A less common route is contamination of surfaces following coughing and sneezing which may lead to self-inoculation via contaminated fingers *(5)*. Both RSV and HPIV can remain viable for several hours on nonporous surfaces *(6, 7)*. These viruses can easily be removed by most common disinfectants.

CLINICAL FEATURES

What are the clinical manifestations of infection with CARVs seen commonly in general practice?

The spectrum of respiratory diseases caused by RSV, HMPV and HPIV is similar. Although infections occur in adults, they are primarily a concern in young children in whom primary infection occurs and is usually symptomatic *(8)*. CARVs are associated with upper (URT) and lower respiratory tract (LRT) illnesses including nasal congestion, rhinorrhoea, otitis media, laryngotracheobronchitis (croup), bronchiolitis and viral pneumonia (8, 9). Respiratory viruses are the most common causes of hospitalisation for pneumonia in children aged < 5 years (10). Bronchiolitis is commonly caused by RSV, HPIV and HMPV. Children present typically with URT findings and a few days later develop LRT illness. The latter is characterised by cough, tachypnea, wheezing, grunting, nasal flaring and retractions (11). Further deterioration may occur due to atelectasis. Croup is typically associated with HPIV infection in children between 6 months and 3 years of age (12). Symptoms of croup may include fever, hoarseness, a barking cough and stridor. In most cases it is a mild, self-limiting illness but the severity of infection depends on the degree of upper airway obstruction and progression to the lower respiratory tract (5, 8). These respiratory viruses cause exacerbations of airway disease in adults with asthma, cystic fibrosis and chronic obstructive airway disease. Furthermore, respiratory viruses were more commonly identified than bacteria as causes of community-acquired pneumonia in adults who required hospitalisation (10).

Does reinfection with these viruses occur in otherwise healthy individuals?

Yes, reinfections are common in childhood and multiple infections are likely needed to induce protection (13).

EPIDEMIOLOGY OF RSV

What is the burden of RSV as a cause of acute respiratory disease?

The burden of RSV infection in young children is significant: data from the United States showed that almost all children are infected with the virus by 2 years of age and RSV is the commonest cause of lower respiratory tract infection and hospitalisation among those aged < 1 year, particularly those < 1 month old (14, 15). RSV infection is also a significant disease burden in elderly adults, those adults with underlying chronic lung and heart disease, and immunocompromised persons (16). Annual epidemics of RSV occur in Europe with first appearance in October followed by peak activity usually in December and waning activity until around April.

PATHOGENESIS

How do viruses like RSV cause bronchiolitis?

Following inhalation of large respiratory droplets infected with RSV during exposure to an infected case, the virus replicates in nasal and pharyngeal epithelial cells causing upper respiratory tract symptoms like coryza, rhinorrhea and poor feeding in young infants. The incubation period of RSV infection is about 4 to 5 days (17). About 3 days later lower respiratory disease may develop. It is presumed that RSV-infected cells from the nasopharynx are aspirated into the lower respiratory tract thereby infecting bronchial epithelium and alveolar pneumocytes (18). A cellular immune response is stimulated by viral replication resulting in the influx into pulmonary tissue of natural killer cells, helper CD4+ and cytotoxic CD8+ T cells thereby causing bronchiolitis *(11)*. Pathological findings include necrosis of ciliated epithelium with peribronchiolar inflammation with lymphocytes, plasma cells, macrophages and granulocytes. This inflammatory process causes intraluminal obstruction of air which is overcome by the negative intrapleural pressure generated on inspiration but is exaggerated on expiration by the combination of positive intrapleural pressure and narrowed lumina of bronchioles in the young *(11, 18)*. All of these pathophysiological changes are manifested clinically by wheezing, hyperinflation of the lungs and atelectasis *(8)*. Bronchiolitis resolves over the following 3 to 4 weeks.

CASE VIGNETTE

A 5-month-old girl was brought to the GP in late February with a 48-hour history of low-grade fever, rhinorrhoea, dry cough and poor feeding. Of note on examination, she was tachypnoeic and had nasal flaring but no retractions - there were inspiratory crackles and expiratory wheeze on auscultation and oxygen saturation was 95%. The GP suspected mild viral bronchiolitis. Eight hours later the GP visited the child at her home, she now had intercostal and supraclavicular retractions and oxygen saturation was 91%. Before she was sent to hospital for review, he collected nasal and throat viral swabs for testing. The child's 7-year-old brother, who had recently completed chemotherapy for leukaemia, was asymptomatic.

What can GPs learn from this case?

LABORATORY DIAGNOSIS

Was laboratory testing for viruses necessary in this case?

Yes but, in general, laboratory confirmation of viral aetiology in bronchiolitis is not necessary as it does not aid in management decisions or predict outcomes *(19)*. The GP wanted to determine if bronchiolitis was influenza-related in this case because antiviral prophylaxis would be given to her immunocompromised brother, who was unvaccinated against influenza.

What was the test result?

RSV RNA was detected at high-level reactivity by real-time reverse transcription polymerase chain reaction (rRT-PCR). Other potential viral pathogens including HPIV, HMPV, influenza A / B, adenovirus, picornaviruses and coronaviruses were not detected.

Were tests performed for bacterial pathogens in this case?

No, there is no evidence that bacteria like *Streptococcus pneumoniae* or *Haemophilus influenzae* have a role in causing bronchiolitis *(11)*. Furthermore, the child did not expectorate.

TREATMENT

Was the young girl treated with an antiviral agent?

No, in hospital she received supportive care, maintaining her hydration and nutritional status and oxygen saturation above 90%. However, for certain immunocompromised patients who are hospitalised with RSV- or HPIV-related LRTI, oral ribavirin may be considered as a therapeutic option *(20, 21)*. Several new antivirals are in development for treatment of RSV infection. These drugs include those that target the fusion (F) protein thereby inhibiting entry of RSV into target cells, and another agent which blocks replication of RSV by inhibiting viral RNA polymerase *(22, 23, 24)*.

Are antiviral agents available currently for treatment of HPIV and HMPV infections?

No but a novel antiviral drug is in development for treatment of HPIV infection. This is a recombinant protein which cleaves sialic acid residues from host respiratory epithelium that act as receptors for viral attachment, thereby blocking viral entry *(25)*. No antiviral agent for treatment of HMPV infection is yet near licensure.

PREVENTION OF RSV

Is it possible to prevent infection of susceptible individuals with RSV?

Yes, immunoprophylaxis with palivizumab is recommended for prevention of RSV disease in children who at high risk of severe respiratory disease. The decision for prophylaxis is made by the paediatrician. Recommendations for use vary by country with many restricting use of this expensive drug because of limited cost-benefit. Palivizumab is a humanised monoclonal antibody that neutralises RSV by binding to the conserved region of the viral fusion protein. It is administered intramuscularly once monthly during the expected RSV season. Those at high risk of complicated RSV-related respiratory disease for whom immunoprophylaxis is recommended include preterm infants with chronic lung disease, infants with haemodynamically significant congenital heart disease, infants with pulmonary or neuromuscular disorders, and others who may be considered for prophylaxis on a case-by-case basis *(26)*. Children < 2 years of age who are recipients of allogeneic haematopoietic stem cell transplantation are also considered for prophylaxis with palivizumab *(20)*. In this case, prophylaxis was not given to her brother who remained asymptomatic.

Are vaccines available against RSV and other community-acquired respiratory viruses?

While no vaccines are currently available, candidate vaccines for RSV, HMPV and HPIV are in various stages of development and evaluation in humans *(27, 28, 29)*. There are several candidate RSV vaccines, however, it is too soon to confirm that they will be effective in protecting against RSV infection in high-risk individuals *(30)*. Even if a vaccine for RSV was identified, it is still possible that circulating virus may undergo mutations at key antigenic epitopes thereby escaping neutralisation by vaccine-induced antibody *(30)*.

Why did previous RSV vaccines fail to prevent RSV infection in the past?

A formalin-inactivated vaccine against RSV was developed in the 1960s but led to severe respiratory disease among some nine vaccine recipients, including two deaths, when they were exposed to natural infection with the virus *(31)*. Initially it was thought that formalin in the vaccine altered the antigenicity of the viral proteins in the vaccine, eliciting antibodies of poor potency *(32)*. However, another contributory factor may have been inadequate Toll-like receptor (TLR) stimulation of B cells thereby inducing immature antibodies of low avidity to RSV antigens which were inadequate to confer protection *(33)*. When inactivated RSV vaccines containing TLR agonists were used in animal models, production of protective antibody was elicited *(33)*. Therefore, the ability of a vaccine to induce a robust neutralising antibody response is important in selection of an inactivated RSV vaccine.

REFERENCES (*useful reviews)

1 G. Boivin *et al.*, *J. Infect. Dis.* **186**, 1330 (2002)

2 B.G. van den Hoogen *et al.*, *Virology.* **295**, 119 (2002)

3 S. Kim *et al.*, *J. Clin. Microbiol.***47**, 1221 (2009)

4 C.B. Hall, R.G. Douglas Jr. *J. Pediatr.* **99**, 100 (1981)

5 K.J. Henrickson. *Clin.Microbiol. Rev.* **16**, 242 (2003)

6 M.T. Brady, J. Evans, J. Cuartas. *Am. J. Infect. Control.***18**, 18 (1990)

7 C.B. Hall *et al.*, *J. Infect. Dis.* **162**, 1283 (1990)

8 C.B. Hall. *N. Engl. J. Med.* **344**, 1917 (2001)

9 B.G. van den Hoogen, D.M. Osterhaus, R.A. Fouchier. *Pediatr. Infect. Dis. J.* **23**Suppl 1, S25 (2004)

10 S. Jain *et al.*, *N. Engl. J. Med.* **372**, 835 (2015)

11 H. C. Meissner. *N. Engl. J. Med.* **374**, 62 (2016)*

12 J.D. Cherry. *N. Engl. J. Med.* **358**, 384 (2008)

13 S. Panda *et al.*, *Int. J. Infect. Dis.* **25**, 45 (2014)

14 C.B. Hall *et al.*, *N. Engl. J. Med.* **360**, 588 (2009)

15 C.B. Hall *et al.*, *Pediatrics.***132**, e341 (2013)

16 A.R. Falsey *et al.*, *N. Engl. J. Med.* **352**, 1749 (2005)

17 E. Simoes. *Lancet.***354**, 847 (1999)*

18 S.J. Hoffman, F.R. Laham, F.P. Polack. *Microbes Infect.* **6**, 767 (2004)

19 F. Stollar *et al.*, *Eur. J. Pediatr.* **173**, 1429 (2014)

20 H.H. Hirsch *et al.*, *Clin. Infect. Dis.* **56**, 258 (2013)

21 J.N. Shah, R.F. Chemaly. *Blood.***117**, 2755 (2011)

22 J.P.DeVincenzo *et al.*, *N. Engl. J. Med.* **371**, 711 (2014)

23 J.P.DeVincenzo *et al.*, *N. Engl. J. Med.* **373**, 2048 (2015)

24 R. Fearns, J. Deval. *Antiviral. Res.* **134**, 63 (2016)

25 R.B. Moss *et al.*, *J. Infect. Dis.* **206**, 1844 (2012)

26 American Academy of Pediatrics Committee on Infectious Diseases.*Pediatrics.***134**, 415 (2014)

27 R.A. Karron *et al.*, *J. Pediatr. Infect .Dis. Soc.* **4**, e143 (2015)

28 https://clinicaltrials.gov/ct2/show/NCT01255410

29 N.I. Mazur *et al.*, *Lancet Respir. Med.* **3**, 888 (2015)

30 C. Griffiths, S.J. Drews, D.J. Marchant. *Clin.Microbiol. Rev.* **30**, 277 (2017)

31` H.W. Kim *et al.*, *Am. J. Epidemiol.* **89**, 422 (1969)

32 B.R. Murphy, E.E. Walsh. *J. Clin. Microbiol.***26**, 1595 (1988)

33 M.F. Delgado *et al.*, *Nat. Med.* **15**, 34 (2009)

HUMAN ADENOVIRUS

What is human adenovirus infection?

Clinical infections associated with human adenoviruses (HAdVs) in immunocompetent individuals, including acute respiratory disease and/or acute gastroenteritis, are usually mild, occurring most commonly in infants and children < 5 years of age *(1)*. However, outbreaks of HAdV-related respiratory infection among young adults in closed settings such as military camps and prisons are well recognized *(2, 3, 4)*. There is recent evidence of severe HAdV-related acute respiratory disease in adults *(5, 6)*. While HAdVs typically cause acute infections, viral shedding may continue well after symptoms have resolved. Furthermore, HAdVs may persist subclinically in sites like the gastrointestinal tract, and reactivate when individuals are severely immunocompromised.

What is the virology of human adenoviruses?

HAdVs are members of the family *Adenoviridae* in the genus *Mastadenovirus (7)*. They are non-enveloped, icosahedral-shaped viruses which contain a linear, double-stranded DNA genome (about 35kb in length).

How many 'types' of HAdVs have been identified?

There are currently 90 types of HAdVs which are classified into seven species designated HAdV-A to HAdV-G *(8)*. Typing of HAdVs was based originally on serological assays, hence the previously common term serotypes *(9)*. Later, a rapid typing scheme was developed based on the sequencing of the ε region of the hexon gene of HAdVs *(10)*. Whole genome sequencing is now recommended for identification of new types of HAdVs *(11)*.

What is the clinical relevance of typing of HAdVs?

Clinical manifestations of HAdV infection can vary with the viral type because some strains have specific tissue tropisms *(12)*. For example, HAdVs of species F (HAdV-F40, -F41) are typically associated with acute gastroenteritis in young children while keratoconjunctivitis is frequently linked to some members of species D (HAdV-D8, -D19, -D37) *(13)*. The common association of HAdV type with specific diseases may have implications for vaccine design; vaccines against HAdV-E4, -B7 were developed for use in the military to prevent respiratory disease *(14, 15)*. While some types show a strong predilection for specific tissues, other HAdV types belonging to different species can still cause similar clinical disease. For example, HAdV-related acute respiratory disease is associated with species B (HAdV-B3, -B7, -B14 and -B55), species E (HAdV-E4) and various types within species C *(16, 17, 18)*. Therefore, molecular diagnostics should be designed to detect all known types of HAdV irrespective of site of clinical disease *(19)*.

CASE VIGNETTE

An otherwise healthy 20-year-old woman, who worked in a crèche, presented to her GP complaining of soreness and mild itchiness in both eyes in the last 48 hours and nasal congestion with a dry nonproductive cough. On examination, the temperature was 37.8⁰C, there was erythema of bulbar and palpebral conjunctiva in both eyes, watery discharge, bilateral lid swelling with follicles on the conjunctiva of the lower lid and slight preauricular lymphadenopathy. The remainder of the examination was normal. She had not attended an ophthalmology clinic recently but several children attending the crèche had either upper respiratory tract illnesses (URTIs) or gastroenteritis recently. The GP suspected viral URTI with viral follicular conjunctivitis.

How was the case managed?

LABORATORY DIAGNOSIS

What pathogens were likely to be involved?

Viral swabs from conjunctiva were collected and sent to the laboratory. The GP requested testing for adenovirus, herpes simplex virus (HSV), varicella-zoster virus (VZV) and enterovirus (enterovirus 70 and Coxsackie 24). He also sent a swab for bacterial culture which was negative. Real-time polymerase chain reaction (PCR) for detection of viral pathogens identified adenovirus DNA, consistent with adenoviral conjunctivitis. Further molecular analysis to identify the type of HAdV was not performed.

ROUTE OF TRANSMISSION OF HAdVs

What was the probable route by which the crèche worker acquired HAdV infection?

HAdVs are typically transmitted from person-to-person through exposure mainly to infected respiratory secretions. The site of infection is usually located at the site of viral inoculation. Respiratory droplets from infected cases are inoculated directly onto the conjunctiva of a close contact or inhaled by close contacts resulting in acute respiratory disease. Adenoviral conjunctivitis can also occur due to direct viral inoculation of conjunctival mucosa through contact with infected eye/nasal secretions via contaminated instruments, eye drops or, indirectly, via contaminated hands of the patient herself (self-inoculation) or of healthcare workers. In addition, when environmental surfaces are contaminated with HAdVs, ingestion of virus via contaminated hands may cause HAdV-related gastroenteritis (20).

Which viral factors favour transmission of HAdVs?

All adenoviruses are nonenveloped which confers hardiness on these viruses and resistance to most disinfectants (21). In fact, they may remain viable on nonporous surfaces for several weeks *(22)*. Therefore, persistence in the environment combined with prolonged shedding of HAdVs, particularly from the gut, in both immunocompetent and immunocompromised individuals, are conducive to ease of transmission of HAdVs with occurrence of outbreaks in the community and healthcare settings *(20, 23)*.

INFECTION CONTROL

What infection control advice was given to the crèche worker with adenoviral conjunctivitis?

She was advised that persons with HAdV-related conjunctivitis are potentially infectious for 14 days after onset of symptoms *(24)*. She was advised to reduce hand-to-eye contact and wash hands using an ethanol-containing disinfectant after such contact, and not to share towels or bed clothes with other family members. Six days after attending the GP, her symptoms resolved and she returned to work but practised frequent hand washing.

What infection control measures should be implemented if a GP is doing an ophthalmological examination of persons with suspected viral conjunctivitis?

Interventions needed include the following; hand hygiene of staff and patient; cohorting patients with suspected viral conjunctivitis in an area separate from others; thorough cleaning of medical equipment and surrounding surfaces using alcohol solutions (85% to 95%) for at least two minutes or sodium hypochlorite for 10 minutes. If a healthcare worker develops viral conjunctivitis, the staff member should be furloughed until symptoms have resolved and should maintain stringent hand hygiene measures, particularly on return to work within 14 days of symptom onset *(25, 26)*.

For how long are individuals with HAdV-related respiratory disease, other than conjunctivitis, potentially infectious?

Immunocompetent persons with adenoviral respiratory tract disease are regarded as infectious when symptomatic *(27)*. However, it is always important to maintain proper hand hygiene when handling body fluids from any patient since even individuals asymptomatically infected with HAdVs can shed virus for weeks or months *(12)*. Individuals in the community with any viral respiratory tract illness should observe good respiratory etiquette; proper disposal of used handkerchiefs, coughing and sneezing into disposal cloth, and hand washing.

CLINICAL FEATURES OTHER THAN CONJUNCTIVITIS

What are the other main clinical presentations of HAdV infections seen in general practice?

In the immunocompetent individual, most HAdV infections are subclinical but when symptomatic they are predominantly mild infections with a self-limited course of illness. Frequent clinical manifestations include upper respiratory tract illness, tracheobronchitis, bronchiolitis and pneumonia (28). Acute HAdV-related gastroenteritis is particularly common in infants, and those with acute HAdV illness may present with general symptoms such as febrile illness, rash and/or general malaise (1). Rare clinical presentations of HAdV-related infection in immunocompetent individuals include pancreatitis, nephritis, acute haemorrhagic cystitis and meningoencephalitis (12).

Are HAdV-related infections usually benign in otherwise immunocompetent individuals?

Yes, but severe and even fatal infections are being reported more frequently in otherwise healthy persons. These may be related to the fact that the predominant circulating type of HAdV disappears over time with its replacement by another strain which either has not circulated for a longtime or has genetically changed (29). For example, HAdV-B14 is a member of species B which was first isolated in 1957 but disappeared until it re-emerged almost 50 years later as a cause of outbreaks of acute respiratory disease of varying severity (30). In addition, molecular analysis showed that it was a genetic variant of the original HAdV-14 type (30). Similarly, the recent re-emergence of HAdV-B7 and its genomic variant type 7d were associated with severe respiratory tract illness in Asia and the United States (6, 16, 31, 32). Furthermore, severe cases of acute respiratory disease in adults in the general population were associated recently with HAdV-E4 (5). Therefore, physicians should test for HAdVs in all patients with severe respiratory tract infections. Molecular characterisation of these viruses, whenever feasible, is important to identify re-emergence of potentially virulent variants of previously circulating HAdVs (6).

TREATMENT

Are antiviral agents recommended for treatment of HAdV-related infections in general practice?

No, most infections seen in the community are mild illnesses which are self-limiting and require supportive care only. Rarely, individuals develop significant end-organ disease which requires hospitalisation in which case use of cidofovir, a cytosine nucleotide analogue with activity against all known types of HAdV, may be considered by the consultant microbiologist (33). This drug is used parenterally for treatment of severe or disseminated infections in immunocompromised individuals and on the rare occurrence of severe disease in immunocompetent persons (34, 35, 36). However, an oral alternative called brincidofovir is currently available on compassionate-use basis for immunocompromised hosts with adenovirus disease.

Is a vaccine against HAdv available in Ireland and the United Kingdom?

No, but there is a HAdV-E4 vaccine available in the United States although its use is confined to military recruits to protect against outbreaks of HAdV-4-related respiratory disease. However, because of recent evidence of severe acute respiratory disease among adult civilians and the likelihood that it is under-diagnosed, there has been a question raised about its use also in this age group, particularly among those living in closed communities like colleges, summer camps and long-term care facilities *(5, 37)*.

HAdV-RELATED INFECTIONS IN IMMUNOCOMPROMISED PERSONS

Why does disseminated HAdV-related disease occur in immunocompromised individuals?

Immunocompromised individuals with suspected HAdV-related disease seen in primary care should be referred to their attending hospital physician. Persons with profound T cell immunodeficiency are at risk of reactivation of HAdV from sites of persistence and development of end-organ disease despite the presence of neutralising antibodies *(38, 39)*. Primary HAdV infection resolves with development of antibody to HAdV and, more importantly, HAdV-specific CD4+ / CD8+ T cells (cellular immunity)which maintains HAdVs in an asymptomatic persistent state in a variety of cell types including lung epithelial cells and lymphoid tissue in the intestine and tonsils *(18, 40, 41)*. When cellular immunity is impaired, for example following iatrogenic immunosuppression for allogeneic haematopoietic stem cell transplantation or solid-organ transplantation, HAdV reactivation in children usually begins in the gut and then disseminates *(18)*. However, reconstitution of HAdV-specific cellular immunity is associated with clearance of virus and resolution of HAdV-related endorgan disease *(42)*.

REFERENCES (*useful reviews)

1 R.J. Cooper *et al.*, *Epidemiol. Infect.* **125**, 333 (2000)

2 M.A. Yusof*et al.*, *Emerg. Infect. Dis.* **18**, 852 (2012)

3 R.N. Potter *et al.*, *Emerg. Infect. Dis.* **18**, 507 (2012)

4 B.J. Parcell *et al.*, *J. Public. Health (Oxf)*.**37**, 64 (2015)

5 A.E. Kajon *et al.*, *Emerg. Infect. Dis.* **24**, 201 (2018)

6 M.K. Scott *et al.*, *Emerg. Infect. Dis.* **22**, 1044 (2016)

7 B. Harrach *et al.*, *Ninth Report of the International Committee on Taxonomy of Viruses.* **2011**, 125 (2011)

8 E. Hage *et al.*, *J. Gen. Virol*.**96**, 2734 (2015)

9 L. Rosen. *Am. J. Hyg.* **71**, 120 (1960)

10 I. Madisch *et al.*, *J. Med. Virol*.**78**, 1210 (2006)

11 D. Seto *et al.*,*J. Virol*.**85**, 5701 (2011)

12 J.P. Lynch III, A.E. Kajon. *Semin. Resp. Crit. Care Med.* **37**, 586 (2016)*

13 J.P. Lynch, M. Fishbein, M. Echavarria. *Semin.Respir. Crit. Care.Med.***32**, 494 (2011)

14 K.L. Russell *et al.*, *Vaccine.* **24**, 2835 (2006)

15 R.A. Kuschner *et al.*, *Vaccine.* **31**, 2963 (2013)

16 Y. Zhiwu *et al.*, *Sci. Rep.* **6**, 37216 (2016)

17 D.M. Lamson *et al.*, *Emerg. Infect. Dis.* **23**, 1194 (2017)

18 T. Lion. *Clin.Microbiol. Rev.* **27**, 441 (2014)*

19 D. Metzgar *et al.*, *J. Clin.Microbiol.***48**, 1397 (2010)

20 H. Jalal *et al.*, *J. Clin. Microbiol.***43**, 2575 (2005)

21 A. Sauerbrei *et al.*, *J. Hosp. Infect.* **57**, 59 (2004)

22 R. Nauheim *et al.*, *Ophthalmology.* **97**, 1450 (1990)

23 J.P. Fox *et al.*, *Am. J. Epidemiol.* **89**, 25 (1969)

24 D. King *et al.*, *MMWR Morb.Mortal.* Wkly. Rep. **62**, 637 (2013)

25 M.E. Killerby *et al.*, *MMWR Morb.Mortal. Wkly. Rep.* **66**, 811 (2017)

26 W.A. Rutal a *et al.*, *Antimicrob. Agents Chemother.***50**, 1419 (2006)

27 J. Coia *et al.*, *J. Hosp. Infect.* **85**, 170 (2013)*

28 I. Tabain *et al.*, *Pediatr. Infect. Dis. J.* **31**, 680 (2012)

29 J. Cook, J. Radke. *F1000Res.* **6**, 90 (2017)

30 A.E. Kajon *et al.*, *J. Infect. Dis.* **202**, 93 (2010)

31S. Zhao *et al.*, *Sci. Rep.***4**, 7365 (2014)

32 O.T. Ng *et al*; *Emerg. Infect. Dis.* **21**, 1192 (2015)

33 F. Morfin *et al.*, *Antivir. Ther.***14**, 55 (2009)

34 M.G. Ison. *Clin. Infect. Dis.* **43**, 331 (2006)

35 S.S. Weigt *et al.*, *Semin. Respir. Crit. Care Med.* **32**, 471 (2011)

36 S.J. Kim *et al.*, *PLOS One.* **10**, e0122642 (2015)

37 R. Narra *et al.*, *J. Clin. Virol.***81**, 78 (2016)

38 L.A. Veltrop-Duits*et al.*, *Clin. Infect. Dis.* **52**, 1405 (2011)

39 T. Feuchtinger *et al.*,*Br. J. Haematol.* **128**, 503 (2005)

40 S. Roy *et al.*, *PLOS One.***6**, e24859 (2011)

41 C.T. Garnett *et al.*, *J.Virol.* **83**, 2417 (2009)

42 M.L. Zandvliet *et al.*, *Haematologica.* **95**, 1943 (2010)

SKIN INFECTION (VIRAL CAUSES)

Vesicular lesions due to

- Enterovirus
- Varicella
- Zoster

Maculopapular rash due to

- HHV6
- Measles
- Parvovirus B19

'Lumps & Bumps' due to

- 'Farmyard pox'
- Molluscum contagiosum
- Warts (nongenital)

ENTEROVIRUSES

What are enteroviruses?

Enteroviruses (EVs) are small, nonenveloped RNA viruses of the genus *Enterovirus* in the family *Picornaviridae*. They cause a wide range of infections in humans and animals. The International Committee on Taxonomy of viruses has classified the genus *Enterovirus* into ten species: four human EVs designated A to D, three human rhinoviruses (A to C) and three EVs infecting animals only [1]. The current classification scheme is based on genetic analysis of the coding region of the gene for the structural viral protein VP1 [2, 3, 4]. There are currently more than 100 serotypes in EV species A to D, identified by molecular sequencing of the gene encoding VP1. Earlier classifications separated human EVs into four biologically distinct subgroups based on disease and host range, including polioviruses, coxsackie A and B viruses, echoviruses and newer enteroviruses designated by serotype numbers.

Within the same family *Picornaviridae*, the *Parechovirus* genus has 14 subtypes of parechovirus; the prototypic subtypes 1 and 2 were originally classified as echovirus 22 and 23 within the *Enterovirus* genus, respectively [5, 6]. However, although parechoviruses have similar epidemiological and clinical features to EVs, they have sufficiently distinct RNA sequences and other biological properties to be classified as a separate genus [5].

EPIDEMIOLOGY OF NON-POLIO EVs

Is polio still a concern to medical practitioners in Europe?

Polioviruses, other than occasional imported oral vaccine strains, are not likely to be found in Europe. In June 2002 the World Health Organisation (WHO) European Region was certified as poliovirus-free. Poliovirus has not been detected in the surveillance programme for enterovirus identification among patients with acute flaccid paralysis (AFP) in Ireland.

What is the typical seasonal and age distribution of EV infections?

Enteroviral infections in temperate climates show marked seasonality with peak activity in summer and early autumn but lower levels throughout the remainder of the year [7]. Most EV infections occur in children < 5 years old with rates of infection much higher in infants < 3 months of age, probably reflecting inadequate hygiene and immunological naïvety in these cohorts [7, 8].

What epidemiological data on EVs are available in Ireland?

While data on EVs can be obtained for notifiable diseases such as viral meningitis and encephalitis in Ireland, the only other source of information is from surveillance for acute flaccid paralysis (AFP). Most EV infections are not notifiable. Furthermore, information on the relationship between EV serotype and disease is also very limited because methods for viral detection have switched from cell culture to molecular assays. While use of polymerase chain reaction (PCR) in routine diagnostics accounts for increased identification of EVs as the aetiology of infection, samples are not always referred for identification by molecular typing *(7, 9)*. Systematic collection of clinical and EV genotype data in all laboratory-confirmed cases is needed to provide comprehensive information on the burden of enteroviral infections, including new emerging viruses, and their patterns of disease.

How are EVs transmitted?

Faecal-oral spread is the main route of transmission of EVs *(10)*. Person to person spread can also occur by contact with saliva, respiratory secretions and vesicular fluid. In addition, EVs can be transferred to the mouth, nasal mucosa and conjunctiva via contaminated fingers, especially after changing children's diapers, or from contaminated surfaces due to survival of virus on inanimate objects *(11, 12)*. Therefore, implementing good hygienic practices in childcare settings, including hand washing by children and carers as well as disinfection of surfaces and fomites, helps to reduce enteroviral transmission *(13)*.

PATHOGENESIS

How do EVs cause disease in humans?

Usually EVs are ingested and, because of their stability at low pH, pass through the stomach to the terminal ileum where they replicate in submucosal lymphoid tissue known as Peyer's patches. Limited viral replication also occurs in the oropharynx. Virus then spreads via blood (primary viraemia) to reticuloendothelial tissues including liver, spleen, bone marrow and regional lymph nodes. Development of a type-specific neutralising antibody response at this stage stops viral replication so that most EV infections are asymptomatic. However, in a minority of infected individuals, significant viral replication continues in the reticulendothelial system (RES) with spillover of virus into blood. Development of illness coincides with onset of this secondary viraemia due to dissemination of virus to organs like skin, heart, lung and central nervous system where tissue damage occurs because of the cytopathic effect of viral replication. Immunopathogenic mechanisms may contribute to chronic diseases such as dilated cardiomyopathy and type 1 diabetes *(14, 15)*. Diseases caused by EVs range from nonspecific febrile illness with or without a rash to hand, foot and mouth disease (HFMD) and herpangina, acute haemorrhagic conjunctivitis, respiratory tract infection, acute flaccid paralysis, aseptic meningitis, brainstem encephalitis and, rarely, poliomyelitis caused by the poliovirus *(16, 17, 18, 19)*.

Why are some patients susceptible to severe and persistent EV infection?

Production of neutralising antibody specific for the EV serotype causing infection is essential for clearance of EV infection *(20)*. Therefore, individuals with humoral immune deficiencies are susceptible to persistent EV infection which may be fatal. Chronic enteroviral meningoencephalitis is a recognised complication of EV infection in agammaglobulinaemic or hypogammaglobulinaemic individuals and sometimes may be accompanied by clinical features of dermatomyositis *(21, 22)*.

CASE VIGNETTE

A 17-month-old boy was brought to the GP by his pregnant mother (10 weeks' gestation) with multiple vesicular skin lesions and lethargy. Of note on examination, the temperature was 38.4°C and he had vesicular lesions on his hands, knees and buttocks without any enanthem. He attended a crèche in which a case of hand, foot and mouth disease (HFMD) had been reported in the last 5 days. The GP suspected HFMD.

What can GPs learn from this case?

LABORATORY DIAGNOSIS

Was there a need for virological confirmation of EV infection in this case?

Yes, although diagnosis of HFMD is primarily clinical when illness is uncomplicated, virological confirmation is necessary when clinical presentation is atypical: for example, the presence of only an exanthem in this suspected case of HFMD. In addition, his mother was pregnant and thought to be nonimmune to varicella-zoster virus (VZV), therefore testing to exclude current VZV infection was done. Laboratory testing to differentiate EV infection from herpes simplex virus (HSV) in suspected eczema herpeticum is advised because the severe cutaneous disease due to coxsackievirus A6 is in the differential diagnosis but is managed differently. Furthermore, laboratory confirmation is also warranted in HFMD and herpangina complicated by concomitant neurological involvement.

How was EV infection confirmed in the laboratory?

Viral swabs from vesicular lesions were collected and EV RNA detected by real-time reverse transcription polymerase chain reaction (rRT-PCR). Further molecular analysis to identify the EV serotype was not performed; it is only available in reference laboratories. HSV and VZV DNA were not detected. In ill patients without lesions, throat swabs and faecal samples may be sent for virological testing but detection of EV RNA in faeces may only reflect viral shedding which occurs for several weeks from this site following symptomatic or asymptomatic EV infection. For most purposes, detection of EV RNA from an upper respiratory site represents strong evidence of causality as EV is typically shed for < 10 days from there.

COMMON DERMATOLOGICAL MANIFESTATIONS OF NON-POLIO EVs

Why was the clinical presentation of HFMD unusual in this case?

Most symptomatic cases of HFMD have both enanthemata and exanthemata but a minority may have only the exanthem, as in this case, or solely an enanthem *(23)*. HFMD usually presents in young children with low-grade fever, malaise and soreness in the mouth and pharynx causing reluctance to eat. Oral lesions, which are maculopapular or vesicular, are usually seen on the tongue and buccal mucosa. Skin lesions vary from macules or maculopapules to vesicles surrounded by a thin halo of erythema and may appear concurrently distributed on the hands, feet, knees or buttocks *(24)*.

What is herpangina?

Herpangina is another common manifestation of EV infection. It is characterised by acute onset of fever, malaise and eruption of papulovesicular lesions with a surrounding red rim which are located typically on the posterior pharynx including the anterior tonsillar pillars, soft palate, uvula or buccal mucosa but, in contrast to HFMD, with rare involvement of the tongue or hard palate *(24)*. The absence of skin involvement distinguishes it from HFMD.

What are the common differential diagnoses of oral ulcers seen in suspected cases of HFMD and herpangina?

Herpes simplex virus (HSV)-induced gingivostomatitis caused by primary HSV type 1 (HSV-1) is an important consideration. Clinical manifestations include painful vesicles on the gingiva causing redness and swelling, and are usually accompanied by ulcers on the buccal mucosa, tongue, hard palate, posterior pharynx and perioral skin. Aphthous ulcers are also painful mouth lesions but have a greyish base unlike the erythematous lesions in HFMD and herpangina.

What was the natural history of this case of HFMD?

There was complete resolution of the lesions within 5 days of their onset at which time he returned to the créche. In patients with HFMD, symptoms usually develop within 3 to 5 days of acquiring the virus followed by complete resolution usually within 7 days of illness onset. Herpangina has a similar incubation period and, like HFMD, is a self-limiting illness with resolution of the lesions within 7 days of onset. However, a more prolonged and severe course of HFMD and herpangina, including a more widespread exanthem and shedding of nails, have been reported recently in children and adults infected with a genetic variant of coxsackievirus A6 (vCA6) *(25, 26, 27)*. Several large outbreaks of atypical HFMD and severe herpangina linked to vCA6 have been reported worldwide since 2008 *(28, 29)*.

What clinical complications may occur in patients with HFMD and herpangina?

Complications requiring hospitalisation rarely develop in immunocompetent children. Dehydration due to dysphagia is the most common problem. Other rarer complications like aseptic meningitis, encephalitis, acute flaccid paralysis and cardiopulmonary disease are mainly associated with enterovirus 71 (EV71) (discussed later).

TRANSMISSIBILITY OF NON-POLIO EVs

What is the typical duration of infectivity in the patient with HFMD or herpangina?

Individuals with these manifestations of EV infection are likely to be most infectious in the first week of illness. Therefore, exclusion of children with current disease from childcare settings should be considered until resolution of lesions, particularly if they are also clinically unwell. After onset of illness, viral shedding from the pharynx persists for about 2 weeks and from gut persists for 4 weeks. Individuals may still be infectious during the asymptomatic convalescence *(30)*. Individuals who never displayed symptoms of EV infection may also shed virus and transmit infection. In childcare facilities, good hygienic practices should always include hand-washing after changing diapers and using the toilet. Appropriate disinfection of inanimate objects and surfaces likely to carry saliva and faecal material is important *(13)*.

NON-POLIO EVs IN PREGNANCY

What were the implications of the son's EV infection for his mother's pregnancy?

None, but she was advised about the need for hand washing on changing his diapers. Enterovirus (EV) infection in pregnancy is not associated with teratogenicity, probably because of negligible transplacental transfer of virus to the fetus *(31)*. However, acute EV infection late in pregnancy can adversely affect the neonate. Most neonates with symptomatic EV infection acquire it from mothers who were acutely ill in the week before delivery *(32)*. These neonatal EV infections can be mild but may progress to fulminant disease, similar in presentation to bacterial sepsis, with severe hepatitis and/or myocarditis *(33)*. Onset of illness usually develops 3 to 5 days postpartum indicating perinatal acquisition probably from maternal genital secretions *(34)*. The time interval between maternal EV infection and delivery affects neonatal outcome *(35)*. When there is sufficient time for passive transfer of maternal EV-specific neutralising antibody to the neonate, systemic infection is usually prevented *(36)*. In contrast, low or absent maternal EV-specific neutralising antibody in the neonate may result in severe infection *(37)*. Furthermore, EV-related herpangina in pregnancy has been associated with adverse outcomes and such cases should be referred to the obstetrician *(38)*.

ANTIVIRAL TREATMENT

Are antiviral agents used currently in the management of EV infections?

At the moment, there is no approved antiviral drug for treatment or prevention of enteroviral infections. Compounds known as capsid inhibitors were developed to target different steps in the replication cycle of EVs. Such capsid inhibitors, administered orally, include pleconaril (no longer available commercially), vapendavir and pocapavir *(39, 40)*. Intravenous immunoglobulin (IVIG) has been used to treat EV infections because it is hypothesised that IVIG contains neutralising antibody to EVs; however, its efficacy remains unproven *(33)*.

OTHER CLINICAL MANIFESTATIONS OF NON-POLIO EVs

What is pleurodynia which is closely associated with EVs in medical textbooks?

Pleurodynia, also known as Bornholm disease, is a myositis of intercostal muscles and those in the upper abdomen caused by enteroviral infection. Clinical presentation is characterised by fever and acute spasmodic pain in the chest or upper abdomen which is exacerbated by inhalation. Minor constitutional symptoms may also be present including headache, rhinorrhoea and loose stools *(41)*. It is a self-limiting illness with resolution within 4-6 days. Coxsackievirus B is classically associated with pleurodynia infection but other EVs may cause it *(42, 43, 44)*.

May EV-related ocular infection be encountered in primary care?

EVs cause acute haemorrhagic conjunctivitis (AHC). Two enteroviruses, enterovirus 70 (EV70) and an antigenic variant of coxsackievirus A24 (CA24v), have caused large outbreaks of AHC worldwide. AHC is characterised by abrupt onset of painful, swollen, red eyes with lacrimation and subconjunctival haemorrhage. The infection is self-limiting with resolution in ≤ 7 days *(45, 46)*. Bacterial super infection may occur and, rarely, neurological complications including radiculomyelitis, have been reported in EV70-related AHC cases *(47)*. Viral AHC is highly contagious being transmitted mainly by direct contact with eye discharges or indirectly via contaminated fomites *(47)*. Epidemics of viral AHC occur predominantly in tropical and subtropical regions *(48)*. Control of spread requires rapid implementation of hygienic measures, including hand-washing and not sharing fomites with infected persons *(49)*.

What is EV-related viral myocarditis?

Myocarditis is an inflammation of the heart muscle *(50)*. Although it has been associated with autoimmune diseases, drug-induced hypersensitivity reactions and toxins, infectious agents including bacteria, fungi, parasites and viruses are also putative causes of the disease *(51)*. In developed countries, viruses are the primary cause of myocarditis with enteroviruses being the classical aetiological agent identified in seroepidemiological studies and molecular investigation of endomyocardial tissue *(50, 52)*. Other viruses identified as causes of myocarditis include adenoviruses and, less frequently, influenza viruses, Epstein-Barr virus, parvovirus, cytomegalovirus and human herpesvirus 6 *(50, 53)*. Human immunodeficiency virus type 1 (HIV-1) RNA has been detected frequently in cardiac tissue from HIV-1-infected persons with dilated cardiomyopathy although it is unclear if it is the primary cause *(54)*. Acute myocarditis may resolve spontaneously or, in a small proportion of cases (10%-20%), may progress to chronic myocarditis and dilated cardiomyopathy with poor outcomes *(50, 55)*.

When should the GP suspect myocarditis?

It is a challenge to recognise myocarditis in primary care, particularly as patients may present with mild disease. Most proven paediatric cases of acute and chronic myocarditis presented with chest pain and dyspnoea and were initially diagnosed with a respiratory illness *(56, 57)*. However, hepatomegaly or radiographic evidence of cardiomegaly and abnormal electrocardiogram are indicative of a cardiac aetiology and should alert the physician to assess the patient for myocarditis *(56, 57)*.

Which virology testing should be performed in suspected cases of myocarditis?

Cases should be referred to the cardiology service. In hospital, nasopharyngeal and faecal samples should be sent for virology testing using molecular assays for enteroviruses, adenoviruses and influenza viruses. Although many viruses linked with myocarditis circulate commonly in the community and therefore viral detection may be coincidental, there is evidence of correlation between positive virological findings in samples collected from peripheral sites and endomyocardial biopsy results *(58, 59)*. However, since clinical presentation may occur weeks after acute viral infection, failure to detect virus does not exclude a viral aetiology *(51, 55)*.

EMERGENT EVs OF CLINICAL SIGNIFICANCE

What is enterovirus D68?

Enterovirus D68 (EV-D68) is an emerging pathogen globally. It is a genetic hybrid of EV and rhinovirus, with the respiratory tract its primary site of infection. Like other EVs, it is seasonal and has the potential to cause CNS disease. The clinical presentation varies widely from mild coryzal symptoms to cough and dyspnoea without systemic manifestations to severe pneumonia requiring mechanical ventilation *(60, 61, 62)*.

What is the timeline for the emergence of EV-D68?

Although EV-D68 was first identified in 1962, it was then one of the most rarely reported serotypes of EV, with only 26 cases reported in the United States between 1970 and 2005 *(63, 64)*. By contrast, in the last decade EV-D68 was identified as the likely cause of small clusters of acute respiratory illness in Europe, Asia and the United States, and in the summer of 2014, the United States experienced a nationwide outbreak of respiratory illness associated with significant morbidity and mortality. EV-D68 was commonly identified as the pathogen in respiratory samples collected during this extensive outbreak *(62)*. Coincidentally, a rise in EV-D68-associated respiratory illness was also documented in other countries in 2014 *(62, 65, 66)*. Molecular data from the Netherlands and Japan showed evidence of significant genetic diversity among EV-D68 isolates, consistent with emergence of a real epidemic in the late 2000s *(67, 68)*.

What are the risk factors for severe EV-D68-associated respiratory tract illness?

Acute lower respiratory tract infection associated with EV-D68 in the 2014 outbreak in the United States occurred predominantly in children with asthma. EV-D68 infection in otherwise healthy children and adults usually present with a mild upper respiratory tract illness. It appears that a more complicated illness may occur in children and adults with a prior history of asthma and wheezing, and also in hosts with chronic obstructive pulmonary disease *(60, 66)*. Immunocompromised individuals are also at risk of severe EV-D68 respiratory infection, particularly those on treatment for haematological malignancy in whom EV-D68 infection can be associated with prolonged hospitalisation and poor outcome *(69, 70)*.

Does EV-D68 cause acute flaccid myelitis (AFM)?

Although still rare, there is increasing evidence of a causative association between EV-D68 infection and development of AFM *(71)*. This atypical neurological condition usually presents with acute onset of limb weakness, cranial nerve involvement usually with bulbar weakness and radiological evidence of lesions in grey matter of the spinal cord and brainstem *(72)*. Among EV-D68-linked AFM cases in the United States between 2012 and 2014, the majority (80%) reported a febrile respiratory tract illness before onset of AFM *(73, 74)*. Emergence of a new strain of EV-D68, known as clade B1, has been temporally associated with an increased incidence of AFM in the United States and Europe *(75, 76, 77)*.

Why is Enterovirus 71 of public health importance?

While the majority of EV71-related infections are subclinical, cutaneous manifestations like HFMD and herpangina occur in the remainder. Severe neurological disease may also occur including aseptic meningitis, acute flaccid paralysis (AFP) and, importantly, brainstem encephalitis (BE), a complication which may progress to cardio respiratory failure and even death *(78, 79)*. Although EV71 was first isolated in the 1960s, in the last two decades it has been recognised as a major cause of outbreaks of HFMD associated with neurological disease and high fatality rates in Malaysia and Taiwan *(80, 81)*. Since then several other large epidemics have been reported across the Asia-Pacific region including Australia *(82, 83)*. EV71 also circulates in Europe and the United States but, unlike reports from the Asia-Pacific region, large outbreaks of severe disease have not occurred to date. However, there is a need for enhanced surveillance of EV71 globally because of recent evidence of its spread within and between distant and neighbouring countries in Europe and recent reports of sporadic cases of severe neurological disease in Europe as well as a large outbreak in Spain associated with neurological disease*(84, 85, 86)*.

What risk factors are associated with acquisition of EV71 infection?

Data from outbreaks in the Asia-Pacific region showed that children aged 6 months to 6 years were found to be at increased risk of EV71 infection and those < 3 years old were at higher risk of severe disease, probably related to lack of protective immunity *(24, 87)*.

Are vaccines available in Europe to protect humans against non-polio enteroviruses?

Not yet but an inactivated enterovirus 71 (EV71) vaccine was shown to induce an effective immune response and protect against EV71-related HFMD and herpangina in Chinese children *(88)*.

REFERENCES (*useful review)

1 http://ictv.org/index.asp

2 M.S. Oberste *et al., J. Virol.* **73**, 1941 (1999)

3 D. Nasri *et al., Expert Rev. Mol. Diagn.* **7**, 419 (2007)

4 W.A. Nix, M.S. Oberste, M.A. Pallansch. *J. Clin. Microbiol.***44**, 2698 (2006)

5 G. Stanway, T. Hyypia. *J. Virol.* **73**, 5249 (1999)

6 G. Stanway *et al., J. Virol.* **68**, 8232 (1994)

7 S.Kadambari *et al.,Clin.Microbiol. Infect.***20**, 1289 (2014)

8 P. Muir. *Medicine.***45**, 794 (2017)*

9 Centers for Disease Control and Prevention.*MMWR Morb.Mortal. Wkly. Rep.* **60**, 1301 (2011)

10 R.B. Couch *et al., Am. J. Epidemiol.* **91**, 78 (1970)

11 Centers for Disease Control and Prevention.*MMWR Morb.Mortal. Wkly. Rep.* **61**, 213 (2012)

12 C.H. Chen, B.M. Hsu, M.T. Wan. *J. Appl. Microbiol.* **104**, 817 (2008)

13 F. Ruan *et al., Pediatrics.* **127**, e898 (2011)

14 N.R. Rose *et al., Ann. N. Y. Acad. Sci.* **475**, 146 (1986)

15 F. Dotta *et al., Proc. Natl. Acad. Sci. USA.* **104**, 5115 (2007)

16 S.H. Wei *et al., BMC Infect. Dis.* **11**, 346 (2011)

17 C.M. Oermann *et al., Annals Am. Thorac. Soc.* **12**, 775 (2015)

18 T. Soloman *et al., Lancet Infect. Dis.* **10**, 778 (2010)

19 R.E. Rhoades *et al., Virology.* **411**, 288 (2011)

20 H.A. Rotbart, A.D. Webster. *Clin. Infect. Dis.***32**, 228 (2001)

21 R.E. McKinney Jr, S.L .Katz, C.M. Wilfert. *Rev. Infect. Dis.* **9**, 334 (1987)

22 A.D. Webster *et al.*, *Clin. Infect. Dis.* **17**, 657 (1993)

23 J.L. Adler *et al.*, *Am. J. Dis. Child.* **120**, 309 (1970)

24 L.Y. Chang *et al.*, *JAMA.* **291**, 222 (2004)

25 E. Gaunt *et al.*, *J. Gen. Virol.***96**, 1067 (2015)

26 E. Ben-Chetrit *et al.*, *J. Clin. Virol.* **59**, 201 (2014)

27 L. Bian *et al.*, *Expert Rev. Anti Infect. Ther.***13**, 1061 (2015)*

28 C. Sinclair *et al.*, *Euro. Surveill.***19**, pii=20745 (2014)

29 T. Fujimoto *et al.*, *Emerg. Infect. Dis.* **18**, 337 (2012)

30 M. Richardson *et al.*, *Pediatr. Infect. Dis. J.* **20**, 380 (2001)

31 M.S. Amstey *et al.*, *Am. J. Obstet. Gynecol.* **158**, 775 (1988)

32 J.F. Modlin. *Rev.Infect.Dis.* **8**, 918 (1986)

33 J.F. Modlin. *J. Pediatr. Infect. Dis. Soc.* **5**, 63 (2016)

34 M.J. Abzug, M.J. Levin, H.A. Rotbart. *Pediatr. Infect. Dis. J.* **12**, 820 (1993)

35 J.F. Modlin, M. Bowman. *J. Infect. Dis.* **156**, 21 (1987)

36 J.F. Modlin *et al.*, *N. Engl. J. Med.* **305**, 368 (1981)

37 P.J. Berry, J. Nagington. *Arch. Dis. Child.* **57**, 22 (1982)

38 Y.H. Chen, H.C.. Lin, H.C. Lin. *Am. J. Obstet. Gynecol.* **203**, 49 (2010)

39 L. Shang, M. Xu, Z. Yin. *Antiviral Res.* **97**, 183 (2013)

40 L. van der Linden, K.C. Wolthers, F.J. van Kuppeveld.*Viruses.***7**, 4529 (2015)

41 W.T. Huang *et al.*, *J. Microbiol. Immunol. Infect.* **43**, 515 (2010)

42 E.J. Bell, N.R. Grist. *Lancet.***1**, 326 (1970)

43 F.S. Kantor, G.D. Hsiung. *N. Engl. J. Med.***266**, 661 (1962)

44 M. Moore *et al.*, *Public Health Rep.* **99**, 515 (1984)

45 V.E. Sklar *et al.*, *Am. J. Ophthalmol.* **95**, 45 (1983)

46 P.W. Wright, G.H. Strauss, M.P. Langford. *Am. Fam. Physician.* **45**, 173 (1992)

47 R. Kono *et al.*, *J. Infect. Dis.* **135**, 706 (1977)

48 L. Zhang *et al.*,*Scientific Reports.* **7**, 45202 (2017)

49 C. Finger. *Lancet.***361**, 1714 (2003)

50 A.M. Feldman, D. McNamara. *N. Engl. J. Med.* **343**, 1388 (2000)

51 C.E. Canter, K.E. Simpson. *Circulation.***129**, 115 (2014)

52 G. Cambridge *et al.*, *Br. Heart J.* **41**, 692 (1979)

53 I.M. Grumbach *et al.*, *ActaCardiol.* **54**, 83 (1999)

54 G. Barboro *et al.*, *N. Engl. J. Med.* **339**, 1093 (1998)

55 C. Kawai. *Circulation.***99**, 1091 (1999)

56 S.B. Freedman *et al.*, *Pediatrics.* **120**, 1278 (2007)

57 Y. Durani*et al.*, *Am. J. Emerg. Med.* **27**, 942 (2009)

58 N. Akhtar *et al.*, *Circulation.* **99**, 2011 (1999)

59 P.E. Daubeney *et al.*, *Circulation.* **114**, 2671 (2006)

60 C.M. Midgley *et al.*, *MMWR Morb.Mortal. Wkly. Rep.* **63**, 798 (2014)

61 Centers for Disease Control and Prevention.*MMWR Morb.Mortal. Wkly. Rep*. **60**, 1301 (2011)

62 C.C. Holm-Hansen, S.E. Midgley, T.K. Fischer.*Lancet Infect. Dis*. **16**, e64 (2016)

63 J.H. Schieble, V.L. Fox, E.H. Lennette. *Am. J. Epidemiol*. **85**, 297 (1967)

64 N. Khetsuriani *et al., Morb.Mortal. Wkly. Rep. Surveill. Summ.***55**, 1 (2006)

65 T. Zhang *et al., Emerg. Infect. Dis*. **21**, 916 (2015)

66 R. Poelman *et al., J. Clin. Virol.***71**, 1 (2015)

67 A. Meijer *et al., Virology*. **423**, 49 (2012)

68 T. Ikeda *et al., Microbiol. Immunol.***56**, 139 (2012)

69 A. Waghmare *et al., Blood*. **125**, 1724 (2015)

70 M.C.Spaeder *et al.,Pediatr. Crit. Care Med*. **16**, 119 (2015)

71 A. Dyda *et al.,* Euro Surveill. **23**, 17-00310 (2018)

72 A. Mirand, H. Peigue-Lafeuille. *Lancet.***385**, 1601(2015)

73 A.L. Greninger *et al., Lancet Infect. Dis*. **15**, 671 (2015)

74 J.J. Sejvar *et al., Clin. Infect. Dis*. **63**, 737 (2016)

75 P. Ayscue *et al., MMWR Morb. Mortal. Wkly. Rep*. **63**, 903 (2014)

76 M. Lang *et al., Euro Surveill*. **19**, pii=20952 (2014)

77 H.C. Pfeiffer *et al., Euro Surveill*. **20**, pii=21062 (2015)

78 C.M. Perez-Velez *et al., Clin. Infect. Dis*. **45**, 950 (2007)

79 M.H. Ooi *et al., BMC Infect. Dis*. **9**, 3 (2009)

80 M.J. Cardosa *et al., Emerg. Infect. Dis*. **9**, 461 (2003)

81 M. Ho *et al., N. Engl. J. Med*. **341**, 929 (1999)

82 Y. Zhang *et al., Virol. J.***7**, 94 (2010)

83 X. Tan *et al., PLoS One*. **6**, e25662 (2011)

84 C. Hassel *et al., Euro Surveill*. **20**, pii=30005 (2015)

85 S.E. Midgley *et al; Euro Surveill.***22**, pii=30565 (2017)

86 R. Gonzalez-Sanz *et al., Euro Surveill*. **24**, pii=1800089 (2019)

87 L.Y. Chang *et al., Pediatrics*. **109**, e88 (2002)

88 F. Zhu *et al., N. Engl. J. Med*. **370**, 818 (2014)

VARICELLA

What is varicella? What is herpes zoster?

Varicella-zoster virus (VZV) is the causal agent of two distinct clinical syndromes: varicella (chickenpox), which occurs during primary infection, and zoster (shingles), which reflects VZV reactivation from its latent state *(1)*. Varicella is a highly contagious disease occurring predominantly among unvaccinated children. On initial infection (varicella), the virus disseminates via blood (viraemia) to many tissues in the host, including skin, with subsequent appearance of a generalised rash. Following recovery from varicella, VZV establishes latency in neurons of the dorsal root and cranial nerve ganglia, and the autonomic nervous system, including the enteric nervous system *(2)*. Reactivation of latent VZV in these ganglia, with unilateral spread along the dermatome innervated by these sensory nerves, causes herpes zoster (shingles), characterised typically by a painful and pruritic vesicular rash.

CASE VIGNETTE

A previously healthy 17-year-old girl presented to her GP with a 48-hour history of a spreading vesicular rash. One day before onset of the rash, she complained of fever, malaise and headache. The rash started on her face, neck and chest. Of note on physical examination was a polymorphic rash with vesicles, pustules and crusting lesions, typical of varicella. About 14 days before onset of illness, she visited her grandmother and nursed weeping vesicles around her right eye (zoster ophthalmicus). The adolescent and her twin sister had no history of varicella or vaccination against the disease. Her twin sister had not visited her grandmother. How was the case managed?

LABORATORY DIAGNOSIS

Was laboratory diagnosis needed to confirm varicella in this case?

No, the GP made the diagnosis on the basis of the vesicular rash and recent history of close contact with a person with active herpes zoster (HZ).

How can VZV-related disease be confirmed in the laboratory?

The method of choice for laboratory diagnosis of varicella and herpes zoster (HZ) is real-time polymerase chain reaction (PCR) for detection of VZV DNA. Testing of skin swabs collected from patients with VZV-related cutaneous disease by PCR has shown the assay to be highly sensitive and specific *(3)*. In addition, cerebrospinal fluid (CSF) samples, fluid from vesicles, scabs from crusted lesions and conjunctival swabs can also be tested reliably by PCR *(4)*.

Is serology useful for diagnosis of varicella?

No, laboratory diagnosis of varicella using serological methods to detect IgM and IgG antibody to VZV (anti-VZV IgM / IgG) is not recommended. Demonstration of anti-VZV IgM and IgG seroconversion, which is needed to confirm varicella serologically, delays diagnosis *(1)*. Rapid diagnosis allows infection control measures to be implemented immediately and, if clinically relevant, antiviral treatment to be started. Moreover, detection of anti-VZV IgM in the presence of anti-VZV IgG does not distinguish between varicella and herpes zoster infection *(1, 3)*.

TRANSMISSION OF VZV

What are the likely routes by which the teenager in this case acquired varicella-zoster virus (VZV)?

Transmission of VZV from patients with varicella occurs predominantly via the airborne route when desquamated superficial skin cells from cutaneous lesions secrete infectious viral particles which become aerosolised and infect susceptible hosts on inhalation *(5, 6)*. Because skin lesions are the main source of virus transmitted via the airborne route, infected cases with high numbers of vesicles are considered very contagious *(7, 8)*. Environmental contamination is unlikely to be of significance in transmission of VZV because of rapid loss of viral infectivity due to its heat lability *(4)*.

When is a person with varicella potentially infectious?

Infectivity of an individual with primary VZV infection ranges from 48 hours before onset of the rash until all skin lesions have crusted. While this usually takes 5 to 7 days, it may be longer in immunocompromised individuals. Transmissibility of VZV by persons with varicella between 1 and 2 days before appearance of the exanthem is based on epidemiological data *(1)*.

CLINICAL FEATURES

Are the clinical features of varicella in this case typical of those seen in general practice?

Yes, in adolescents and adults a prodrome of fever, myalgia, anorexia and headache occurs frequently about 1-2 days before onset of the exanthem, while, in contrast, varicella in children is not usually preceded by a prodromal illness *(1)*. The incubation period in varicella is usually between 10–21 days, as in this case. A generalised, pruritic, vesicular rash concentrated mainly on the face, scalp and trunk with lesser involvement of the limbs is typical of varicella *(9)*. The rash starts as small, erythematous macules which progress to papules followed by the appearance of clear vesicles on erythematous papules, known as 'dewdrops on a rose petal'. New lesions appear over the next 3-5 days leading to the characteristic clinical feature of varicella which is the presence of papules, vesicles, pustules and crusted lesions at the same time in any area of skin *(10)*. Later the vesicles become cloudy and subsequently crust over *(1)*. Lesions may be seen on mucous membranes, including the palate, conjunctiva and introitus of the genital tract *(1)*. The disease lasts for 5-7 days with as many as 100 to 300 vesicles in otherwise immunocompetent individuals. Hypopigmentation may be seen on healing of lesions but scarring is rare *(10)*. Varicella can be classified clinically by the number of cutaneous lesions present: mild (< 50 lesions), mild/moderate (50-249) lesions, moderate (250-499 lesions) or severe (≥ 500 lesions) *(11)*.

What complications of varicella, in otherwise immunocompetent persons, may be seen in general practice?

Secondary bacterial infection of skin lesions may commonly be seen in otherwise healthy children with varicella. The pruritic nature of the exanthem causes scratching of lesions which is a predisposing factor to super infection with streptococci and staphylococci from contaminated fingers, causing cellulitis and erysipelas *(9)*. Neurological complications may occur in the course of varicella or shortly after its resolution. Cerebellar ataxia, which is self-limiting and seen mainly in those < 15 years of age, occurs at a frequency of 1 in 4,000 cases. In contrast, encephalitis can be fatal and occurs in 1 in 10,000 cases of varicella among previously healthy children and adults *(1)*. Angiitis of small or large blood vessels may cause strokes in children *(9, 12)*. Adults with varicella, including pregnant women, are at a higher risk of viral pneumonia with more significant morbidity and mortality than seen in children *(13)*.

VARIATIONS IN CLINICAL PRESENTATION OF VARICELLA SEEN IN GENERAL PRACTICE

Can otherwise healthy individuals develop varicella even if they have a past history of varicella or serological evidence of immunity to VZV?

Yes, symptomatic varicella reinfection, which is usually mild, may occur in immunocompetent and immunocompromised persons who were previously infected with VZV *(14, 15, 16)*. One study in the United States showed that varicella reinfection in individuals with physician-diagnosed clinical episodes of disease occurred at a frequency of 4.5% and 13.3% of reported varicella cases in 1995 and 1999, respectively *(17)*.

What is breakthrough varicella?

Some individuals immunised with live varicella vaccine may develop varicella following exposure to an index case, hence the term breakthrough varicella (BTV). It refers specifically to varicella occurring in a person who received at least one dose of varicella vaccine ≥ 42 days prior to onset of disease *(18)*. The time gap of 42 days is used to define

BTV cases due to wild-type VZV because the live attenuated varicella vaccine may also occasionally cause a generalised rash in the 6 weeks following immunization *(19)*.

What is the typical clinical course of BTV?

The clinical course is usually mild with fewer skin lesions (< 50 compared to about 300 in unvaccinated persons) which are mainly maculopapular and may not evolve into vesicles *(19)*. Although BTV is also known as 'mild varicella-like syndrome', about 25% of cases present clinically in a similar manner to unvaccinated cases with varicella. Complicated BTV disease may occur in both immunocompetent and immunocompromised hosts albeit uncommonly *(19)*. Physicians should consider BTV in the differential diagnosis of children presenting with a maculopapular rash or vesicular rash ≥ 42 days after immunisation with varicella vaccine.

What about infectivity in a person previously vaccinated against varicella who develops breakthrough disease?

As in varicella due to wild-type VZV, those with a vesicular rash are potentially infectious until lesions have crusted. However, some patients with BTV only develop macules and papules in which case they are only regarded as infectious for 24 hours after the last appearance of new lesions of this type *(20)*.

TREATMENT

Was antiviral treatment considered by the GP in this case of varicella?

Yes, because varicella is more severe in otherwise healthy adolescents (≥ 13 years of age) than in younger children. Treatment with oral aciclovir (800 mg four times daily for five days) should be started within 24 hours of onset of the rash to be most beneficial. This approach was shown to reduce significantly time to defervescence and crusting of lesions as well as the number of vesicles present (21). Similar findings were observed with early treatment with oral aciclovir (800 mg five times daily for five days) in otherwise healthy adults with uncomplicated varicella *(22)*.

Since the girl presented > 24 hours after onset of the rash, did the GP give antiviral treatment?

No, because initiation of oral aciclovir between 24 hours and 72 hours after rash onset in otherwise healthy adults with uncomplicated varicella was shown previously to have no impact on the course of disease *(22)*. However, some physicians would still prescribe oral aciclovir if fresh lesions were appearing after 24 hours. In this case, the patient's clinical illness resolved without any complications within 10 days of onset of prodrome.

Should otherwise healthy children with uncomplicated varicella receive antiviral treatment?

In general, treatment with oral antivirals is only recommended in children older than 12 months with a history of chronic cutaneous or pulmonary disorders, including those receiving oral or inhaled steroids (9). Varicella is usually self-limiting in otherwise immunocompetent children with uncomplicated disease. It can be managed with antipyretics (other than acetylsalicylates or non-steroidal anti-inflammatory agents), rehydration and antihistamines or calamine lotion for pruritus (9). Treatment with oral aciclovir (20 mg/kg four times daily for five days) in healthy children aged 2 to 12 years with varicella was shown to have modest benefits in reducing the severity of illness including the number of skin lesions, duration of fever and other constitutional symptoms when treatment was started within 24 hours of rash onset (23). However, the rate of disease complications in the study was too low to allow an impact of antiviral treatment on reducing their occurrence to be seen.

What about antiviral treatment in otherwise healthy persons with complicated varicella or immunocompromised individuals with varicella?

These patients should be referred to hospital for clinical assessment and intravenous aciclovir (10 mg/kg three times daily) for 7 days or longer, depending on the clinical course of the illness.

PREVENTION OF VARICELLA

What measures did the GP take to prevent varicella in the patient's twin sister?

Active immunisation with varicella vaccine was given to her sister as post exposure prophylaxis (PEP). She did not develop varicella. Vaccination with varicella vaccine is an effective option for prevention or attenuation of varicella in non-pregnant and otherwise immunocompetent persons with no evidence of immunity to varicella, as long as administered within 72hours of exposure (24, 25). It should be noted that any individual given a dose of varicella vaccine as post exposure prophylaxis (PEP) may still develop mild disease. While some recommend vaccination for up to 5 days post exposure, there are limited data to support its effectiveness at this late stage (25, 26). Although most data are derived from studies in children, PEP with varicella vaccine can be considered for adolescents and adults. A second dose at a four-week interval is advised for contacts who already received their first dose of vaccine as PEP and did not develop varicella.

What are the other options for prophylaxis against varicella following exposure?

Passive immunity can be given using plasma products containing high titres of VZV-specific neutralising antibody (VZIG) and is only recommended for susceptible pregnant women, infants and immunocompromised hosts following significant exposure. Referral to hospital is advised for VZIG administration. In general, there is no recommendation on the use of aciclovir as PEP either for immunocompetent or immunocompromised hosts because of limited data including lack of randomised controlled trials *(27, 28)*.

In general, when should the general practitioner consider the need for prophylaxis following exposure to varicella?

Post exposure prophylaxis (PEP) is considered necessary for nonimmune individuals who have had a significant exposure to VZV *(28, 29)*.

Exposure to an index case with varicella or with exposed VZV lesions like zoster ophthalmicus/zoster oticus or with disseminated zoster or with localised zoster in an immunocompromised individual due to shedding of high VZV load.

Exposure during the time of infectivity in the index case which is 48 hours before onset of the rash in varicella or disseminated zoster or at the onset of the rash in other types of zoster until the lesions have crusted over.

Type of exposure to the index case with VZV-related disease listed above such as household contact or being in the same room/hospital ward for > 15 minutes or face-to-face contact.

REFERENCES (*useful reviews)

1 A.M. Arvin. *Clin.Microbiol. Rev.* **9**, 361 (1996)

2 J. Chen *et al.*, *J. Neurovirol.* **17**, 578 (2011)

3 J. Leung *et al.*, *Clin. Infect. Dis.* **51**, 23 (2010)

4 A.A. Gershon, M.D. Gershon.*Clin.Microbiol. Rev.* **26**, 728 (2013)*

5 J.J. Chen *et al.*, *Cell.* **119**, 915 (2004)

6 M. Tsolia *et al.*, *J. Pediatr.* **116**, 184 (1990)

7 J.F. Seward *et al.*, *JAMA.* **292**, 704 (2004)

8 J.D. Siegel *et al.*, *Am. J. Infect.Control.***35**Suppl 2,S65 (2007)

9 U. Heininger, J.F. Seward. *Lancet.***368**, 1365 (2006)*

10 J.W. Ely, M. Seabury Stone. *Am. Fam. Physician.* **81**, 726 (2010)*

11 A.S. Lopez, J. Zhang, M. Marin. *MMWR Wkly. Rep.* **65**, 902 (2016)

12 R. Askalan *et al.*, *Stroke.* **32**, 1257 (2001)

13 A. Mirouse *et al.*, *Crit Care.* **21**, 137 (2017)

14 A.A. Gershon *et al.*, *J. Infect. Dis.* **149**, 137 (1984)

15 A.K. Junker, E. Angus, E.E. Thomas. *Pediatr. Infect. Dis. J.* **10**, 569 (1991)

16 J.A. Johnson, K.C. Bloch, B.N. Dang.*Clin. Infect. Dis.***52**, 907 (2011)

17 S. Hall *et al.*, *Pediatrics.***109**, 1068 (2002)

18 S. Weinmann *et al.*, *J. Infect. Dis.* **197**, Suppl 2 S132 (2008)

19 J. Leung, K.R. Broder, M. Marin. *Expert Rev. Vaccines*. **16**, 391 (2017)*

20 American Academy of Pediatrics. Red Book. 2012; 774

21 H.H. Balfour Jr *et al.*, *J. Pediatr*. **120**, 627 (1992)

22 M.R. Wallace *et al.*, *Ann. Intern. Med*. **117**, 358 (1992)

23 L.M. Dunkle *et al.*, *N. Engl. J. Med*. **325**, 1539 (1991)

24 M.J. Ferson.*Commun. Dis. Intell*. **25**, 13 (2001)

25 K. Macartney, A. Heywood, P. McIntyre. *Cochrane Database Syst. Rev*. **23**, CD001833 (2014)

26 M. Brotons *et al.*, *Pediatr. Infect. Dis. J*. **29**, 10 (2010)

27 Y Asano *et al.*, *Pediatrics*. 92, 219 (1993)

28 M. Marin *et al.*, *MMWR Recomm. Rep*. **56** (RR-4), 1 (2007)

29 Department of Health UK. The Green Book; 2014

VARICELLA VACCINE

What is the varicella vaccine?

This is a live vaccine composed of an attenuated strain of VZV, designated vOka. The vaccine strain of virus was first isolated from a 3-year-old Japanese boy in 1972 *(1)*. In 1974, a Japanese group attenuated the virus by serial passage in cell culture using human embryonic lung cells and guinea-pig fibroblast cells. The passaged virus was then administered to 71 hospitalised children as a measure to control an outbreak of varicella *(2)*. Varicella vaccine was licensed for clinical use in the United States in 1995.

What schedule for varicella vaccination is used?

Two doses of vaccine are administered at least 3 months apart in children aged 12 months to < 13 years while in persons aged ≥ 13 years, two vaccine doses are given at least 1 month apart. In Ireland, varicella vaccine is not yet part of the routine immunisation programme.

Which criteria are used to define immunity to varicella?

Immunity may be indicated by laboratory evidence (detection of VZV-specific IgG or previous laboratory confirmation of varicella or herpes zoster), a past clinical diagnosis of varicella or herpes zoster made by a healthcare provider, or evidence of immunisation with two doses of varicella vaccine *(3)*.

Who should be considered for varicella vaccination when it is not in the routine immunization schedule?

Individuals in whom pre-exposure vaccination should be considered include the following:

Healthcare workers and family members who do not have evidence of immunity to varicella and are likely to have close contact with individuals at risk of severe disease. While medical and nursing staff are candidates for the varicella vaccine, others who should also be considered are those who attend wards and have the potential to transmit VZV including cleaners, catering staff and ward clerks.

Those at risk for exposure to VZV and with potential to transmit to those at risk of severe disease include staff and residents in institutions such as residential units for disabled children, staff in crechés, teachers and nonpregnant women of childbearing age.

Can varicella vaccination be used for prophylaxis following exposure to VZV?

Yes, varicella vaccination as soon as possible after exposure may prevent or attenuate natural infection by stimulating a robust VZV-specific immune response early in the incubation period (10 to 21 days after contact). The vOka strain of VZV induces an antibody and cell-mediated immune response to the virus within 3 to 5 days of immunization *(4)*.

Can immunocompromised individuals be immunised with the varicella vaccine?

Yes, however, varicella vaccination of severely immunocompromised persons is not recommended. For those on low-level immunosuppression, varicella vaccination may be considered including the following:

HIV-infected patients who are not severely immunocompromised and have CD4+ T cells ≥ 200 mm^{-3}; those receiving < 20 mg daily of prednisone or equivalent for ≥ 14 days (< 2 mg/kg if < 10 kg weight); on methotrexate ≤ 0.4 mg/kg/week, azathioprine ≤ 3 mg/kg daily or 6-mercaptopurine ≤ 1.5 mg/kg daily *(5)*.

What is the recommended interval between administration of varicella vaccine and starting immunosuppression?

For recipients of any live vaccine, it is recommended that there should be a delay of ≥ 4 weeks before starting an immunosuppressive regimen *(5)*. This delay likely represents the time needed to induce immunity and control replication of the vaccine virus while the patient is still immunocompetent. Concomitant use of anti-herpetic antivirals should be avoided during this time interval.

Why is vaccination against varicella not recommended in children aged less than 12 months?

Because it is likely that circulating maternal VZV-specific antibody will reduce the ability to induce an immune response to the vaccine.

Does it matter if a child aged less than 12 months of age is inadvertently vaccinated?

Yes, vaccination before 12 months of age can be ineffective due to the interfering effect of maternal antibody to VZV. Therefore, when the child is ≥ 12 months old, revaccination should be started with two doses of varicella vaccine, ideally 12 weeks apart.

A child was given the first dose of varicella vaccine at 13 months of age and the second dose six weeks later. Is that acceptable?

Yes, even though ideally there should be a 12-week gap between the vaccine doses in those aged 12 months to < 13 years, a minimum interval of four weeks is acceptable.

Is it necessary to test for VZV-specific IgG following two-dose varicella vaccination?

No, there is no recommendation to test vaccine recipients because they are regarded as immune once they have received two doses of varicella vaccine. In addition, commercial assays are often unable to detect antibody in those vaccinated successfully *(6)*.

A healthcare worker with documented evidence of immunisation with two doses of varicella vaccine was tested for antibodies and found to be negative for VZV-specific IgG. Should the person be revaccinated?

No, two doses of varicella vaccine given at least 28 days apart confers immunity. The absence of VZV-specific IgG most probably reflects the insensitivity of commercial assays for this marker *(6)*.

An 11-year-old girl developed a varicella-like rash 7 days after receiving a dose of varicella vaccine following recent exposure to a sibling with varicella, should she receive the second dose of vaccine?

Yes, while it is likely that this is 'breakthrough' varicella with wild-type virus, it could be a vaccine-associated rash. However, it is not possible to differentiate rapidly between wild-type VZV and the vaccine strain (vOka) in the routine diagnostic laboratory. There is no safety concern with giving the second dose three months later even if she acquired varicella after the exposure.

In the above case, can the child attend school?

Because the rash developed only seven days after vaccination, it is likely due to wild type virus, therefore the child should not attend school. There is no rapid test to differentiate wild-type and vaccine-associated VZV (vOka strain). Contact with pregnant women and immunocompromised persons should be avoided *(7)*.

What are the common side-effects of varicella vaccination seen in general practice?

In general, the varicella vaccine is safe and well-tolerated with severe morbidity being rare *(7, 8)*. Severe disease may occur in varicella vaccine recipients due to unmasking of undiagnosed natural killer cell or T-cell immunodeficient states *(9)*. Breakthrough varicella is discussed in the clinical features section of the chapter on varicella. Other adverse effects include the following:

Vaccine-associated rash

Development of vesicular varicella-like rashes within 42 days of vaccination may occur in about 5% of otherwise healthy vaccine recipients, usually at the injection site but can be generalised *(6)*. Those appearing in the first 14 days after vaccination are likely to be due to natural VZV infection while those developing between 15 and 42 days are usually due to vaccine-related VZV *(7)*. When vaccine-associated rashes are vesicular, the cases should be regarded as potentially infectious to nonimmune contacts *(7)*. Although the risk of transmission from otherwise healthy vaccine recipients with a vaccine-associated rash is very low, advice should be sought from the local microbiologist regarding management of close contacts who are nonimmune pregnant women or immunocompromised.

Vaccine-associated Herpes Zoster

Vaccine-associated HZ is uncommon and is usually clinically manifest in the cervical and lumbar dermatomes corresponding to the sites of immunisation with varicella vaccine *(10)*. However, the overall incidence of HZ is significantly reduced in children immunised with the varicella vaccine *(11)*.

VARICELLA VACCINATION AND PREGNANCY

What is the recommended time gap between administration of varicella vaccine and attempting to conceive?

Women should avoid pregnancy for one month after vaccination *(12)*. This delay likely represents the time needed to induce immunity and control replication of the vaccine virus, thereby preventing infection of the fetus with live vaccine virus.

Is there a role for active immunisation with varicella vaccine as post exposure prophylaxis in pregnancy?

No, administration of varicella vaccine is contraindicated during pregnancy *(12)*.

What advice would you give a pregnant woman who is inadvertently given the varicella vaccine?

Current evidence does not suggest that the accidental use of varicella vaccine during pregnancy causes teratogenicity, or the congenital varicella syndrome *(12)*.

Is breast feeding allowable after varicella vaccination of the mother postpartum?

Yes, there is no evidence of the secretion of the vaccine strain of VZV in breast milk following immunisation of the mother postnatally *(12, 13)*.

REFERENCES (*useful reviews)

1 A.A. Gershon.*Int. J. Infect. Dis.* **1**, 130 (1997)

2 M. Takahashi *et al.*, *Lancet.* **2**, 1288 (1974)

3 M. Marin *et al.*, *MMWR Recomm. Rep.* **56**, (RR4): 1 (2007)*

4 M.J. Ferson. *Commun. Dis. Intell.* **25**, 13 (2001)

5 L.G. Rubin *et al.*, *Clin. Infect. Dis.* **58**, e44 (2014)*

6 A.A. Gershon, M.D. Gershon.*Clin.Microbiol. Rev.* **26**, 728 (2013)*

7 S.A. Galea *et al.*, *J. Infect. Dis.* **197**Suppl 2, S165 (2008)

8 S.S. Chaves *et al.*, *J. Infect. Dis.* **197**Suppl 2, S170 (2008)

9 O. Levy *et al.*, *J. Infect. Dis.* **188**, 948 (2003)

10 S. Weinmann *et al.*, *J. Infect. Dis.* **208**, 1859 (2013)

11 R. Civen *et al.*, *Pediatr. Infect. Dis. J.* **35**, 1132 (2016)

12 E. Wilson *et al.*, *J. Infect. Dis.* **197**Suppl 2, S178 (2008)

13 K. Bohlke *et al.*, *Obstet. Gynecol.* **102**, 970 (2003)

HERPES ZOSTER

What is zoster?

As is well known, zoster is caused by the same virus as that causing varicella (i.e., chickenpox), and represents reactivation of that virus, usually in older patients and typically presenting with a unilateral rash. Zoster can be associated with significant pain, and some forms are especially concerning such as ophthalmic zoster and zoster in the immunocompromised patient which may lead to disseminated cutaneous and/or visceral disease.

CASE VIGNETTE

A 71-year-old man, otherwise healthy, presented to his GP with a 48-hour history of painful vesicles and pustules distributed in a dermatomal manner (T2) on the left side of his back. The rash was preceded by paraesthesia. The GP diagnosed herpes zoster. What can GPs learn from this case?

LABORATORY DIAGNOSIS

Is laboratory diagnosis of herpes zoster necessary in this case?

In general, a clinical diagnosis of herpes zoster (HZ) is sufficient, however, because the patient in this case lived in the same household as his pregnant daughter who had no history of varicella, a viral swab was collected from a vesicle and tested by real-time polymerase chain reaction (PCR) for VZV DNA and confirmed VZV-related disease. HSV 1 & 2 DNA were not detected. His daughter was immune to VZV (a fresh serum sample was anti-VZV IgG positive).

TREATMENT

Did the GP treat the patient in this case with an antiviral agent?

Yes, the GP prescribed valaciclovir (1 g every 8 hours) until the lesions crusted. Antiviral treatment is recommended in people aged > 50 years or if the rash is severe and painful or when there is ocular disease or other HZ-related complications *(1)*. However, some physicians do recommend antiviral treatment in those aged <50 years with uncomplicated HZ *(1, 2)*.

Is there a time limit within which to start antiviral treatment for HZ?

Trials of antivirals for treatment of HZ were designed to start aciclovir, valaciclovir or famciclovir within 3 days of rash onset *(1)*. Therefore, treatment as early as possible, within 72 hours after onset of rash, seems best *(3)*. However, if new crops of vesicles continue to appear more than 3 days after onset of the rash or if HZ-related complications develop, patients may still benefit from treatment *(4)*.

INFECTION CONTROL

What infection control advice was given to the patient in this case?

He was advised that transmissibility of VZV to susceptible contacts begins with appearance of the rash and ends when the lesions have crusted. Transmission of VZV from immunocompetent individuals with unilateral dermatomal zoster is thought to occur mainly via direct contact with vesicles so that only contact precautions are recommended together with covering of the lesion *(5, 6, 7)*. His pregnant daughter was shown to be immune and no immunocompromised person lived in the same household. In contrast, airborne and contact precautions are generally recommended for hospitalised individuals with disseminated cutaneous zoster and for immunocompromised persons with localised HZ *(7)*. These precautions are taken because aerosolisation of viral particles from multiple skin lesions with high viral loads contributes significantly to transmission of VZV *(1)*.

RISK FACTORS FOR HZ

What was the most likely risk factor for this patient developing HZ?

His predisposition for HZ relates to his age. There is a sharp rise in the incidence of HZ among those aged 50 years to 60 years. For example, it is about 10 per 1,000 person-years for 60-year-olds *(8)*. The lifetime risk of HZ is approximately 25% *(2)*. The mechanism predisposing the elderly to HZ is likely to involve decline in VZV-specific cell-mediated immunity, referred to as immunoscenescence *(9)*.

What other risk factor commonly predisposes to HZ?

Immunosuppression is a key factor leading to HZ: individuals with profound cellular immunodeficiency due to acquired or iatrogenic immunosuppression, such as persons on chemotherapy for malignancy or immunomodulatory agents for inflammatory diseases, are at risk of HZ *(1)*. Immunosuppression also increases the risk of severe complications, which are otherwise uncommon.

Is it true that lack of exposure to children with varicella is a risk factor for HZ in the elderly?

No, the absence of exposure to varicella (exogenous exposure) was shown not to increase their risk of HZ. It is thought that subclinical reactivation of VZV in sensory ganglia in an individual, known as endogenous boosting, confers protection against VZV reactivation *(10)*.

CLINICAL FEATURES

Are the clinical features of HZ in this case typical of HZ in otherwise immunocompetent persons?

Yes, as in this case, individuals usually report tingling, pain and/or pruritus in the affected dermatome a few days before onset of the exanthema *(1)*. The rash progresses rapidly from an erythematous maculopapular phase to clusters of vesicles which continue to appear for the next 3-4 days *(5)*. Vesicles then evolve through pustular, ulcerative and crusting phases over the next 10 days or so *(1)*. The rash is typically unilateral, following the dermatome of the segmental nerve and does not usually cross the midline. While only a single dermatome is usually involved in otherwise healthy persons, adjacent dermatomes may be affected in 20% of cases due to normal variation in innervation patterns *(2)*.

What are the typical clinical features of HZ in immunocompromised individuals?

New lesions may continue to appear for several weeks in immunocompromised hosts with development of an extensive rash known as disseminated cutaneous HZ, defined by the presence > 20 skin lesions beyond the primary or adjacent dermatomes, and may evolve into disseminated visceral zoster *(1, 5)*. Although disseminated cutaneous HZ occurs mainly among those with cellular immune deficiency, it may develop occasionally in individuals who are not on immunosuppression, particularly the elderly *(11, 12)*.

Can the painful manifestations of HZ occur in the absence of a rash?

Yes, this condition, known as *zoster sine herpete*, is a clinical variant of HZ characterised by a unilateral, dermatomal distribution of radicular pain without a rash. It is believed to be caused by chronic active ganglionitis due to VZV replication *(13)*. However, definite diagnosis requires detection of VZV DNA in CSF or evidence of intrathecal production of anti-VZV IgG *(14)*.

COMMON COMPLICATIONS OF HERPES ZOSTER SEEN IN GENERAL PRACTICE
POSTHERPETIC NEURALGIA

What is postherpetic neuralgia?

Postherpetic neuralgia (PHN) is pain in a dermatomal distribution that persists > 90 days after onset of the rash *(15)*. It may manifest as allodynia (when an innocuous stimulus is perceived as painful) or hyperaesthesia (when a weak pain stimulus is perceived as very painful) or dysaesthesia (when spontaneous pain is felt in the absence of any stimulus) *(16)*. The risk of progressing to PHN greatly increases among those aged > 50 years, affecting 10% to 50% of cases with HZ *(1)*. PHN is relatively uncommon among persons younger than the age of 50 years.

Did the elderly man with HZ in this case develop PHN?

No, he did develop acute herpetic neuralgia but it resolved quickly. PHN should be distinguished from two other phases of pain related to HZ: acute herpetic neuralgia, occurring in the first month after onset of the rash, and subacute herpetic neuralgia, which is pain in the affected dermatome persisting between one month and three months (17).

What are the potential treatment options for postherpetic neuralgia?

Treatment is aimed at pain relief. There are several options, listed below, which have been shown to be effective for PHN, and combination therapy rather than monotherapy seems to be the more effective. Nonetheless, caution is advised due to adverse effects of medication. Referral to a pain specialist may be necessary for those with PHN that is refractory to treatment (1).

Tricyclic antidepressants (TCAs), such as amitryptiline, nortriptyline and despiramine, are commonly used for PHN (18). Calcium channel α2-δ ligands, gabapentin and pregabalin, are effective in reducing PHN-related pain by approximately 50% (19). Topical capsaicin cream (0.075%) applied 3-4 times daily has also been used for PHN (19). Similarly, use of lidocaine patches (5%) has been shown to reduce pain and decrease allodynia, particularly in the elderly (20). Opioids, including oxycodone, morphine, methadone and tramadol, were shown to be effective for pain relief in PHN but are second- or third-line options because of their side-effect profiles (21). The following dual therapy has been found to be useful when monotherapy with either alone was ineffective: lidocaine 5% patch and pregabalin; gabapentin with nortriptyline and the use of gabapentin with morphine (21, 22).

OCULAR DISEASE AND STROKE

Why is ocular involvement an important clinical complication of herpes zoster?

Herpes zoster ophthalmicus (HZO) is a sight-threatening condition caused by reactivation of VZV in the trigeminal nerve ganglion. The ophthalmic branch (VI) of the trigeminal nerve (V) is involved and this manifests clinically as erythematous macules, papules, vesicles and crusts in a unilateral dermatomal distribution on the nose, upper eyelid, frontal, parietal and temporal areas (2, 23). Conjunctivitis and episcleritis may also occur (5). Another key clinical feature is the presence of lesions on the skin or mucosa at the tip of the nose. This indicates involvement of the nasociliary branch of the ophthalmic division of the trigeminal nerve and, is known as Hutchinson's sign. It is associated with a high risk of intra-ocular involvement (24). The GP should consider referring patients with HZO or Hutchinson's sign for ophthalmological review and management with antivirals (aciclovir, valaciclovir or famciclovir) with or without the use of corticosteroids (1).

Is there an association between herpes zoster and stroke?

Yes, epidemiological studies have shown an increased risk of stroke after an episode of herpes zoster (HZ) compared to age-matched controls (25). In a large, population-based study in Taiwan, there was a 31% increased risk of stroke, while among those with herpes zoster ophthalmicus (HZO) an approximately four times higher risk of stroke within one year of onset of HZ compared with a matched cohort of controls (26). Studies in Denmark and the United Kingdom (UK) support this finding and also show a higher risk of transient ischaemic attack (TIA) following HZ, particularly after HZO (27, 28, 29). The risk of stroke is greater shortly after an episode of HZO or non-ophthalmic HZ and then declines over time; but it remains significant for the first year (30). There are insufficient data to confirm that treatment of HZ with an antiviral reduces the risk of stroke (29, 30).

When should the GP suspect VZV-related vasculopathy?

Patients with a recent history of HZO or HZ may present with headache and abnormal mentation with or without a focal neurological deficit (31). However, it should be noted that one-third of VZV vasculopathy cases do not report a history of HZ rash (25). Diagnosis involved detection of VZV DNA in CSF or evidence of intrathecal production of anti-VZV IgG. Once VZV vasculopathy is suspected, the patient should be hospitalised immediately. In general, treatment includes intravenous aciclovir 10 mg/kg three times daily for at least 14 days, and oral prednisone (1 mg/kg once daily for 5 days)(14).

PREVENTION OF HERPES ZOSTER AND ITS ASSOCIATED COMPLICATIONS

What vaccines available to prevent herpes zoster? How do they work?

There are two vaccines licensed for prevention of shingles. The rationale for immunisation with zoster vaccine is to boost VZV-specific CD4+ T cell-mediated immunity, thereby preventing VZV reactivation or attenuating disease if it develops (32).

The first to be licensed was a live attenuated vaccine, designated zoster virus live (ZVL), which contains the vOka strain used also in the varicella vaccine. The dose of vOka virus used in the live zoster vaccine (ZVL) is 14-fold higher than in the live varicella vaccine, reflecting the degree of antigenic stimulation needed to induce a robust cell-mediated immune response in those previously exposed to VZV (3). This vaccine should not be used in those lacking a history of varicella or zoster and when in doubt VZV IgG positivity in serum should be determined. More recently, a recombinant adjuvanted HZ vaccine, designated recombinant zoster vaccine (RZV), has been approved for use in adults aged ≥ 50 years in the United States (US), Europe and Japan. This vaccine is composed of glycoprotein E, an immunogenic surface viral protein, and a single adjuvant system which helps to induce a robust immune response.

Why is the recombinant zoster vaccine (RZV) more suitable for clinical use?

This inactivated vaccine was shown to retain high protective efficacy against zoster and postherpetic neuralgia (PHN), unlike ZVL which has lower and shorter-lived efficacy *(33)*. RZV is preferred for use in clinical practice in the United States *(34)*. The efficacy of RZV against shingles was found to be > 90% in adults ≥50 years old, including those aged ≥ 70 years *(35, 36)*. The overall incidence of PHN among RZV vaccine recipients was reduced with a protective efficacy ranging from 88% to 91% *(36)*.

REFERENCES (*useful reviews)

1 J.I. Cohen. *N. Engl. J. Med.* **369**, 255 (2013)*

2 J.W. Gnann, R.J. Whitley. *N. Engl. J. Med.* **347**, 340 (2002)

3 A.A. Gershon, M.D. Gershon.*Clin.Microbiol. Rev.* **26**, 728 (2013)

4 M.J. Wood *et al.*, *J. Infect. Dis.* **178** Suppl 1, S81 (1998)

5 D.H. Dworkin *et al.*, *Clin. Infect. Dis.* **44** Suppl 1, S1 (2007)

6 J.A. Johnson, K.C. Bloch, B.N. Dang. *Clin. Infect. Dis.* **52**, 907 (2011)

7 J.D. Siegel *et al.*, *Am. J. Infect. Control.***35** Suppl**2**, S65 (2007)

8 G. Mick. *Expert Rev. Vaccines.* **9** Suppl 3; 31 (2010)

9 S.C. Castle. *Clin. Infect. Dis.* **31**, 578 (2000)

10 J. Gaillat *et al.*, Clin. Infect. Dis. **53**, 405 (2011)

11 E. Gomez, I. Chernev. *Infect. Dis. Rep.* **6**, 5513 (2014)

12 E.A. O'Toole, E.E. Mooney, J.B. Walsh. *Ir. J. Med. Sci.* **166**, 141 (1997)

13 M. Birlea *et al.*, *Neurology.* **82**, 90 (2014)

14 M.A. Nagel, D. Gilden. *Curr.Opin. Neurol.* **27**, 356 (2014)

15 R.H. Dworkin *et al.*, *J. Pain.* **9**Suppl 1, S37 (2008)

16 J. Fashner, A.L. Bell. *Am. Fam. Physician.* **83**, 1432 (2011)*

17 Y.H. Jeon. *Korean J. Pain.***28**, 177 (2015)

18 C.E. Argoff. *Postgrad. Med.***123**, 134 (2011)

19 N. Garroway *et al.*, *J. Fam. Pract.***58**, 384d (2009)

20 R. Casale *et al.*, *J. Pain Res.* **7**, 353 (2014)

21 T. Mallick-Searle, B. Snodgrass, J.M.Branti.*J. Multidiscip. Healthc.***9**, 447 (2016)

22 S. Nalamucha, P. Morley-Forster. *Drugs Ageing.***29**, 863 (2012)

23 C. Makos *et al.*, *Internet J. Neurol.* **13**, 1 (2010)

24 M. von Dyk, D. Meyer. *SAMJ.***100**, 172 (2010)

25 M.A. Nagel, D. Gilden. *Curr. Neurol. Neurosci. Rep.* **16**, 12 (2016)

26 J.H. Kang *et al.*, *Stroke.* **40**, 3443 (2009)

27 N. Sreenivasan *et al.*, *PLOS One.* **8**, e69156 (2013)

28 J. Breuer *et al.*, *Neurology.* **82**, 206 (2014)

29 S.M. Langan *et al.*, *Clin. Infect. Dis.* **58**, 1497 (2014)

30 F. Marra, J. Ruckenstein, K. Richardson. *BMC Infect. Dis.* **17**, 198 (2017)

31 M.A. Nagel *et al.*, *Neurology.***77**, 364 (2011)

32 A. Weinberg *et al.*, *J. Infect. Dis*. **200**, 1068 (2009)

33 K.M. Neuzil, M.R. Griffin. *N. Engl. J. Med*. **375**, 1079 (2016)

34 K.L.Dooling *et al.*, *MMWR Morb. Mortal. Wkly. Rep*. **67**, 103 (2018)

35 H. Lal *et al.*, *N. Engl. J. Med*. **372**, 2087 (2015)

36 A.L. Cunningham *et al.*, *N. Engl. J. Med*. **375**, 1019 (2016)

HUMAN HERPESVIRUS TYPE 6 (HHV-6)

BACKGROUND

What is HHV-6?

Human herpesvirus type 6 (HHV-6) is a DNA virus and member of the family of human herpes viruses, *Herpesviridae (1)*. Symptomatic primary HHV-6 infection occurs most frequently in children 2 years of age and younger, and is a common cause of presentation to primary care clinics.

VIROLOGY

Is there more than one species of HHV-6?

Yes, HHV-6 was recently classified as two separate viruses, designated HHV-6A and HHV-6B (HHV-6A/B), based on molecular and antigenic differences *(2)*.

Can the genome of HHV-6A/B integrate into human chromosomes?

Yes, HHV-6A/B may establish latency by integration of their whole genomes into telomeres of human chromosomes *(3)*. Integration of the HHV-6A/B genome may occur into the telomeric region of any human chromosome in any infected cell.

Can chromosomally integrated HHV-6 (ciHHV-6) be inherited?

Yes, inherited chromosomally integrated HHV-6 (iciHHV-6) occurs in approximately 1% of healthy blood donors in the UK and USA *(4)*. While HHV-6B infection is ubiquitous among children, the virus establishes latency in a minority of cells in each individual. However, in some cases it infects gametes with integration of the viral genome into the host germline and transmission in a Mendelian manner to 50% of offspring *(5)*. Individuals with iciHHV-6 are likely to carry at least one copy of the complete viral genome integrated into a host chromosome in every nucleated cell *(5, 6)*.

EPIDEMIOLOGY

Which cohorts in the general population acquire HHV-6?

Like all known herpes viruses, HHV-6B is ubiquitous. Primary HHV-6B infection occurs usually in the first two years of life as shown by HHV-6B seroprevalence globally of almost 100% in children within that age group *(7, 8, 9)*. The peak age of HHV-6B acquisition occurs between 9 and 21 months reflecting the time of loss of protective maternal antibody *(8, 9)*. Current serological assays cannot differentiate between antibody to HHV-6A and HHV-6B variants because of their antigenic similarity. However, using molecular and immunological techniques, HHV-6B was shown to account for most symptomatic primary infections in infants in many developed countries *(10, 11, 12)*. In contrast, very little is known about the horizontal transmission of HHV-6A. It is speculated that HHV-6A is acquired subclinically *(10, 13)*.

What is the main route of transmission of HHV-6B?

The salivary glands are the main site of HHV-6B replication and of shedding with subsequent transmission via saliva to close contacts *(5, 13)*. As with other herpes viruses, HHV-6B establishes latency after resolution of primary infection. It can however come out of latency at anytime and replicate at a low level with asymptomatic shedding of infectious virus *(6)*. It is most likely that asymptomatic adults who are shedding the virus in saliva transmit it to children. Furthermore, it may be transmitted from sibling to sibling since, following primary infection in children, HHV-6 DNA was still detectable in saliva 12 months later *(9, 13)*.

CLINICAL MANIFESTATIONS

What are the common clinical manifestations of primary HHV-6B infection seen in general practice?

Primary infection with HHV-6B occurs predominantly in young children and is usually symptomatic, resulting in attendance at the family practice or emergency department. This is unlike other human herpes viruses for which newly acquired infections are typically subclinical *(9, 14)*. HHV-6B is a significant cause of acute febrile illness with or without a rash in children under 2 years of age attending emergency departments *(15)*. Primary HHV-6B infection is characterised by high fever (≥ 40°C) which may last several days and is markedly higher than that seen in other illnesses *(15)*. However, fever is not always a feature of primary HHV-6B infection since a significant number of cases were afebrile in a population-based study which used molecular diagnostics to confirm viral infection *(9)*. In addition, although primary HHV-6B infection causes roseola infantum (also known as exanthemsubitum), only a minority of children with recently acquired HHV-6 infection are reported to develop the disease *(9, 15, 16)*. The condition typically presents as a febrile illness lasting a few days, followed by the abrupt appearance of a macular non-pruritic rash on the trunk, neck and lower extremities. The sudden onset of the rash accounts for the term exanthemsubitum, the Latin for 'sudden' being 'subitum' *(17)*. Other commonly reported features of primary HHV-6 infection in children include fussiness, rhinorrhoea, cough, and diarrhoea *(9, 15)*. Primary HHV-6B infection has long been associated with febrile seizures (FS) in children under 2 years old. While the frequency of seizures is low (< 10%), the infection is almost universal *(9, 13, 15)*.

What are the less common clinical features of primary HHV-6B infection in children and adults?

While most cases of febrile seizures (FS) are transient, some may be prolonged and fulfil the criteria for status epilepticus, though febrile status epilepticus (FSE) accounts for only a small proportion (5%) of cases *(18, 19, 20)*. FSE may result in hippocampal injury and ultimately temporal lobe epilepsy *(20, 21)*. Other infrequent presentations seen in otherwise immunocompetent children and adults with delayed primary HHV-6B infection include infectious mononucleosis-like illness, acute lymphadenitis and hepatitis *(13, 14)*.

LABORATORY DIAGNOSIS

Should virological tests be used for otherwise healthy children with suspected HHV-6 disease seen in general practice?

No, clinical findings are usually suggestive of HHV-6 infection in children. However, if clinical presentations are atypical or the host is immunosuppressed or there is a severe complication like encephalitis, then laboratory confirmation is justified. In addition, the features of roseola infantum may be difficult to differentiate from an allergic drug reaction or development of a rash following recent MMR vaccination *(22)*.

Which laboratory test can be performed for HHV-6 when that is necessary?

HHV-6 DNA detection by real-time polymerase chain reaction (PCR) in samples of plasma, serum, whole blood, saliva or cerebrospinal fluid (CSF) is available.

What is the clinical significance of detection of HHV-6 DNA in a sample collected from any site?

While detection of HHV-6 DNA indicates infection, it does not distinguish between acute infection, reactivation, which may occur asymptomatically in immunocompetent children, and inherited chromosomally integrated HHV-6 (iciHHV-6). Therefore, results should be always be interpreted in combination with clinical findings, knowledge of the immune status of the individual and exclusion of other potential pathogens *(22)*.

EXAMPLE

An otherwise healthy 6-year-old boy who had a 48-hour history of malaise and a disseminated maculopapular rash attended the GP with his mother who was pregnant (18 weeks' gestation). The GP sent a salivary viral swab for investigation of suspected erythema infectiosum (EI) and roseola infantum. RT-PCR was performed for parvovirus B19 DNA and HHV-6 DNA. Low-levels of parvovirus B19 DNA and HHV-6 DNA were detected. How would you interpret the result?

Acute parvovirus B19 infection was subsequently confirmed. The low level of HHV-6 DNA detected in saliva probably reflected coincidental HHV-6 reactivation in the nasopharynx or salivary gland. Because of the implications of exposure to parvovirus B19 for the pregnant mother, who was known to be susceptible to parvovirus B19 (booking blood at 12 weeks was B19 IgG negative), a serum sample was collected from the boy a few days later: parvovirus B19 IgM was positive and B19 DNA > 10^8 IU/mL confirming current EI. HHV-6 DNA was not detected in serum.

Can the inherited chromosomally-integrated HHV-6 (iciHHV-6) status of a patient lead to misdiagnosis of HHV-6 infection?

Yes, samples such as whole blood, leucocytes and hair follicles, when collected from individuals with iciHHV-6, will invariably have high HHV-6 DNA (usually $\geq 10^6$ copies/ml) reflecting the 1:1 ratio of viral genome to human cells in these specimens (23, 24). Among iciHHV-6 carriers, even samples with few cells such as cerebrospinal fluid, serum and plasma usually have detectable HHV-6 DNA due to *ex vivo* cell breakdown with release of cellular nucleic acids containing integrated viral DNA (24).

EXAMPLE

HHV-6 DNA (> 10^5 copies/mL) in cerebrospinal fluid (CSF) collected from a 40-year-old male with suspected viral meningitis – white cells were 510/mm³, 98% mononuclear cells. Is HHV-6 the causative agent of the meningitis?

The virology result alone is insufficient to conclude that HHV-6 is the aetiology in this case. Caution is needed in interpretation of HHV-6 DNA levels in any sample, particularly CSF (24). Inherited chromosomally-integrated HHV-6 (iciHHV-6) occurs in about 1% of the population globally and means that every nucleated cell in these individuals carries the complete HHV-6 genome on any of its chromosomes (5). In contrast, most individuals with resolved primary HHV-6 infection in childhood carry the viral genome in an occasional peripheral blood mononuclear cell (PBMCs) (1 copy per 10^4 to 10^5 PBMCs), a recognised site of latency of HHV-6 (25, 26). To determine the significance of HHV-6 in this case, HHV-6 DNA was quantified in whole blood to exclude or confirm iciHHV-6 carrier status. The HHV-6 DNA level (5 x 10^6 copies/mL) indicated ≥ 1 copy of HHV-6 DNA/leucocyte, consistent with iciHHV-6 (24). Therefore, the HHV-6 DNA result in CSF was regarded as a 'red-herring' and other causes sought. The patient's meningeal symptoms resolved within 3 days without antiviral treatment. Measurement of HHV-6 DNA in whole blood 6 weeks after hospital discharge yielded a similar viral load (8 x 10^6 copies/mL) indicating persistence of high-level HHV-6 DNA, characteristic of healthy individuals with iciHHV-6 (5).

ANTIVIRAL TREATMENT

Is there a role for use of antiviral agents in management of HHV-6 infections seen in general practice?

Specific antiviral therapy is not warranted in the great majority of HHV-6 infections due to their self-limited nature in immunocompetent children. While ganciclovir, foscarnet and cidofovir are antivirals with known *in vitro* activity against both variants of HHV-6, controlled trial data are lacking *(14, 27)*. Therefore, their use is limited to the hospital setting involving immunocompromised patients with evidence of endorgan disease or immunocompetent individuals with severe complications such as meningoencephalitis *(28)*.

REFERENCES (*useful reviews)

1 D.Ablashi *et al.*, *Arch. Virol.***129**, 363 (1993)

2 M.J. Adams, A.M. King, E.B. Carstens. *Arch. Virol.* **157**, 1411 (2012)

3 J.H. Arbuckle *et al.*, *Proc. Natl. Acad. Sci. USA.* **107**, 5563 (2010)

4 S.D. Hudnall *et al.*, *Transfusion.***48**, 1180 (2008)

5 P.E. Pellett *et al.*, *Rev. Med. Virol.* **22**, 144 (2012)*

6 L. Flamand. *Clin. Infect. Dis.* **59**, 549 (2014)

7 K.N. Ward *et al.*, *J. Med. Virol.* **39**, 131 (1993)

8 T. Okuno *et al.*, *J. Clin. Microbiol.***27**, 651 (1989)

9 D.M. Zerr *et al.*, *N. Engl. J. Med.* **352**, 768 (2005)

10 S. Dewhurst *et al.*, *J. Clin.Microbiol.***31**, 416 (1993)

11 F.Z. Wang *et al.*, *J. Med. Virol.* **57**, 134 (1999)

12 S.N. Pantry, P.G. Medveczky. *Viruses.***9**, 194 (2017)

13 L. De Bolle, L. Naesens, E. De Clercq.*Clin.Microbiol. Rev.* **18**, 217 (2005)

14 H. Agut, P. Bonnafous, A. Gautheret-Dejean.*Clin.Microbiol. Rev.* **28**, 313 (2015)*

15 P. Pruksananonda *et al.*, *N. Engl. J. Med.* **326**, 1445 (1992)

16 K. Yamanishi, T. Okuno.*Lancet.***1**, 1065 (1988)

17 C. Prober. *N. Engl. J. Med.* **352**, 753 (2005)

18 D.C. Hesdorffer *et al.*, *Ann. Neurol.* **70**, 93 (2011)

19 S. Shinnar *et al.*, *Epilepsia.***38**, 907 (1997)

20 L.G. Epstein *et al.*, *Epilepsia.* **53**, 1481 (2012)

21 Y. Kawamura *et al.*, *J. Infect. Dis.* **212**, 1014 (2015)

22 K.N. Ward. *J. Clin. Virol.***32**, 183 (2005)

23 D.A. Clark *et al.*, *J. Infect. Dis.* **193**, 912 (2006)

24 K.N. Ward *et al.*, *J. ClinMicrobiol.* **45**, 1298 (2007)

25 D.A. Clark *et al.*, *J. Gen. Virol.* **77**, 2271 (1996)

26 J.H. Ohyashiki *et al.*, *Leuk. Res.* **23**, 625 (1999)

27 C. Manichanh *et al.*, *Cytometry.* **40**, 135 (2000)

28 E. Denes *et al.*, *Emerg. Infect. Dis.* **10**, 729 (2004)

MEASLES

What is measles?

Measles is a highly contagious acute febrile exanthematous illness caused by measles virus.

What is measles virus?

Measles virus (MeV) is a spherical, enveloped RNA virus belonging to the genus *Morbillivirus* in the family *Paramyxoviridae (1)*. Although there are 24 recognised genotypes of the virus, MeV appears to be monotypic, in other words immunity to one genotype confers protection against all known strains *(2)*.

From which groups in the general population is measles notified?

The number of measles cases in Ireland has greatly declined since the introduction of measles, mumps and rubella (MMR) vaccination in 1988. For example, the incidence diminished from 8.4 cases per 100,000 to 0.7 cases per 100,000 in a decade, reflecting an uptake of MMR vaccine among 2-year olds of 80% in 2002 and of 93% in 2014 *(3)*. However, there are still gaps in immunity to measles among children and young adults and these allow measles outbreaks *(4, 5)*. Outbreaks are clustered among certain subpopulations who have low uptake of MMR vaccine due to social exclusion, including the Traveller and Roma communities, and the children of parents who refuse the vaccine on religious or philosophical grounds. When measles spreads among members of these unvaccinated subpopulations, susceptible individuals in the general population are placed at risk. Such outbreaks may begin when unvaccinated or partially vaccinated individuals visit measles-endemic areas and return to Ireland with active infection *(5)*. To prevent sustained measles transmission in the community, the national rate of MMR vaccine uptake should be at least 95% *(4, 6)*. All children who have not had two doses of MMR by the age of 5 years should be offered immunisation opportunistically to close immunity gaps *(7)*.

PATHOGENESIS

How does MeV cause disease?

MeV is very infectious and is transmitted between individuals mainly when respiratory droplets containing the virus are inhaled. The virus initially infects immune cells in the respiratory tract including alveolar macrophages, dendritic cells and T lymphocytes. These cells carry the protein molecule CD150 on their cell surface which acts as an entry receptor for MeV *(8)*. Infected immune cells then migrate to local lymphatic tissue and regional lymph nodes and, finally, disseminate by blood to other tissues, including lung where MeV is transferred to respiratory epithelial cells *(9)*. Replication of MeV in respiratory epithelium is followed by the release of many virions into the airways with potential transmission to other hosts by coughing.

CASE VIGNETTE

A 16-year old patient presented to his GP with a 3-day history of fever, malaise, sore throat, dry cough, headache, sore eyes, rhinorrhoea and a rash that developed 24 hours prior to presentation, beginning on the trunk, spreading to the back and arms. The GP noted that the patient had not received MMR vaccination. On examination, the temperature was 38°C and a blanching, maculopapular rash was noted on the patient's chest, back and upper limbs. He had mild pharyngitis and Koplik spots were seen on his buccal mucosa. The GP suspected measles infection and notified public health.

What can GPs learn from this case?

LABORATORY DIAGNOSIS

Which laboratory tests were used to confirm measles in this case?

Both serological and molecular tests confirmed current measles in this unimmunised individual. Detection of MeV RNA by real-time reverse transcription PCR (rRT-PCR) in oral fluid (saliva collection system) and throat swabs, confirmed current measles. Oral fluid samples can also be tested forMeV-specific IgM, which was negative in this case. MeV-specific IgM/IgG were positive in a serum sample collected 5 days later. The diagnostic yield of tests for MeV is influenced significantly by the timing of sample collection relative to rash onset. Oral fluid samples for MeV-specific IgM should ideally be taken ≥ 5 days after rash onset and IgM usually remains detectable for a month *(5, 10)*. MeV-specific IgM may be undetectable in serum when samples are collected in the first 72 hours after appearance of the rash *(11)*. Ideally, oral fluid samples should be collected ≤ 7 days after rash onset and tested for MeV RNA by rRT-PCR *(10)*.

CLINICAL FEATURES

When should the GP suspect measles?

As shown in this case, measles should be suspected in patients who present with a febrile illness accompanied by cough, coryza or conjunctivitis followed by a maculopapular rash. It should be considered especially if the patient is unvaccinated, or in any person who travelled recently to a community with current transmission of measles or has had contact with travellers to these areas. Other individuals at risk are those who have not been vaccinated including infants who may have lost passively-acquired maternal antibody before the age of routine vaccination.

Was the clinical presentation typical of measles?

Yes, the measles prodrome is characterised by fever, malaise and the classic triad (the 3C's) of cough, coryza and conjunctivitis *(12)*. It starts 3-4 days before onset of the rash. Koplik's spots, which are pathognomic of measles, usually appear 1-2 days before the rash. These small spots look like 'grains of sand' on a reddened background and are located on the buccal mucosa. Following the prodrome, a maculopapular rash begins usually on the forehead, side of the neck and postauricularly and spreads downwards to the trunk and extremities. In the meantime, the rash regresses from face to feet and disappears typically within 5 – 7 days of its onset.

What complications may be seen in measles?

One or more complications occur in up to 40% of measles cases *(12)*. Respiratory tract complications, including otitis media, laryngotracheobronchitis and secondary bacterial pneumonia occur frequently, the latter causing fatalities in infants and toddlers *(13)*. In individuals with cellular immune deficiency, giant cell pneumonitis caused by measles virus can occur *(14)*. Many children with measles develop stomatitis and diarrhoea and, among those with vitamin A deficiency, keratoconjunctivitis and corneal ulceration may lead to blindness *(15)*.

What are the central nervous system complications of measles?

Around 0.1% of measles cases develop central nervous system (CNS) complications such as acute disseminated encephalomyelitis (ADEM). This occurs once the rash begins to disappear and is characterised clinically by the sudden recurrence of fever with seizures and altered mental status *(16)*. ADEM is a demyelinating disease probably reflecting a post-infectious autoimmune response to antigens on neural cells. A further complication which usually presents 7-10 years after acute measles infection is subacute sclerosing panencephalitis (SSPE). This is a rare but fatal degenerative disease caused by persistent infection of the CNS with a mutated version of wild type MeV *(17)*. Primary MeV infection in children < 5 years old is a risk factor for developing SSPE, particularly when infection occurs before 12 months of age when the estimated risk in one study was as high as 1:609 *(18)*. However, immunisation with MMR vaccine protects against SSPE *(19)*. Another fatal CNS complication is measles inclusion body encephalitis (MIBE) which occurs several months after exposure to measles. MIBE has been reported in patients with significant cellular immune deficiency and may reflect uncontrolled viral replication in neural and glial cells *(20)*.

Are there clinical variants of measles?

Modified measles may occur in persons with pre-existing immunity to MeV following either previous MMR vaccination or past measles infection or receipt of plasma products containing antibody to measles virus around the time of viral exposure. The clinical presentation is short-lived and mild, characterised usually by rash and fever, although sometimes with respiratory involvement such as cough and coryza, which resolve quickly *(21, 22)*. Atypical measles may be seen in those immunised with formalin-inactivated measles vaccine between 1963 and 1967. There is usually a brief prodromal illness followed by a maculopapular rash which, in contrast to classic measles, begins on the extremities and spreads centripetally. In addition, severe respiratory distress can sometimes develop *(23, 24)*.

MANAGEMENT

How are measles cases managed?

Clinical management of measles is mainly supportive including maintenance of good hydration, as in this case, oral vitamin A supplementation and treatment of secondary bacterial infections *(25, 26)*. No specific antiviral agent is recommended for treatment of uncomplicated measles *(12)*. While ribavirin has *in vitro* activity against MeV, there are no randomised control trial data available to prove its therapeutic value. However, in patients with significant end-organ disease such as severe measles pneumonitis, therapy with intravenous ribavirin has been used *(12)*. There is no established treatment for SSPE although there are reports in the literature that various combinations of oral inosiplex, intraventricular interferon-α2b and intravenous or intraventricular ribavirin may slow progression of the disease but do not halt it *(27, 28)*.

TRANSMISSION AND INFECTIVITY

By which route was MeV acquired in this case?

Transmission of MeV occurs by contact, droplet as well as airborne spread. Small-particle aerosols (< 3μm in diameter), generated from the respiratory tract of an infected patient particularly on coughing, can remain suspended in air for up to 2 hours *(15, 29)*. Even if the infected patient is no longer present in an area, transmission to others may still occur. Patients with measles are infectious 4 days before the onset of the rash and for 4 days thereafter. The median incubation period between infection and onset of prodromal symptoms and signs is about 12 days *(30)*. The source of infection in this case was not identified.

How infectious is a case of measles?

Measles is highly contagious as indicated by its basic reproduction number (R_0), meaning the average number of people who would be infected by a single primary infectious case with classical clinical features in a fully susceptible population *(6)*. Its R_0 value of 12 to 18 means that every case results in 12 to 18 other cases in a fully susceptible population *(31, 32)*. The secondary attack rate in susceptible exposed household contacts is > 90% *(6)*. Herd immunity, which is the threshold level of immunity needed to prevent sustained transmission of an infectious agent in the community, can be calculated as $R_0 - 1/R_0$. For measles, this means that almost 95% immunity is needed to eliminate virus transmission, which is higher than the values for all other vaccine-preventable infections *(33)*. However, epidemiological findings suggest that patients with modified measles i.e. fever and rash but without measles-related respiratory symptoms like cough, coryza or sneezing, are considerably less infectious than cases with classical clinical features *(34)*.

How can transmission of measles in the community be prevented?

Because measles is so infectious its control requires high-level herd immunity achieved by intense immunisation coverage with two doses of measles-containing vaccine *(35)*. The MMR vaccine is highly effective, with the measles component conferring immunity in 92%-95% of individuals after a single dose *(36)*. However, because of primary vaccine failures of approximately 5% in children immunised at $\geq$ 12 months of age, a second dose of MMR vaccine for school-aged children is recommended globally *(37)*. Moreover, protective levels of antibody to measles virus induced by vaccination persist for a mean of 26-33 years after immunisation *(38)*.

PUBLIC HEALTH ASPECTS

When is an individual presumed to be immune to measles?

Presumptive evidence of measles immunity includes documentation of receipt of two doses of live measles-containing vaccine at least 28 days apart with the first dose given at > 12 months of age, laboratory evidence of immunity or laboratory confirmation of past measles infection *(3)*. Although persons born before 1978 are likely to have been infected with wild-type MeV, in an outbreak setting they may be considered nonimmune, particularly if they have no history of measles.

What post-exposure prophylaxis (PEP) was recommended for other patients in the waiting area of the GP practice?

Public health authorities were notified immediately. Fortunately, the case was seen by the GP and practice nurse (both of whom were immune) at the end of the day's surgery. No person was allowed to enter the clinical examination room for two hours after it was vacated by the suspected measles case because of potential transmission to other susceptible individuals. No nonimmune contacts were found (in particular those who had an increased risk of severe illness and complications such as pregnant women, immunocompromised hosts or those < 12 months of age). If such contacts had been identified, PEP by passive immunisation with subcutaneous or intravenous human normal immunoglobulin within 6 days of exposure would have been administered, if the contact was susceptible to measles.

Can MMR vaccine be used as PEP when a contact has no presumptive evidence of measles immunity?

In principle, active immunisation with MMR vaccine may attenuate the clinical course of measles if administered within 72 hours of initial contact with the index case because it induces an immune response more rapidly than following natural measles infection *(39)*. However, MMR vaccine is not indicated in infants < 12 months of age (< 6 months in outbreak situations), pregnant women and immunocompromised hosts (see above).

Should a contact be given a dose of MMR vaccine as PEP even if it is more than 72 hours after exposure to an index case of measles?

Yes, while the recommended timing of MMR vaccination in a contact is within 72 hours of exposure, the clinical course of infection will not be exacerbated if the contact is incubating or develops measles during or within days of vaccination. Furthermore, this dose of MMR vaccine may protect the individual if exposed to measles in the future.

Can measles be acquired by persons previously immunised with two doses of MMR?

Yes, but it occurs rarely. For example, measles infection was reported in six healthcare workers following exposure to unvaccinated primary cases or patients with unknown vaccination status, yet the healthcare workers had documented proof of two-dose MMR vaccination *(34)*. The illness course in each case was mild, typical of modified measles. Intense exposure of previously vaccinated persons to index cases with typical symptomatic measles is an important risk factor for infection *(40)*. It is hypothesised that levels of protective measles antibody can wane sufficiently over time so that exposure via the airborne route to a large measles inoculum may cause symptomatic illness *(41, 42)*. The rapid anamnestic immune response following measles exposure, mediated by humoral and cellular arms of the immune system, probably controls viral replication thereby attenuating the clinical course of infection resulting in modified measles *(43)*. The reduced severity or even absence of respiratory symptoms in these patients also may lower their infectivity *(21, 43)*.

Would you be concerned if a child developed fever and measles-like rash within 1–2 weeks of MMR vaccination?

It is useful from a public health viewpoint to collect oral fluid for molecular confirmation of measles infection and, if measles RNA is detected, to perform genotyping to differentiate between vaccine and wild-type strains of MeV *(44)*. The MeV in MMR vaccine belongs to genotype A which has not been documented currently to cause natural measles *(2)*. While the measles component of MMR vaccine may be detected in oral fluid, recent vaccine recipients are not infectious to others *(45)*. However, fever and rash in recent MMR vaccine recipients are not necessarily due to the vaccine; they may still be caused by wild-type MeV and other viral infections such as parvovirus, enterovirus and HHV6 which can give similar clinical presentations *(46)*. While it has been reported that the absence of cough and coryza as well as rash-onset within 6 to 14 days following vaccination are typical features of vaccine-associated measles, these features do not exclude a mild case of natural measles *(47)*.

For more information on MMR vaccinesee reference 39 and
https://www.hse.ie/eng/health/immunisation/hcpinfo/guidelines/chapter12.pdf

REFERENCES (*useful reviews)

1 Y. Yanagi, M. Takeda, S. Ohno. *J. Gen. Virol.* **87**, 2767 (2006)

2 P.A. Rota *et al.*, *J. Infect. Dis.* **204**Suppl 1, S514 (2011)

3 Health Protection Surveillance Centre (HPSC). Measles Annual Report. Dublin: HPSC, 2015

4 S. Gee *et al.*, *Euro. Surveill.***15**, pii=19500 (2010)

5 P. Barrett *et al.*, *Euro. Surveill.***21**, pii=30277 (2016)

6 G. De Serres, N.J. Gay, C.P. Farrington. *Am. J. Epidemiol.* **151**, 1039 (2000)

7 D.N. Durrheim, N.S. Crowcroft, P.M. Strebel. *Vaccine.***32**, 6880 (2014)

8 H. Tatsou *et al.*, *Nature.* **406**, 893 (2000)

9 M.D. Mühlebach *et al.*, *Nature.* **480**, 530 (2011)

10 R.F. Helfand *et al.*, *Epidemiol. Infect.* **123**, 451 (1999)

11 W.J. Bellini, R.F. Helfand. *J. Infect. Dis.* **187**Suppl 1, S283 (2003)

12 W.J. Moss. *Lancet.***390**, 2490 (2017)*

13 L.J. Wolfson *et al.*, *Int. J. Epidemiol.* **38**, 192 (2009)

14 T.M. Moussallem *et al.*, *Hum. Pathol.***38**, 1239 (2007)

15 C.I. Paules, H.D. Marston, A.S. Fauci. *N. Engl. J. Med.* **23**, 2185 (2019)

16 R.T. Johnson *et al.*, *N. Engl. J. Med.* **310**, 137 (1984)

17 W.J. Bellini *et al.*, *J. Infect. Dis.* **192**, 1686 (2005)

18 K.A. Wendorf *et al.*, *Clin. Infect. Dis.* **65**, 226 (2017)

19 H. Campbell *et al.*, *Int. J. Epidemiol.* **36**, 1334 (2007)

20 B.K. Rima, W.P. Duprex. *J. Pathol.* **208**, 199 (2006)

21 L.F. Yeung *et al.*, *Pediatrics.* **116**, 1287 (2005)

22 K.P. Coleman, P.G. Markey. *Epidemiol.Infect.* **138**, 1012 (2010)

23 D.E. Griffin, C.H. Pan. *Curr.Top.Microbiol.Immunol.***330**, 191 (2009)

24 F.P. Polack, G. Crijeiras, D.E. Griffin.*Nat. Med.* **9**, 1209 (2003)

25 Y. Huiming, W. Chaomin, M. Meng. *Cochrane Database Syst. Rev.* **4**, CD001479 (2005)

26 WHO. *Wkly. Epidemiol. Rec.* **143**, 3442 (2010)

27 T. Solomon *et al.*, *J. Child. Neurol.* **17**, 703 (2002)

28 M. Hosoya. *Nihon Rinsho.* **70**, 625 (2012)

29 R.T. Chen *et al.*, *Am. J. Epidemiol.***129**, 173 (1989)

30 J. Lessler *et al.*, *Lancet Infect. Dis.* **9**, 291 (2009)

31 H.A. Kelly, M.A. Riddell, R.M. Andrews. *Med. J. Aust.* **176**, 50 (2002)

32 Centers for Disease Control and Prevention. *Morb.Mortal. Wkly. Rep.* **61**, 30 (2012)

33 W. Orenstein, K. Seib. *N. Engl. J. Med*. **371**, 1661 (2014)*

34 J.S. Rota *et al.*, *J. Infect. Dis*. **204**Suppl 1, S559 (2011)

35 J. Seward, W.A. Orenstein. *Clin. Infect. Dis*. **55**, 403 (2012)

36 Centers for Disease Control. MMWR Recomm. Rep. **62,** 1 (2013)

37 WHO position paper.*Wkly. Epidemiol. Rec*. **84**, 349 (2009)

38 M.S. Dine *et al.* ,*J. Infect. Dis*. **189**Suppl 1, S123 (2004)

39 https://www.gov.uk/government/publications/measles-the-green-book-chapter-21

40 F.A. Lievano *et al.*, *J. Infect. Dis*. **189**, S165 (2004)

41 P. Aaby *et al.*, *J. Infect. Dis*. **154**, 858 (1986)

42 M. Paunio *et al.*, *Am. J. Epidemiol*. **148**, 1103 (1998)

43 J.B. Rosen *et al.*, *Clin. Infect. Dis*. **58**, 1205 (2014)

44 C.Y. Ting, N.W. Tee, K.C. Thoon. *ActaPaediatr*.**104**, e232 (2015)

45 S.L. Katz, J.F. Enders, A. Holloway. *N. Engl. J. Med*. **263**, 159 (1960)

46 I. Davidkin *et al.*, *J. Infect. Dis*. **178**, 1567 (1998)

47 V. Dietz *et al.*, *Bull. World Health Org*. **82**, 852 (2004)

HUMAN PARVOVIRUS B19

What is human parvovirus B19?

Human parvovirus B19 (hereafter, B19V) is a member of the family *Parvoviridae* and sub-family *Parvovirinae*. The latter is subdivided into eight genera, including *Erythroparvovirus* of which B19V is the only member so far *(1)*. The virus is small (23 - 26nm in diameter), nonenveloped and has a linear single-stranded DNA genome (about 5,600 nucleotides). Erythema infectiosum, occurs in children with acute B19V infection while adults usually present with acute or chronic arthropathy. Transient aplastic crisis can occur in those with low haematological reserve due to underlying chronic haemolytic anaemia, while pure red blood cell aplasiadue to chronic B19V infection typically occurs in immune suppressed individuals. Fetal loss, including hydrops fetalis, may develop following acute maternal B19V infection *(2)*.

Explain the etymology of B19V.

The name is derived from the Latin word parvum, implying it is one of the smallest DNA viruses. While using a technique known as counter current immunoelectrophoresis to detect hepatitis B surface antigen in serum samples, Yvonne Cossart discovered the virus serendipitously in a sample on panel B of the assay plate at position number 19, hence the name human parvovirus B19 *(3)*.

COMMON CLINICAL MANIFESTATIONS OF B19V INFECTION SEEN IN GENERAL PRACTICE

What is erythema infectiosum?

Erythema infectiosum (EI) is a childhood exanthem, also known as 'slapped cheek disease' or fifth disease, characterised by a rash which appears initially like a 'slapped cheek' before spreading to the trunk and extremities. In children it is the most common clinical manifestation of acute infection with B19V. In the 1900s, a series of common childhood exanthems were numbered in the order in which they were reported. These included measles, scarlet fever, rubella, Duke's disease, fifth disease and roseola (sixth disease) *(2)*.

EPIDEMIOLOGY

In which cohorts in the general population is EI most frequently seen?

B19V infection is common worldwide: approximately 50% of children are seropositive for B19V by 15 years of age with 60% and 90% seroprevalence rates in 30 year olds and elderly adults, respectively *(4,5,6)*. The annual seroconversion rate in nonimmune pregnant women is estimated at 1.5% *(7)*. Acute B19V infections show seasonality with most cases occurring in winter and spring, and with cyclic epidemics about every 3 to 4 years *(8)*. A significant risk factor for B19V acquisition in adults is daily contact with school-age children at home and in primary schools, as shown by annual seroconversion rates to B19V as high as 5.6% and 5.2%, respectively *(9)*.

How is B19V transmitted when circulating in the community?

Transmission of B19V is mainly via the respiratory route. This is supported by the finding that B19V DNA was detected in respiratory secretions during the viraemic phase of infection in the week before onset of rash or arthropathy *(10)*. Furthermore, secondary transmission of B19V is high, consistent with respiratory transmission. For example, in schools, the secondary attack rates among children and teachers during community epidemics of erythema infectiosum can be as high as 50% and 30%, respectively *(11, 12)*. In addition, B19V is stable in the environment because it lacks an outer lipid envelope, thereby conferring resistance to detergents and potentially facilitating transmission by inanimate objects or hand contact *(13)*. Moreover, nosocomial transmission of B19V was reported among hospital staff who did not adopt strict hand washing procedures after contact with infected patients *(14)*.

PATHOGENESIS

What is the likely pathogenesis of EI and arthropathy?

Deposition of immune complexes in the skin, formed as a consequence of a robust antibody response to B19V, may cause the rash *(2)*. Similarly, arthritis and arthralgia, which occur mainly in adults with acute B19V infection, may be related to immune complex deposition in joints *(15)*. About 6 days after B19V infection via the respiratory route, the host develops a viraemia which lasts about one week. B19V DNA can also be detected in respiratory secretions at this time *(10)*. Development of IgM antibody to B19V begins around day 10 after exposure and is followed by anti-B19V IgG around 2 weeks postinfection. There is a temporal relationship between the appearance of anti-B19V antibodies and onset of the rash in children and arthropathy in adults *(2)*.

CLINICAL FEATURES

What is the typical clinical course of EI in children?

A week after exposure to B19V, prodromal symptoms including fever and/or nonspecific influenza-like illness may occur, corresponding to the viraemic phase of infection *(10)*. The exanthematous rash, which begins on the cheeks with circumoral pallor, usually occurs about 2 weeks after exposure, around the time of development of anti-B19V humoral response. A second phase occurs 1 to 4 days later, characterised by a maculopapular rash on the trunk and limbs which changes into a reticular lace-like pattern due to fading in the central areas of maculae. The rash may recur in the subsequent weeks induced by exercise or stress or even environmental stimuli like heat and sunlight *(2, 7)*. Arthropathy in children presenting with erythema infectiosum is uncommon (< 10%) *(12, 17)*.

What is the course of symptomatic acute B19V infection in otherwise healthy adults?

While most infections are probably asymptomatic, when there are clinical manifestations in healthy adults the most common is acute arthropathy involving joints of the hands, wrists, knees and ankles. It predominantly affects women in contact with children and can last for weeks *(18)*. It does not cause tissue damage in joints *(19)*. Skin manifestations of acute B19V infection are infrequent in adults and can be atypical: for example, the eruption of papular, purpuric lesions on the hands and feet, known as 'gloves and socks' syndrome, has been reported *(20, 21)*.

Can acute B19V infection occur subclinically?

Asymptomatic B19V infection occurs commonly in both children and adults *(1, 2)*. As many as 50% of acute B19V infections may not develop any features of EI or report any arthropathy even when there is serological evidence of recent infection. However, those infected asymptomatically with B19V may still be infectious to susceptible contacts *(9, 22)*.

CASE VIGNETTE

A 10-year-old boy presented to his GP with a 72-hour history of a febrile illness and a rash on his cheeks. His mother was concerned because her 12-year-old daughter, who had chemotherapy for a haematological malignancy, was discharged home from hospital 24 hours before her brother developed the rash. The GP suspected erythema infectiosum as several cases occurred in the community already.

What was the approach to this case?

LABORATORY DIAGNOSIS

Is laboratory confirmation of EI always necessary?

No, the presumptive diagnosis is made on clinical grounds based on febrile illness with an exanthematous malar rash. However, if the presentation is atypical such as 'gloves and socks' syndrome or there is an arthropathy of unknown cause, laboratory confirmation is helpful in clinical management.

Was it necessary to confirm the diagnosis of B19V-related EI in this case?

Yes, because if acute B19V infection was confirmed, the boy was potentially infectious in the week before onset of the rash and horizontal transmission of B19V to his sister could have occurred. Acute B19V infection in immunocompromised individuals may cause transfusion-dependent chronic pure red cell aplasia. Fortunately in this case, a serum sample from the girl was anti-B19V IgG positive confirming her existing immunity to the virus.

What laboratory test was requested by the GP?

IgM antibodies and IgG antibodies to B19V (anti-B19V IgM / IgG)were positive in a serum sample. Anti-B19V IgM / IgG are detected in almost all cases of EI on presentation and persist for at least 3 months after acute infection *(2)*. Demonstration of anti-B19V IgG seroconversion in paired samples (from anti-B19V IgG negative to IgGpositive) confirms infection *(1)*.

Is detection of B19V DNA by PCR recommended for diagnosis of EI?

No, in immunocompetent persons the viral load decreases dramatically within the first month of B19V infection but low-level viral DNA may persist for longer than a year in serum despite the presence of neutralising antibodies *(23)*. Therefore, detection of B19V DNA alone does not always indicate current infection *(24)*. Furthermore, there are three genotypes (1,2 and 3) of B19V with similar biological and clinical properties, however, they show 10% to 20% nucleotide divergence and therefore PCR assays must be designed to detect all genotypes of B19V *(1)*.

EMERGENT HUMAN PARVOVIRUSES

Are parvoviruses other than B19V associated with disease in humans?

Human bocavirus 1 (HBoV1), PARV4 and bufavirus (BuV) are parvoviruses that are emerging as potential pathogens in humans, but proof of their virulence is still awaited. These viruses belong to different genera in the family *Parvoviridae*. Furthermore, their reported clinical manifestations do not overlap with those of B19V. There is evidence that primary infection with HBoV1 causes upper and lower respiratory tract infections predominantly in children < 5 years of age *(25)*. PARV4 appears to be transmitted parenterally by contaminated needles but is of uncertain clinical significance *(26)*. BuV is a parvovirus detected infrequently in faeces of children and adults with acute gastroenteritis but not in stool samples of healthy persons *(27)*.

REFERENCES (*useful reviews)

1 J. Qiu, M. Söderlund-Venermo, N.S. Young. *Clin.Microbiol. Rev.* **30**, 43 (2017)*

2 N.S. Young, K.E. Brown. *N. Engl. J. Med.* **350**, 586 (2004)*

3 Y.E. Cossart *et al.*, *Lancet.* **1**, 72 (1975)

4 L.J. Anderson *et al.*, *J. Clin. Microbiol.***24**, 522 (1986)

5 B.J. Cohen, M.M. Buckley. *J. Med. Microbiol.* **25**, 151 (1988)

6 H.A. Kelly *et al.*, *Epidemiol. Infect.* **124**, 449 (2000)

7 W.C. Koch, S.P. Adler. *Pediatr. Infect. Dis. J.* **8**, 83 (1989)

8 M.J. Anderson *et al.*, *Lancet.* **329**, 738 (1987)

9 S.P. Adler *et al.*, *J. Infect. Dis.* **168**, 361 (1993)

10 M.J. Anderson *et al.*, *J. Infect. Dis.* **152**, 257 (1985)

11 S.M. Gillespie *et al.*, *JAMA.* **263**, 2061 (1990)

12 E.D. Heegaard, K.E. Brown. *Clin.Microbiol. Rev.* **15**, 485(2002)

13 J.S. Garner. *Infect. Control Hosp. Epidemiol.* **17**, 53 (1996)

14 C. Seng *et al.*, *Epidemiol. Infect.* **113**, 345 (1994)

15 T.L. Moore.*Curr.Opin.Rheumatol.***12**, 289 (2000)

16 J.T. Servey, B.V. Reamy, J. Hodge. *Am. Fam. Physician.* **75**, 373 (2007)

17 J.J. Nocton *et al.*, *J. Pediatr.* **122**, 186 (1993)

18 A.D. Woolf *et al.,Arch. Intern. Med.* **149**, 1153 (1989)

19 I. Speyer, F.C. Breedvelt, P. Hannonen. *Clin. Exp. Rheumatol.* **16**, 576 (1998)

20 P.Mackowiak *et al.*, *Clin. Infect. Dis.* **41**, 1529 (2005)

21 L. Harel*et al.*, *Clin. Infect. Dis.* **35**, 1558 (2002)

22 S.M. Gillespie *et al.*, *JAMA.* **263**, 2061 (1990)

23 L. Mouthon, L. Guillevin, Z. Tellier. *Autoimmune Rev.* **4**, 264 (2005)

24 A. Corcoran, S. Doyle. *J. Med. Microbiol.* **53**, 459 (2004)*

25 C.M. Nascimento-Carvalho *et al.*, *J. Med. Virol.* **84**, 253 (2012)

26 P. Simmonds *et al.*, *Emerg. Infect. Dis.* **13**, 1386 (2007)

27T. Chieochansin *et al.*, *Arch. Virol.* **160**, 1781 (2015)

ACUTE PARVOVIRUS B19 INFECTION IN THOSE WITH UNDERLYING CHRONIC HAEMOLYTIC ANAEMIA

What is transient aplastic crisis?

Transient aplastic crisis (TAC) is a self-limiting condition involving mainly suppression of red blood cell production in marrow of persons with underlying chronic haemolytic anaemia and is usually linked to acute parvovirus B19 (B19V) infection. In general, supportive care and blood transfusion are sufficient to manage the crisis until the person's immune response suppresses viral replication with gradual recovery of marrow function.

PATHOGENESIS

How does TAC occur in B19V-infected patients with underlying chronic haemolytic anaemia?

TAC is characterised by sudden onset of anaemia due to abrupt cessation of erythropoiesis for 10 to 15 days caused by acute B19V infection. B19V preferentially infects rapidly dividing erythroid precursor cells, including pronormoblasts in which high-level viral replication occurs, thereby leading to their destruction by cytotoxic apoptosis and lysis (1). TAC occurs in individuals in whom erythrocyte survival is decreased due to increased destruction, such as hereditary spherocytosis or sickle cell disease, and in those with decreased red cell production caused, for example, by iron deficiency anaemia or α- and β-thalassaemias (2, 3). Inhibition of erythropoiesis occurs in all individuals with acute B19V infection, even in otherwise healthy volunteers, as shown by the absence of reticulocytes (immature erythrocytes) in blood, however, anaemia does not usually occur because erythrocyte production is only halted transiently and circulating erythrocytes have a long life span (4). In contrast, in persons with shortened erythrocyte survival or in whom there is an increased demand for red cells, even a temporary halting of erythrocyte production may precipitate a crisis (2, 3). Although red cell aplasia occurs predominantly, there are occasional reports of concurrent thrombocytopenia, neutropenia and pancytopenia in patients with chronic haemolytic anaemia and B19V-related TAC (3).

CASE VIGNETTE

A 14-year-old African boy, who was diagnosed with hereditary spherocytosis (HS) when two years old, presented to the GP with a 48-hour history of fever, fatigue and abdominal pain. On examination, the temperature was 38.3°C, the skin and conjunctivae were pale, pulse rate was 98 beats / minute, respiratory rate 22 breaths /

minute and the spleen palpable 3 centimeters below the left costal margin, while other physical findings were normal. He had annual testing for full blood count (FBC) by the GP since time of diagnosis with HS. The GP sent a blood sample urgently for FBC: of note was haemoglobin 4.2 g/dL (baseline 8.5 g/dL to 9.0 g/dL) and reticulocyte count 0.1% (baseline 10%) indicating significant reticulocytopenia. The GP referred the patient to hospital immediately with suspected viral-induced aplastic crisis. What can GPs learn from this case?

LABORATORY DETECTION OF B19V

What virological tests were performed?

On hospital admission, a serum sample was tested for anti-B19 IgM / IgG which were both negative. However, the same sample was tested by real-time polymerase chain reaction (PCR) for B19V DNA which was detected at a high load (10^{10} IU/mL) indicating high level viral replication in acute B19V infection.

NATURAL HISTORY OF TAC

What was the course of B19V-related TAC in this child?

The boy received two units of packed red blood cell transfusions and other supportive care. He showed marked clinical improvement and was discharged seven days later. As shown in this case, the most frequent clinical presentation in those with TAC is fever, pain and pallor sometimes with acute splenic sequestration and acute chest syndrome (5). Anaemia is potentially fatal and urgent red blood cell transfusion is necessary. In the acute phase of aplastic crisis, such as in the current case, B19V replicates intensely as shown by serum B19V DNA levels of 10^{10} to 10^{13} IU/mL(6). This patient was regarded as highly infectious at this stage (B19V DNA 10^{10} IU/mL and anti-B19V IgM/IgG negative) and was isolated with implementation of respiratory precautions while hospitalised (7, 8). Similar to the current case, the reticulocyte count in blood, which is usually raised in patients with chronic haemolytic anaemia, decreases to almost nil and is diagnostic of a B19V-induced aplastic crisis (2, 3). Erythrocyte production recovers within 1 to 2 weeks, coinciding with development of an anti-B19V IgM and IgG response (10). In the current case, anti-B19V IgM / IgG were positive in a serum sample collected 11 days after diagnosis. B19V DNA was not retested since the boy had developed an anti-B19V antibody response and haematological laboratory findings indicated recovery.

REFERENCES (*useful reviews)

1 A. Corcoran, S. Doyle. *J. Med. Microbiol.* **53**, 459 (2004)*

2 E.D. Heegaard, K.E. Brown. *Clin.Microbiol. Rev.* **15**, 485 (2002)*

3 N.S. Young, K.E. Brown. *N. Engl. J. Med.* **350**, 586 (2004)*

4 M.J. Anderson *et al.*, *J. Infect. Dis.* **152**, 257 (1985)

5 K. Smith-Whitley *et al.*, *Blood.* **103**, 422 (2004)

6 A. Ishikawa *et al.*, *J. Med. Virol.* **86**, 2102, (2014)

7 L.M. Bell *et al.*, *N. Engl. J. Med*. **321**, 485 (1989)

8 T.L. Chin *et al.*, *J. Hosp. Infect.* **87**, 11 (2014)

9 U.M. Saarinen *et al.*, *Blood.* **67**, 1411 (1986)

10 T. Takano, K. Yamada.*Pediatr. Int.* **49**, 459 (2007)

'FARMYARD' POX VIRUSES

What is 'farmyard pox'?

This term embraces orf, milker's nodule and bovine papular stomatitis, common parapoxvirus infections of skin and oral mucosa that occur in sheep, goats and cattle throughout the world and can be transmitted to humans. They usually cause self-limiting noduloulcerative skin lesions (1, 2).

VIROLOGY

What are parapoxviruses?

Parapoxviruses belong to the genus *Parapoxvirus* in the family *Poxviridae*. Members of this genus primarily infect animals and can then be transmitted to humans, 'zoonotic' transmission (3). The most common parapoxviruses causing infection in humans are orf virus, pseudocowpox or paravaccinia virus (also known as milker's nodule virus) and bovine papular stomatitis virus (4). Other genera in the family *Poxviridae* of medical interest include *Molluscipoxvirus* (molluscum contagiosum), *Yatapoxvirus* (tanapox reported in Africa only) and the *Orthopoxviruses* (smallpox, cowpox and monkeypox) (2).

Which parapoxviruses are common causes of 'farmyard pox'?

Parapoxviruses causing human infections vary according to the animal source (2). Orf virus is the cause of ecthymacontagiosum (also known as 'sore mouth' or 'scabby mouth' or 'contagious pustular dermatitis') in sheep and goats (3). Orf virus does not infect cattle. Milker's nodule virus (pseudocowpox or paravaccinia virus) typically infects teats of cows while bovine papular stomatitis virus causes oral mucosal lesions in cattle (2). These distinct viruses cause identical clinical disease in humans (2).

EPIDEMIOLOGY

What is the incidence of 'farmyard pox' infections in humans?

It is unknown since many individuals in the farming community recognise the typical appearance and self-limiting nature of orf-like lesions, and therefore do not seek medical attention (5). Those infected may even seek clinical advice from veterinarians (6).

Which human populations are particularly at risk of acquiring parapoxvirus infections?

Those who have occupational or recreational exposure to farm animals such as veterinarians, farmers, wool shearers and abbatoir workers are at risk of parapoxvirus infection (2). In the United Kingdom, human orf cases acquired from contact with sheep were reported to occur more commonly than parapoxvirus infections from other animals *(5)*. Those at risk of orf infection include persons under 20 years of age living on farms, direct contact with infected animals and contact with flayed skin of sick animals *(7)*. Cases of orf may occur in urban households due to manipulation of skin and raw meat of sheep or participation in ritual sacrifices as part of religious customs *(8, 9)*. During ritual sacrifices of sheep, the struggling animal is held with bare hands while it bleeds to death, thereby facilitating potential contamination of participants with or virus if the animal is infected. Veterinary students, whose hands contact the mouths of infected cattle while medicating or inserting endotracheal tubes, are prone to skin infections with bovine papular stomatitis virus *(10)*. Similarly, inexperienced milkers of cows are at risk of infection with milker's nodule virus (pseudocowpox virus) from infected teats of cattle *(11)*.

TRANSMISSION

How are parapoxviruses transmitted to humans?

Humans are infected by direct inoculation of virus into cuts or skin abrasions following contact with infected lesions on animals *(12)*. However, there is evidence that asymptomatic parapoxvirus infections occur in animals and can be a source of transmission to humans *(13)*. Because parapoxviruses are hardy and persist in the farm environment for months to years, indirect transmission to humans by contaminated equipment or soil can occur *(14, 15)*.

NATURAL HISTORY

What is the clinical course of 'farmyard pox'?

The course of disease is benign and self-limiting in immunocompetent hosts, typically lasting 6–10 weeks *(16)*. In humans with milker's nodule or bovine papular stomatitis infections, their clinical presentation is identical to orf. Therefore, differentiation between orf and the other parapoxvirus infections is determined from the patient's history of animal contact, sheep and goats versus cattle *(2)*. Lesions are typically solitary (2 – 3 cm in diameter) or a few lesions on the fingers, hands and forearms but can rarely be found on the face and eye *(17, 18)*. The lesions usually progress through six clinical stages, each lasting about 6 days *(19)*. Initially, a maculopapular lesion appears 3 – 7 days after inoculation and develops into a targetoid lesion which is nodular with a red centre, with a halo and red base. This is followed by an acute phase characterised by an erythematous weeping nodule. In the regenerative phase, the nodule is dry with black dots on the surface due to dilated hair follicles filled with debris. In the next stage, papillomas appear on the surface. A week later there is spontaneous regression with the appearance of a dry scab and healing usually without scarring.

What complications occur with parapoxvirus infections?

Secondary bacterial infection, lymphangitis and lymphadenopathy are uncommon complications of orf *(20)*. Orf-induced immunobullous disease and erythema multiforme, albeit infrequent, have been reported 2-4 weeks after onset of lesions *(21)*. Parapoxvirus infections in immunocompromised patients can be persistent, with development of large lesions ('giant orf'), and located at unusual sites such as the face *(4, 6)*.

Can reinfection occur in individuals previously infected with a parapoxvirus?

Yes, the immune response to parapoxvirus infections appears to be short-lived, and prior infection does not seem to confer immunity against reinfection *(22)*. A history of smallpox vaccination does not confer protection against parapoxvirus since the viruses belong to different genera of poxviruses *(23)*.

What is the differential diagnosis of orf-like lesions in humans?

The differential diagnosis of lesions on the distal upper extremities is broad and includes non-infectious causes like pyogenic granuloma, keratoacanthoma and cutaneous malignancy *(6, 24)*. Infectious considerations include atypical mycobacterial infections, sporotrichosis (fungal disease), bacillary angiomatosis and syphilitic chancre. Cutaneous leishmaniasis, cutaneous anthrax and tularaemia should be considered in travellers from endemic areas *(2, 6)*.

CASE VIGNETTE

A 21-year-old male veterinary student presented to the GP with an enlarging, painless, red lesion on the metacarpal-phalangeal joint of the right index finger that first appeared 8 days earlier. He incurred a minor cut in the same area while intubating a sheep without wearing gloves 10 days before he first noticed the lesion. He did not recall any recent insect or animal bites. On examination, the lesion was a 3-cm, fluctuant, erythematous nodule which was oozing slightly. It was nontender to touch and there was no surrounding erythema, lymphangitis or lymphadenopathy. The professor of veterinary medicine diagnosed it as orf and the GP agreed. The lesion had resolved completely one month later without any intervention.

How is 'farmyard pox' infection diagnosed in clinical practice?

Typical clinical findings and history of contact with farm animals are sufficient for a diagnosis *(2, 4)*.

When is laboratory confirmation needed?

Laboratory confirmation of parapoxvirus infection is important when a lesion is atypical or the infection is suspected in an individual with no obvious risk factor. Definite diagnosis excludes life-threatening zoonoses, such as cutaneous anthrax, which have significant public health implications *(4)*.

Do rapid laboratory tests exist for diagnosis of parapoxvirus infections?

There are two approaches, electron microscopy (EM) with negative staining of material from the vesicle is useful if done in the first two weeks of infection *(16)*. Parapoxviruses appear as large (260 nm x 160 nm) ovoid or brick-shaped particles with a core surrounded by an outer membrane in which are protein tubules arranged in a criss-cross pattern like a 'ball of yarn'. However, EM cannot differentiate or virus from other parapoxviruses. Polymerase chain reaction (PCR) methods can identify parapoxviruses in vesicular material. Parapoxviruses have high amounts (> 60%) of the nucleosides guanosine (G) and cytosine (C) while, in contrast, orthopoxviruses have a lower proportion of GC (< 40%). A molecular assay was developed which differentiates between poxviruses based on whether the target virus has a low or high GC content *(25)*. To further differentiate between parapoxviruses, real-time PCR assays are available to identify orf virus, pseudocowpox virus and bovine papular stomatitis virus *(26)*.

How is 'farmyard pox' managed in general practice?

No specific antiviral treatment is recommended for parapoxvirus infections which are self-limiting in otherwise healthy persons. Supportive care with application of local antiseptics is commonly used. However, in immunocompromised individuals who have large and persistent lesions, several treatment strategies may be considered. Topical imiquimod, an imidazoquinoline which activates and recruits plasmacytoid dendritic cells into skin thereby enhancing antiviral immunity, has been used successfully to treat orf in immunosuppressed patients *(6, 27)*. There are also anecdotal reports of successful treatment of orf with topical cidofovir (1%) applied for 5 days followed by a 5-day holiday for a total of 5 cycles *(28)*. Reduction in immunosuppressive drugs may also be beneficial *(6)*. Surgical approaches such as excision and cryotherapy are other options *(29)*.

How can 'farmyard pox' be prevented?

The use of nonpermeable gloves and strict hand hygiene are recommended for persons handling animals or those in contact with farmyard environments if they have damaged skin or are immunocompromised *(30, 31)*. Furthermore, those who slaughter animals and handle raw meat as part of religious or cultural traditions should also be educated on prevention of parapoxvirus infections *(9)*.

REFERENCES (*useful review)

1 W.B. Shelley, E.D. Shelley. *Br. J. Dermatol.***108**, 725 (1983)

2 D.G. Diven. *J. Am. Acad. Dermatol.* **44**, 1 (2001)

3 D.M. Tack, M.G. Reynolds. *Animals*.**1**, 377 (2011)

4 M. Hosamani *et al., Expert Rev. Anti Infect. Ther*.**7**, 879 (2009)*

5 D. Baxby, M. Bennett. *J. Med. Microbiol*. **46**, 17 (1997)

6 E.R. Lederman *et al., Clin. Infect. Dis*. **44**, e100 (2007)

7 Y. Bayinder *et al., New Microbiologica*. **34**, 37 (2011)

8 M. Uzel *et al., Epidemiol. Infect*. **133**, 653 (2005)

9 Centers for Disease Control and Prevention, *Morb.Mortal. Wkly. Rep*. **61**, 245 (2012)

10 K.F. Bowman *et al., JAMA*. **246**, 2813 (1981)

11 C.E. Wheeler, E.P. Cawley. *Arch. Dermatol*. **75**, 249 (1957)

12 E.R. Lederman *et al., Pediatr. Infect. Dis. J*. **26**, 740 (2007)

13 E.R. Lederman *et al., Animals*. **3**, 142 (2013)

14 U.W. Jr. Leavell *et al., JAMA*. **204**, 657 (1968)

15 B. Steinhart. *CJEM*.**7**, 417 (2005)

16 J.V. Johannessen *et al., J. Cutan. Pathol*.**2**, 265 (1975)

17 M.S. Gurel *et al., Eur. J. Dermatol*. **12**, 183 (2002)

18 S.J. Key *et al., J. Craniofac. Surg*. **18**, 1076 (2007)

19 J.L. Zimmerman.*JAMA*.**266**, 476 (1991)

20 E. Schmidt *et al., J. Eur. Acad. Dermatol. Venereol*.**20**, 612 (2006)

21 K.P. White *et al., J. Am. Acad. Dermatol*. **58**, 49 (2008)

22 A.J. Robinson, G.V. Petersen. *N.Z. Med. J*. **96**, 81 (1983)

23 D.L. Yirrell, J.P. Vestey, M. Norval. *Br. J. Dermatol*. **130**, 438 (1994)

24 N. Chahidi, S. de Fontaine, B. Lacotte. *Br. J. Plast. Surg*. **46**, 532 (1993)

25 Y. Li *et al., J. Clin. Microbiol*.**48**, 268 (2010)

26 L. Gallina*et al., J. Virol. Methods*.**134**, 140 (2006)

27 M. Ara *et al., J. Am. Acad. Dermatol*. **58**Suppl 2, S39 (2008)

28 K. Geerinck *et al., J. Med. Virol*. **64**, 543 (2001)

29 C. Degraeve *et al., Dermatol*. **198**, 162 (1999)

30A.A. Roess *et al., N.Engl. J. Med*.**363**, 2621 (2010)

31 L.U. Osadebe*et al., Clin. Infect. Dis*. **60**, 195 (2015)

MOLLUSCUM CONTAGIOSUM

What is molluscum contagiosum?

It is a benign skin tumour caused by chronic localised infection with the mollusum contagiosum poxvirus. Like all poxviruses, it is a brick-shaped virus with a large double-stranded DNA genome. It is the only member of the genus *Molluscivirus* in the family *Poxviridae (1)*. It is classified into four subtypes by molecular analysis: MCV-1, MCV-1a, MCV-2 and, the rare genotype MCV-3 *(2)*. MCV-1and MCV-2 are associated with infection in both children and adults globally but MCV-2 is the less frequent.

EPIDEMIOLOGY

What is the incidence of molluscum contagiosum?

Fewer than 5% of children in the United States present with clinically apparent disease *(3)*. However, a seroprevalence study in Australia showed an overall seropositivity rate of 23% in subjects aged 1 year to 69 years *(4)*. A recent seroprevalence study showed seroprevalence rates of 14.9% and 30.3% in German and United Kingdom populations, respectively *(5)*. Overall, these findings imply that subclinical or very mild infections are common.

How is molluscum contagiosum transmitted?

Infection requires inoculation of virus into breaches in the epidermis. Routes of transmission include direct skin-to-skin contact as seen in participants of contact sports like wrestling, and during sexual intercourse *(3, 6)*. Autoinoculation by scratching a lesion and transferring the virus to another site also occurs frequently *(7)*. Fomites are implicated in transmission as shown by higher rates of infection among children sharing bath sponges and towels *(8)*.

Which groups are at high risk of molluscum contagiosum?

This is mainly an infection of childhood (1 – 14 years) *(4)*. Almost half of those households in which lived a child with molluscum contagiosum reported transmission to other resident child contacts *(9)*. Sexually active young adults are at risk of genital molluscum contagiosum (5). Cell-mediated immunity is important in viral control, therefore individuals with low numbers of CD4 T-cells, as occurs in HIV infection or in those on potent immunosuppression, predisposes to severe molluscum contagiosum infection *(10)*. In children with atopic dermatitis, molluscum contagiosum can be extensive and persistent, probably because damage to the skin barrier predisposes to autoinoculation and decreased cell-mediated immunity caused by the use of topical immunosuppressants *(11)*.

Is communal use of swimming pools a risk factor for molluscum contagiosum?

Although an association between swimming pool use and molluscum contagiosum was first documented in 1910, the route of transmission is probably via fomites rather than use of the pool itself *(12, 13)*. The anatomical distribution of lesions suggested that contact with kickboards used during swimming classes, sitting on seats around the pool or sharing bath towels and sponges were likely sources of infection *(8, 14, 15)*.

Should children with nongenital molluscum contagiosum be allowed to attend school and participate in contact sports?

No restrictions are needed but lesions should be covered with clothing or waterproof bandages. Sharing of towels and bath sponges should be avoided.

CLINICAL FEATURES

What are the typical clinical features of molluscum contagiosum on presentation?

The lesions are usually small (3-5mm in diameter), pearly white or flesh-coloured papules with central umbilication *(16)*. On average there are 11-20 lesions present on examination but, in one study, 25% of children had severe disease with ≥ 21 papules *(9)*. Furthermore, most children had lesions in > 1 anatomic site, mainly arms and torso, but not on palms of hands, soles of feet or oral mucosa. Lesions are infrequently found on genital and conjunctival mucosal surfaces *(16)*. In sexually transmitted disease the lesions are distributed around the genitalia, proximal thighs and lower abdomen but this is rare in children before sexual debut *(16)*. In immunocompromised individuals with molluscum contagiosum there can be hundreds of lesions *(17)*.

Molluscum contagiosum has been described as 'the bump that rashes'. Explain.

Molluscum dermatitis, which is a localised eczematous area surrounding the lesion, occurs frequently (30% of cases) *(16)*. Pruritus associated with molluscum dermatitis increases the risk of autoinoculation by scratching of lesions and inoculating virus into surrounding skin. The eczema disappears with resolution of molluscum contagiosum. Inflamed lesions may be confused with bacterial infection but should not be treated with antibiotics as they are likely to resolve spontaneously *(18)*.

Explain the term 'giant' molluscum?

In severely immunosuppressed patients, including HIV-infected individuals with low CD4 T-cell counts, molluscum contagiosum disseminates extensively and lesions may coalesce to form giant nodules (> 1 cm diameter)*(19)*.

What is the natural history of molluscum contagiosum?

An individual lesion may resolve spontaneously within 8 weeks, however, because of autoinoculation new lesions appear as old ones resolve thereby prolonging the condition. It was shown that approximately 50% of individuals had complete resolution within 12 months of onset while 30% and 13% still had lesions at 18 months and 24 months, respectively *(9, 20)*. Furthermore, time to resolution of the infection was not influenced by the number of lesions at presentation, number of infected sites and underlying atopic dermatitis. In addition, treatment did not reduce time to resolution.

DIAGNOSIS

How is molluscum contagiosum diagnosed?

The presence of small umbilicated skin-coloured papules are pathognomic to the attending clinician. However, at least 40 types of dermatoses share similar morphology, for example, in immunosuppressed hosts fungal infections like crytococcosis, penicilliosis, coccidiomycosis and histoplasmosis are in the differential diagnosis *(21)*.

What methods can be used to support the clinical diagnosis of molluscum contagiosum?

Dermoscopy can visualise the presence or absence of orifices and the pattern of blood vessels which aids the diagnosis of molluscum contagiosum *(21)*. Vascular features in this disease include crown, radial, mixed flower and, most commonly in inflamed lesions, punctiform patterns. Lesions sampled by biopsy and examined histologically are characterised by giant cells containing large eosinophilic intracytoplasmic inclusions known as molluscum bodies or Henderson-Paterson bodies *(22)*. Molecular diagnostic methods are now available *(23)*.

TREATMENT

Should children with nongenital molluscum contagiosum be treated?

There is insufficient evidence currently to support any definitive treatment *(24)*. However, treatment by a dermatologist should be considered when there are many lesions (≥ 21), and for those in whom the condition is causing physical and psychological discomfort impacting adversely on their quality of life *(9, 16)*.

What treatments are commonly used for nongenital molluscumc ontagiosum?

Cantharidin, an extract from the blister beetle, is useful in treatment of individual lesions *(17)*. It acts by inducing intraepidermal blistering through acantholysis *(25)*. Scarring is generally not a problem but it should be applied skilfully to the lesion and removed within 2 hours – 6 hours. Application to genital and facial lesions should be avoided. Cryotherapy is rapid and effective but children may not tolerate the pain. Similarly, curettage is effective but requires local anaesthesia. However, curettage is recommended in Europe and reduces lesions to zero instantaneously with a high chance

(> 80%) of complete success when applied in patients with small numbers of lesions *(26, 27)*.

Is there a role for imiquimod for treatment of nongenital molluscum contagiosum?

Recent evidence suggests that imiquimod is inactive against MCV probably because the virus actively inhibits the Toll-like receptor response *(28)*. Moreover, recent trial data showed a lack of efficacy of imiquimod for treatment of MCV infection and it is proposed that it should not be used for this purpose *(29)*.

What options are available for treating severe molluscum contagiosum in immunocompromised individuals?

The patient should be referred to an Infectious Diseases service. Cell-mediated immunity needs to be restored to resolve this infection: the number of lesions correlates with CD4 T-cell count and resolution of lesions was achieved successfully in HIV-infected patients using highly active antiretroviral therapy to restore cellular immunity *(30)*. Another option is cidofovir, a nucleotide analogue with activity against DNA viruses. It can be applied topically, intralesionally and intravenously for treatment of giant molluscum contagiosum *(31)*. Intralesional and systemic interferon-α were used for treatment in immunodeficient patients *(32)*.

REFERENCES (*useful reviews)

1 W.L. Epstein. *Semin.Dermatol.***11**, 184 (1992)

2 C.H. Thompson. *J. Med. Virol.***53**, 205 (1997)

3 M.A. Dohil*et al., J. Am. Acad. Dermatol.* **54**, 47 (2006)

4 J. Konya, C.H. Thompson. *J. Infect. Dis.* **179**, 701 (1999)

5 S. Sherwani *et al.*, *PLOS ONE.* **9**, e88734 (2014)

6 S.T. Brown, J. Weinberger. *J. Am. Vener. Dis. Assoc.* **1**, 35 (1974)

7 A. Braue *et al.,Pediatr. Dermatol.***22**, 287 (2005)

8 K.Y. Choong, L.J. Roberts.*Australas. J. Dermatol.* **40**, 89 (1999)

9 J.R. Olsen *et al.,Lancet Infect. Dis.***15**, 190 (2015)

10 K. Birthistle, D. Carrington. *J. Infect.* **34**, 21 (1997)*

11 K. Damevska, A. Emurlai. *N Engl J Med.***377**, e30 (2017)

12 N. Walker. *Br. J. Dermatol.* **22**, 284 (1910)

13 B. Oren, S.O. Wende. *Infection.***19**, 159 (1991)

14 K. Niizeki *et al.,Dermatologica.* **169**, 197 (1984)

15 K. Weismann. *UgeskrLaeger.* **135**, 2151 (1973)

16 N.B. Silverberg. *Adv. Dermatol.***20**, 23 (2004)

17 N.B. Silverberg, R. Sidbury, A.J. Mancini. *J. Am. Acad. Dermatol.* **43**, 503 (2000)

18 N. Butala, E. Siegfried, Weissler A. *Pediatrics.* **131**, e1650 (2013)

19 J.J. Schwartz. *J. Am. Acad. Dermatol.* **27**, 583 (1992)

20 H. Basdag, B.M. Rainier, B.A. Cohen. *Pediatr.Dermatol.***32**, 353 (2015)

21 M. Ianhez *et al., An. Bras. Dermatol.***86**, 74 (2011)

22 R.J. Reed, R.P. Parkinson. *Am. J. Surg. Pathol.* **1**, 161 (1977)

23 Y. Li *et al., J. Clin. Microbiol.***48**, 268 (2010)

24 Editorial Office. *Evid Based Child Health.* **6**, 1600 (2011)

25 R. Eldridge, J.E. Casida. *Toxicol. Appl. Pharmacol.***130**, 95 (1995)

26 D. Hanna *et al., Pediatr.Dermatol.***23**, 574 (2006)

27 X. Chen, A.V. Anstey, J.J. Bugert. *Lancet Infect .Dis.* **13**; 877 (2013)*

28 C.M. Randall, J.L.Shisler. *Future Virology.***8**, 561 (2013)

29 K.A. Katz. *Lancet. Infect. Dis.* **14**, 372 (2014)

30 D. Calista, A. Boschini, G. Landi. *Eur. J. Dermatol.* **9**, 211 (1999)

31 C. Erickson, M. Driscoll, A. Gaspari. *Arch. Dermatol.* **147**652 (2011)

32 J. Hourihane *et al., Arch. Dis. Child.* **80**, 77 (1999)

NONGENITAL CUTANEOUS WARTS

What are nongenital cutaneous warts?

Benign epithelial proliferations caused by infection of skin with human papillomaviruses.

What are human papillomaviruses (HPVs)?

These are viruses with circular double-stranded DNA genomes about 8kb in length in the family *Papillomaviridae*. The viruses are non-enveloped with icosahedral capsids. HPVs are very diverse with > 160 different types *(1, 2)*.

How are HPVs broadly subdivided?

HPVs infect squamous epithelium in the majority of cases and can be classified clinically into types which infect <u>nongenital</u> skin and those which infect <u>anogenital</u> skin and mucous membranes. Furthermore, HPV types can be classified as *'low-risk'* or *'high-risk'* depending on their potential to become cancerous. For example, HPV types encountered commonly are HPV 1, 2, 27 and 57 which commonly cause benign cutaneous warts while HPV 6 and 11 are transmitted sexually and cause condylomataacuminata (genital warts) of the anogenital skin and mucosae. These too are generally benign. In contrast, sexually transmitted types HPV 16 and 18 have high oncogenic potential and may progress to high-grade precancerous lesions and neoplasia, particularly in the cervix *(3, 4)*. Furthermore, at least 11 other high-risk HPV types are linked to cancer in other sites including vulva, vagina, penis, anus and head-and-neck *(5, 6)*.

EPIDEMIOLOGY

What are the risk factors for acquiring cutaneous warts?

Warts are ubiquitous in the general population, particularly among schoolchildren in whom the prevalence varies from 4% - 33%, but only a small proportion of children with warts present to general practitioners, usually cases with larger and inconvenient warts *(7, 8)*. Risk factors include the presence of a family member with warts and high prevalence (≥ 40%) of skin warts in the school class, both of which presumably reflect exposure of children to viral loads sufficiently high to cause skin infection *(7, 9)*. While the use of public swimming pools and communal showers is regarded as a risk factor for transmission of warts, evidence supporting this route is limited and contradictory *(7, 10)*. Warts occur more frequently on the hands of butchers and other meat and fish handlers than among other adults in the general population, possibly related to a constituent present in animal flesh which preferentially promotes replication of HPV 7 in human skin *(11)*. Decreased cellular immunity predisposes to development of persistent and extensive skin warts in immunocompromised individuals such as HIV-positive patients with low CD4 counts and solid organ transplantation recipients *(12, 13)*. Similarly, rapid spread and persistence of warts occur in individuals with epidermodysplasia verruciformis (EDV). This rare genetic condition is usually inherited in an autosomal recessive manner. EDV patients have defective cell-mediated immunity and an increased risk of non-melanoma skin cancer *(14)*.

TRANSMISSION

By what route are cutaneous warts acquired?

It appears that individuals with warts are the main source, and those with persistent subclinical infection are a source of continuing HPV transmission. Human papillomavirus (HPV) virus infects skin by direct contact. Breaches in the epidermis predisposes individuals to inoculation with HPV as does mascerated skin; both probably allow viral transmission *(15)*. Autoinoculation is the usual route of transmission to other body sites, for example, transfer of hand warts to other locations by scratching. In addition, transmission of HPV via fomites and environmental surfaces has been hypothesised. HPV is shed from skin in dehydrated squames and may remain infectious within these cells for 7 days at room temperature, raising the possibility for HPV transmission via contaminated environmental surfaces *(16, 17)*. However, robust epidemiological evidence of indirect transmission of HPV via fomites or environmental contamination is lacking.

What advice should be given to individuals with skin warts to reduce potential transmission?

While there is no formal advice from public health authorities, common sense measures would be to avoid scratching lesions thereby reducing autoinoculation, and covering warts with a plaster, both at home and in school class where warts seem primarily to be transmitted *(9)*.

CLINICAL FEATURES

How are nongenital cutaneous warts subtyped clinically?

Cutaneous warts can be subtyped by their morphology and location *(15, 18)*. Common warts (verrucae vulgaris) are rough hyperkeratotic papules, 3 to 10 mm in diameter seen most commonly on the dorsum of hands and less frequently on the knees and other body sites such as skin around nails (periungal warts). Plantar warts are common warts located on the sole of the foot which characteristically have thick overlying skin (callus) which can be painful at pressure points. Mosaic warts are clusters of plantar warts usually covered by a callus. Gentle paring of skin on the sole will confirm plantar warts if there are pinpoint areas of bleeding indicating the presence of capillaries which are not found in calluses. Flat warts (verrucae plana) are usually located on the face, neck and dorsum of the hand. They differ from common warts by their smooth, flat topped, flesh or tan-coloured papular appearance and smaller size (2 to 4 mm in diameter). Occasionally, flat warts on the hand appear as linear streaks, a consequence of trauma to warts and spread of infection in the line of trauma (Köbner phenomenon). Filiform warts are long, thread-like warts with a narrow base and verrucous tip. Digitate warts are filiform warts arranged in a finger-like pattern. While filiform warts may be seen on the face of children, digitate warts are common on the scalp.

What is the differential diagnosis?

Warts can be mistaken for other keratotic lesions on the hands, feet or the face seen commonly in clinical practice such as thin actinic keratoses, knuckle pads, calluses, corns, lichen planus, seborrhoeic keratoses and, rarely, squamous cell carcinomas or melanocytic lesions. Conversely, malignant melanomas may have a verrucous and depigmented appearance and squamous cell carcinomas may resemble warts. Therefore, biopsy of lesions should be considered if a typical warty lesion shows altered biological behaviour or an unusual response to therapy.

TREATMENT OF NONGENITAL CUTANEOUS WARTS

When should nongenital cutaneous warts be treated in healthy individuals?

Patients will commonly request treatment when warts are painful and impair function or when there are cosmetic concerns and associated social stigma. Most warts resolve spontaneously without treatment within a few years (19, 20). Therefore, reassurance should be the mainstay of management in asymptomatic cases.

Which treatments are commonly used in primary care for common and plantar warts?

There is no definitive cure for human papillomavirus. In addition, definitive recommendations on treatment of nongenital cutaneous warts are limited by paucity of quality studies of therapeutic interventions. Topical salicyclic acid and cryotherapy are the most common treatments for common and plantar warts (21). Salicyclic acid acts by exfoliating the infected epithelium and probably stimulates a local immune response. It is useful for hyperkeratotic lesions such as periungal and plantar warts. The lesions should be soaked in warm water for 5 minutes, then pared down and the skin dried before application of the agent (21). Application to facial and anogenital lesions should be avoided due to severe irritation and scarring (22). Cryotherapy involves application of liquid nitrogen to warts with a cotton bud or a spray gun. It is painful and should be avoided in young children. However, treatment with cryotherapy alone is of questionable value since a 2012 Cochrane review of randomised trials did not find a statistically significant benefit of cryotherapy over placebo (23). Salicylic acid was shown to be superior to placebo for treatment of cutaneous warts with no difference in outcome between common and plantar warts *(23)*. Three cycles of cryotherapy while continuing salicylic acid is recommended as the second line treatment for warts which are not responding to salicylic acid alone although of unproven efficacy *(21, 23, 24, 25)*.

How are plane warts and filiform warts usually treated in primary care?

Plane (flat) warts, which occur on the face and dorsum of the hands, are mainly a cosmetic problem and will regress spontaneously *(21)*. Salicylic acid and cryotherapy are unsuitable for treatment of facial warts because they may cause scarring. In addition, there are limited efficacy data on treatment of plane warts with salicylic acid, cryotherapy and other treatments such as dithranol, imiquimod, 5-fluoruracil and tretinoin *(26, 27, 28, 29)*. Because of the small pedunculated nature of filiform warts, surgical removal and cryotherapy can be used *(21)*.

When should patients with nongenital cutaneous warts be referred to a dermatologist?

Referral to a dermatology clinic should be considered if treatments used in primary care are unsuccessful after 12 weeks, or when the diagnosis is uncertain or there are extensive lesions and patient concern for cosmesis or the patient is immunocompromised *(24)*.

What potential therapeutic options for nongenital warts may be used by dermatologists?

The antiviral agent cidofovir, which inhibits viral and cellular DNA polymerases leading finally to apoptosis of proliferating epithelium, has been used topically and intralesionally for HPV lesions and is well tolerated *(30, 31)*. Bleomycin is a glycopeptide antibiotic used to treat recalcitrant cutaneous warts. It has antiviral and antimitotic properties and is applied topically or intralesionally with response rates varying from 16% to 94% *(23)*. Like bleomycin, 5-fluorouracil is an antimitotic agent shown to be beneficial in treatment of cutaneous warts when applied topically or by intralesional injection *(32, 33)*. Immunotherapy with topical imiquimod acts by stimulating a robust antiviral immune response *(34)*. While it is an established treatment for genital warts, its effectiveness against nongenital cutaneous warts is unclear due to a lack of randomised controlled trials. Other potential treatments include pulsed dye laser and laser treatment with CO_2 *(35, 36)*.

REFERENCES

1 H.U. Bernard *et al.*,*Virology*. **401**,70 (2010)

2 R.D. Burk, A Harani, Z Chen. *Virology*.**445**, 232 (2013)

3 J.M Walboomers. *J.Pathol.* **189**, 12 (1999)

4 B.X. Bosch *et al.,J.Clin.Pathol.***55**, 244(2002)

5 J.Doorbar. *J.Clin.Virol.***32S**, S7(2005)

6 A.Psyrri, D DiMaio. *Nat.Clin.Pract.Oncol.***5**, 24 (2008)

7 F.M. van Haalen *et al.*, *Br. J. Dermatol.* **161**, 148 (2009)

8 R.S. Mohammedamin *et al.*, *Eur. J. Gen. Pract.***14**, 34 (2008)

9 S.C. Bruggink *et al.,Pediatrics.***131**, 928 (2013)

10 M.V.Rigo *et al.*, *Aten Primaria.***31**, 415 (2003)

11M. Keefe et al., *Br. J.Dermatol.* **130**, 9 (1994)

12 P. Barbosa.*Clin.Podiatr. Med. Surg.***15**, 317 (1998)

13 S.Jablonska *et al.,Clin.Dermatol.***15**, 309 (1997)

14 S.Majewski, S Jablonska. *Arch.Dermatol.* **138**, 649 (2002)

15 N.B. Silverberg. *AdvDermatol.* **20**, 23 (2004)

16 R.B.Roden, D.R. Lowy, J.T. Schiller. *J. Infect. Dis.* **176**, 1076(1997)

17 A.M.Surovy, R.E. Hunger. *N. Engl. J. Med.* **365**, 548 (2011)

18 R. Young *et al.*, *J. Cut. Med. Surg.* **2**, 78 (1997)

19 E.M. Massing, W.L. Epstein.*Arch.Dermatol.* **87**, 306 (1963)

20 H.C. Williams, A. Pottier, D. Strachan. *Br. J.Dermatol.* **128**, 504 (1993)

21 J.C. Sterling *et al.*, *Br. J.Dermatol.* **171**, 696 (2014)

22 A. Rivera, S.K.Tyring. *DermatolTher.* **17**, 441 (2004)

23 C.S. Kwok *et al.,Cochrane Database Syst. Rev.* **9**, CD001781 (2012)

24 J. Lynch, M.D. Cliffe, R. Morris-Jones. *BMJ.***348**, g3339; doi: 10. 1136/bmj.g3339 (2014)

25 K. Steele, W.G. Irwin. *J. R. Coll. Gen.Pract.***38**, 256 (1988)

26 V.Mirceva *et al.*, *AktuelleDermatol.***34**, 428 (2008)

27 M.B. Kim *et al.*, *J. Eur. Acad.Dermatol.Venereol.***20**, 1349 (2006)

28 S. Lee, J.G. Kim, SI Chun. *Dermatologica.***160**, 383 (1980)

29 M. al Aboosi. *Int. J. Dermatol.***33**, 826 (1994)

30 G.L. Padilla *et al.*, *Dermatol. Ther.***27**, 89 (2014)

31 P.Broganelli *et al.*, *Dermatol.Ther.***25**, 468 (2012)

32 A.Iscimen *et al.*, *J. Eur. Acad.Dermatol.Venereol.***18**, 455 (2004)

33 A.Yazdanfar *et al.,Dermatol. Surg.***34**, 656 (2008)

34 S.K.Tyring, I.Arany, M.A. Stanley. *J. Infect. Dis.***2**, 551 (1998)

35 T.Passeron *et al.*, *Ann.Dermatol.Venereol.***134**, 135 (2007)

36 T.Mitsuishi *et al.*, *Dermatol. Surg.***36**, 1401 (2010)

TRAVEL-RELATED VIRAL INFECTIONS

Arboviruses

- Dengue virus
- West Nile virus
- Zika virus
- Chikungunya virus

Rabies

ARBOVIRUSES

Recent data suggest that between 43-79% of travellers to Africa and Asia acquire a travel-related illness during or after visiting these regions, of which diarrhoeal disease is the commonest *(1)*. An important challenge for GPs is the presentation of a returned traveller with fever without a focus. Dengue virus (DENV), chikungunya virus (CHIKV), West Nile virus (WNV) and Zika virus (ZIKV) are common causes of undifferentiated febrile illnesses in returned travellers. These viruses are transmitted to humans through bites of infected mosquitoes and are termed arthropod-borne viruses (arboviruses). These vector-borne diseases are imported into Ireland by travellers returning from endemic areas. Other common causes of acute systemic febrile illness in returned travellers include malaria and typhoid fever *(2)*. A thorough history, physical examination and laboratory tests are important in determining the aetiology of any suspected case of tropical disease.

What are the common arboviruses?

DENV, WNV and ZIKV are RNA viruses belonging to the genus *flavivirus* within the family *Flaviviridae*. There are four serotypes of DENV, 1 to 4. Infection with one serotype confers lifelong immunity but does not provide protection against the other serotypes. CHIKV is an alphavirus belonging to the family *Togaviridae*. DENV, ZIKV and CHIKV are primarily transmitted to humans from day-biting mosquitoes, *Aedesaegypti* and *Aedesalbopictus*. WNV is transmitted by bites from mosquitoes of the *Culex*species.

DENV

What are the common clinical features likely to be seen in general practice?

Most people infected with DENV remain asymptomatic, although mild presentations as transient 'influenza-like illnesses' are common. Among clinical cases, the typical incubation period is 4-8 days (maximum 14 days). Dengue fever usually presents with abrupt onset of fever, retro-orbital headache, severe myalgia (hence the term 'breakbone fever'), arthralgia, nausea and sometimes a transient macular rash. Petechiae may occur at sites of compression such as with a tourniquet, and bruising can be seen at venipuncture sites. Laboratory findings usually include leukopenia and thrombocytopenia, with mildly raised liver function tests. Most patients recover clinically within 7 days and laboratory parameters return to normal. In a proportion of patients who recover, a second self-limiting maculopapular rash may appear *(3)*.

What is severe dengue fever?

Severe dengue fever can arise in a small proportion of patients after the initial phase of infection, although this is rarely seen in travellers *(4)*. This phase of the disease is characterised by haemorrhagic manifestations, thrombocytopenia and capillary leak syndrome (haemoconcentration, serosal effusions and/or hypoproteinaemia). Previous exposure to one serotype of DENV (primary infection) seems to predispose to severe dengue fever when a person is subsequently infected with a different serotype (secondary infection), known as antibody-dependent enhancement *(5)*.

What virology tests are recommended for diagnosis of suspected DENV infection?

Serum can be tested for the DENV antigen, non-structural protein 1 (NS1), and IgM/IgG antibody to DENV (anti-DENV IgM /IgG). NS1 antigen is usually detectable in the first 7-9 days after onset of fever *(6)*. Anti-DENV IgM and IgG become detectable in blood around day 5 and day 9, respectively, after illness onset in primary infection.

WNV

What are the clinical features of WNV infection?

WNV may be acquired in tropical areas but is also endemicin the United States *(17)*. The incidence in the US peaks annually between July and September. It is estimated that symptomatic disease develops in about 25% of those infected *(18)*. The incubation period ranges from 2 to 14 days. The clinical course is usually characterised by sudden onset of a self-limited influenza-like illness with appearance of a maculopapular, non-pruritic rash around the time of defervescence. Less than 1% of all cases develop neuroinvasive disease including meningitis, encephalitis, acute flaccid paralysis and other neurological illnesses like Parkinsonism and Guillain-Barré syndrome *(19)*. WNV-related neuroinvasive disease is associated with long-term morbidity and has a fatality rate of 5-10%. Treatment of neuroinvasive disease is supportive care. There is no licensed human vaccine currently. Preventive measures include use of insecticides to reduce mosquito populations and personal protection against insect bites by use of insect repellants and wearing long-sleeved shirts and trousers *(17)*.

What virology test is recommended for diagnosis of suspected WNV infection?

In non-neuroinvasive disease, serum can be tested for IgM antibody to WNV (anti-WNV IgM). WNV RNA can be detected in urine for several weeks and should be tested in addition to serology *(20)*. In neuroinvasive disease, serum and cerebrospinal fluid (CSF) should be tested for anti-WNV IgM / IgG. Detection of anti-WNV IgM in CSF is highly suggestive of neuroinvasive disease. WNV RNA is detected transiently in serum and CSF, and is usually absent on clinical presentation.

ZIKV

In which geographical areas is ZIKV endemic?

An outbreak of ZIKV infection began in Brazil in May 2015 and spread throughout the

Americas. Transmission of ZIKV by the *Aedes* mosquito is endemic in the Caribbean and most countries in Central and South America. (For areas of risk for ZIKV infection see reference *(7)*).

What are the common clinical features of ZIKV infection as seen in general practice?

Most infected persons will not develop clinical illness. In those who do become ill, the incubation period ranges from 3-14 days. Symptoms are similar to those of dengue fever but usually milder; fever, arthralgia, myalgia, an itchy maculopapular rash and non-purulent conjunctivitis *(8)*. ZIKV is a cause of a number of neurological disorders including Guillain-Barré syndrome in adults and, in fetuses and newborns, structural brain abnormalities, including microcephaly and the congenital Zika syndrome *(9, 10)*. Birth defects occur most frequently in fetuses and neonates born to mothers infected with ZIKV early in pregnancy *(11)*. Women should avoid travel to ZIKV-endemic areas, particularly in early pregnancy.

What are the implications for heterosexual couples of sexual transmission of ZIKV?

ZIKV can be transmitted by sexual intercourse. It is more likely to occur from male to female than female to male *(12)*. Most sexual transmissions of ZIKV occur within 19 days of symptom onset in the male *(13)*. Late sexual transmission, 44 days after illness onset in the male partner, suggests persistence of ZIKV in semen *(14)*. Recent evidence suggests that most men clear ZIKV RNA from semen within 4 months of symptom onset *(15)*. Current advice for males is to use condoms or abstain from sex for at least 3 months after illness onset or last possible exposure (if asymptomatic). For women who were infected with ZIKV or exposed to it, they should wait at least 8 weeks from onset of illness or last possible exposure (if asymptomatic) before attempting to conceive *(16)*.

What virology tests are recommended currently for diagnosis of suspected ZIKV infection?

Serum or plasma and urine should be sent for ZIKV RNA testing in symptomatic persons with suspected ZIKV infection who develop illness within 4 weeks of returning from an endemic area or after last possible exposure. In addition, request IgM / IgG antibody to ZIKV (anti-ZIKV IgM / IgG). If ≥ 4 weeks since onset of illness or last possible exposure, send serum for anti-ZIKV IgM / IgG only.

CHIKV

What is the etymology of CHIKV?

The name chikungunya is derived from the language of the Makonde, a tribe living in Tanzania, and means 'that which bends up', referring to the stooped posture of patients with severe arthralgia caused by CHIKV infection *(21)*.

What are the common clinical features likely to be seen in general practice?

The typical incubation period in CHIKV infection is 2-4 days (maximum 14 days). Although unrelated taxonomically to DENV and ZIKV, CHIKV causes similar clinical features such as abrupt onset of fever, myalgia, headache, rash, nausea and vomiting, with characteristically disabling arthralgias. Symmetrical polyarthralgia involving the small and medium joints (interphalangeal joints, ankles, knees and wrists) is the most common clinical manifestation of CHIKV infection (22). Unlike dengue, haematological findings of leukopenia and thrombocytopenia are less pronounced in chikungunya fever and a bleeding diathesis is rare, however, raised serum creatinine kinase levels and hypocalcaemia may be found. An array of mucocutaneous lesions may occur in 40-50% of those with chikungunya fever, in particular aphthous-like ulcers and/or morbilliform eruptions (23). Joint problems may persist from weeks to years in a proportion of patients (25%-52%) following CHIKV infection, ranging from mild arthralgia to full-blown arthritis (24). Mortality is rare in CHIKV infection and usually due to an underlying comorbidity.

What virology tests are available for diagnosis of suspected CHIKV infection?

IgM/IgG antibody to CHIKV (anti-CHIKV IgM/IgG) usually become detectable in serum > 5 days are onset of symptoms. A convalescent serum should be tested if an initial serum sample, collected < 5 days after illness onset in a suspected case, is anti-CHIKV IgM/IgG negative (25). CHIKV RNA can be detected by real-time reverse transcription polymerase chain reaction in serum/plasma ≤ 5 days after onset of illness but is currently unavailable here.

Is there an antiviral agent available to treat infection due to the above arboviruses?

There is no specific antiviral drug licensed for treatment of DENV, CHIKV, ZIKV and WNV infections. Management is entirely supportive. Bed rest and adequate hydration are recommended. Acetaminophen is recommended for analgesia and as an antipyretic. Aspirin and nonsteroidal anti-inflammatory drugs (NSAIDs) should be avoided because of their anticoagulant properties and the risk of Reye syndrome. For CHIKV-infected persons with persistent arthralgia, NSAID use may be considered and, when arthralgia is refractory to other analgesics, hydroxychloroquine is an option (26).

CASE VIGNETTE

A 32-year-old female presented to her GP with acute onset of fever, malaise, myalgia, arthralgia, headache and nausea. She had returned from an 8-day honeymoon to the Caribbean 48 hours before onset of illness. On examination, her vital signs were normal except for a temperature of 39.1°C and she had a confluent erythematous rash, with areas of unaffected skin on her abdomen and lower limbs. The GP suspected a tropical infection causing a febrile illness without a focus.

What questions did the GP ask to determine her exposure risks while abroad?

Was she bitten by insects (mosquitoes, ticks, flies, mites or lice) while in the Caribbean?

She was bitten multiple times by mosquitoes.

Did she have pretravel vaccinations and malaria prophylaxis?

She received typhoid fever and hepatitis A vaccines. She took malaria prophylaxis as recommended.

Did she have any comorbidity such as diabetes or was she taking immunosuppressants?

She was otherwise healthy. She was not pregnant.

Did she consume improperly cooked food?

She did not eat salads or raw foods. She drank bottled water.

Did she have exposure to fresh water?

She swam in the hotel swimming pool. She did not participate in water sports (kayaking, canoeing) in rivers or lakes.

Did she have unprotected sexual intercourse with multiple partners?

She was in a monogamous relationship.

Had she close contact with ill persons or with animals including pet birds?

No.

Which common pathogens cause tropical diseases with short incubation periods (< 14 days) in returned travellers from the Caribbean and other geographic regions?

Caribbean: DENV, CHIK, ZIKV, WNV, malaria (mostly *Plasmodium vivax*) and leptospirosis.

Central America: DENV, CHIK, ZIKV, WNV, malaria (mostly *P. vivax*) and leptospirosis.

South America: DENV, CHIK, ZIKV, WNV, malaria (mostly *P. vivax*) and leptospirosis.

South Central Asia: DENV, CHIK, ZIKV, WNV, malaria (non-falciparum), typhoid fever and leptospirosis.

Southeast Asia: DENV, CHIK, ZIKV, WNV, malaria (non-falciparum), rickettsia and leptospirosis.

Sub-Saharan Africa: DENV, CHIK, ZIKV, WNV, malaria (mainly *P. falciparum*) and tickborne rickettsia.

For more information see *(27)*.

Which laboratory investigations did the GP request?

A blood sample (EDTA bottle) was sent for haematology profile which showed a low white cell count: neutrophils 0.8 mm^{-3} and lymphocytes 0.6 mm^{-3}, and thrombocytopenia (platelets 81 x 10^3 mm^{-3}). Haematocrit was normal (40%). The GP requested a malaria screen also; malaria antigen was negative and confirmed by thick and thin blood films. A repeat blood sample collected several days later was also negative for malaria. **Malaria should be excluded in all travellers with a febrile illness returning from endemic areas even if they adhered to prophylaxis** *(28)*. A serum sample sent for biochemistry, including electrolytes and liver function tests, was normal. Another serum was sent for 'further investigations'.

Which virology tests did the laboratory perform?

Based on the travel history and clinical details, the serum sample for 'further investigations' was tested for DENV NS1 antigen and anti-DENV IgM/IgG, and anti-CHIKV IgM/IgG. DENV NS1 antigen was positive and anti-DENV IgM/IgG were negative, consistent with an early primary DENV infection. A repeat serum sample tested 10 days after onset of illness was anti-DENV IgM/IgG positive, confirming seroconversion to DENV. Anti-CHIKV IgM/IgG were negative. Serum and urine were sent to test for ZIKV RNA by the real-time reverse transcription polymerase chain reaction (rRT-PCR) assay; viral RNA was not detected. Testing for WNV is only done for patients with negative results for the above arboviruses and for travellers with clinical details of abnormal neurological findings. Leptospirosis IgM antibody in serum was negative.

MANAGEMENT

What clinical follow-up was performed in this case?

The GP prescribed acetaminophen (paracetamol). The patient was referred to the Infectious Diseases clinic. She was evaluated daily with a full blood count to monitor haematocrit and platelet values. Six days after presenting to the GP she was clinically much improved and laboratory parameters were normal.

What warning signs would indicate the need for hospital admission?

Persistent fever (> 5 days), any bleeding subcutaneously or through any orifice, decreased urine output, hypotension and/or confusion should alert the physician to the possibility of severe dengue. Laboratory findings including an increase in haematocrit, decrease in platelet count and unstable haemodynamic status portend onset of severe illness *(29)*.

The woman and her husband avoided conception for 3 months after returning from the ZIKV-endemic area, as recommended. The couple wanted to attempt conception. They asked the GP for a virology test for ZIKV to reassure them. What did he advise?

The GP collected a serum sample for anti-ZIKV IgM / IgG. Antibody results were negative indicating no recent infection with ZIKV. If the anti-ZIKV IgM/IgG are negative in serum collected ≥ 4 weeks after returning from an endemic area or last possible exposure, then recent ZIKV infection is very unlikely.

Is there a vaccine available for pre-travel immunisation against DENV?

Not yet. The only licensed DENV vaccine increases the risk for serious DENV fever and hospitalisation in patients with no previous exposure to the virus. The vaccine is efficacious and safe in individuals with serological evidence of previous exposure to DENV (30). Since most travellers are from countries in which DENV is not endemic, they should not receive this vaccine. It is thought that the vaccine acts like a primary infection in previously unexposed individuals, potentially exacerbating subsequent infection following natural exposure to a different viral serotype (31).

REFERENCES (*useful reviews)

1 K.M. Angelo *et al.*, *J. Travel Med.* **24**, doi:10.1093/jtm/tax046 (2017)

2 K. Leder*et al.*, *Ann. Intern. Med.* **158**, 456 (2013)

3 C.P. Simmons *et al.*, *N. Engl. J. Med.* **366**, 1423 (2012)

4 V. Johnston *et al.*, *J. Infect.* **59**, 1 (2009)

5 S. Yasmin, M. Mukerjee.*Scientific American.***4**, 38 (2019)

6 V. Tricou *et al.*, *BMC Infect. Dis.* **10**, 142 (2010)

7 https://www.cdc.gov/zika/index.html

8 L.R. Petersen *et al.*, *N. Engl. J. Med.* **374**, 1552 (2016)

9 N. Brout et *et al.*,*N. Engl. J. Med.* **74**, 1506 (2016)

10 C.A. Moore *et al.*,*JAMA Pediatr.***171**, 288 (2017)

11 B. Hoen *et al.*, *N. Engl. J. Med.* **378**, 985 (2018)

12 M.J.Counotte *et al.*,*PLoS Med.* **15**, e1002611 (2018)

13 G. Venturi*et al.*, *Euro. Surveill.***21**, pii=30148 (2016)

14 J.M. Turmel *et al.*, *Lancet.* **387**, 2501 (2016)

15G. Paz-Baily *et al.*, *N. Engl. J. Med.* **379**, 1234 (2018)

16 K.D. Polen *et al.*, *MMWR Morb. Mortal. Wkly. Rep.* **67**, 868 (2018)

17 E.J. Curren *et al.*, *MMWR Morb. Mortal. Wkly. Rep.* **67**, 1137 (2018)

18 S. Zou *et al.*, *J. Infect Dis.* **202**, 1354 (2010)

19 J. Hart Jr *et al.*, *BMC Infect. Dis.* **14**, 248 (2014)

20 V. Parkash *et al.*, *Emerg. Infect. Dis.* **25**, 367 (2019)

21Centers for Disease Control.*Emerg. Infect. Dis.* **12**, 1772, (2006)

22 K.B. Gibney *et al.*, *Clin. Infect. Dis.* **52**, e121 (2011)

23 D. Bandyopadhay, S.K. Ghosh. *Indian J. Dermatol.***55**, 64 (2010)

24 A.Y. Chang *et al.*, *Arthritis Rheumatol.* **70**, 578 (2018)

25 S.C. Weaver, M Lecuit. *N. Engl. J. Med.***372**, 1231 (2015)

26 http://www.who.int/iris/handle/10665/205178

27   https://wwwnc.cdc.gov/travel/yellowbook/post-travel-evaluation/general-approach-to-the-returned-traveler

28 G.E. Thwaites, N.P.J. Day. *N. Engl. J. Med.* **376**, 548 (2017)*

29 http://www.wpro.who.int/mvp/documents/handbook_for_clinical_management_of_dengue.pdf

30 S. Sridhar *et al.*, *N. Engl. J. Med.* **379**, 327 (2018)

31 A. Wilder-Smith. *J. Travel Med.* **25**, doi:10.1093/jtm/tay057 (2018)

RABIES

What is rabies?

Rabies is an acute progressive encephalitis transmissible from certain animals to humans (zoonosis) with a reported fatality rate of almost 100%. The virus commonly causing rabies in humans is rabies virus (RABV) which is the prototype of the lyssavirus genus. Rabies causes almost 60,000 deaths annually, mainly in Africa and Asia with infected domestic dogs being the most common source of viral transmission (1). Other RABV-related lyssaviruses are all species in the genus *Lyssavirus* other than the prototypical RABV. They are also capable of causing fatal encephalitis in mammals, and a small number of human cases have been documented (2, 3). Rabies is not endemic in Western Europe and Australia. As regards North America, domestic animals are, where appropriate, fully vaccinated, but wild animal species may carry rabies. Travellers to Asia and Africa from Ireland and the UK should, however, be aware of the real risk to them from animal species especially dogs, and so modify their usual behaviour towards such animals. Travellers should be advised to avoid contact with wild or domestic animals, not to attract stray animals by offering food or by being careless with litter, and to be aware that certain activities may attract dogs (e.g. running, cycling). There is no specific antiviral treatment for rabies and prevention relies on the assessment of risk following or anticipating a possible exposure.

POSTEXPOSURE PROPHYLAXIS

In countries where animal rabies is endemic, bites from any mammalian species must be promptly reviewed with a view to offer prophylaxis. Post-exposure prophylaxis (PEP) against rabies is very effective when used straight away. Prophylaxis with active and passive immunisation is facilitated by the relatively long incubation period of rabies. There are three important components of PEP:

Prompt local treatment of the wound by abundant washing and flushing it with soap or detergent to reduce the viral load at the inoculation site (4).

Infiltration of all wounds with rabies immune globulin (RIG) early after exposure. Thisneutralises RABV at the wound site before it enters neurons.

Complete vaccination according to recommended schedules. This induces production of rabies-specific virus neutralising antibodies which, like RIG, neutralise the virus extra-neurally.

What is a potential exposure to RABV?

Any penetration of the skin by a bite or scratch from an animal known to have rabies or exhibiting rabid behaviour.

When saliva or other potentially infectious material (tears, cerebrospinal fluid or neural tissue) is introduced into mucous membranes or an open wound on the skin.

When there is direct contact with a bat and bites or scratches from the animal cannot be ruled out.

NB - It is not always possible to confirm exposure in which case the potential for an exposure having occurred has to be assessed.

What other factors are relevant when considering use of PEP against rabies because a bite has been reported?

Country where exposure occurred: to check if a country is rabies-endemic www.who-rabies-bulletin.org

Has the individual exposed to rabies been vaccinated previously (relevant to schedule of PEP)?

If animal was apparently healthy at time of exposure, did it become ill or change its behaviour in the following 10 days?

Was the animal known to have been vaccinated, risk of rabies is very low but should be considered?

Any unprovoked attack by a mammal in a rabies-endemic area, especially a dog bite, is of concern for rabies.

Who should be contacted when exposure to RABV is suspected?

The local Public Health Team should be contacted at
www.hpsc.ie/hpsc/NotifiableDiseases/Whotonotify/File,13160,en.pdf

What schedule is used when PEP against rabies is indicated?

The regimen for PEP against rabies in those who were previously unvaccinated consists of one dose of rabies immune globulin (RIG) and four doses of rabies vaccine on days 0, 3, 7 and 14 (for immunocompromised persons an extra dose is given on day 30) *(5)*. The RIG should only be infiltrated into all wounds caused by the animal attack. The RIG is not given after day 7 of the PEP vaccination series because an antibody response to vaccine is likely to have occurred *(6)*. If the exposed person had prior vaccination, only two doses of vaccine are needed on days 0 and 3.

What type of rabies vaccine is available in Ireland?

Two types of rabies vaccine are licensed for use here. One vaccine is produced in human diploid cell culture and the other is produced in chick embryo cell culture *(7)*. Each is inactivated. Each can be used interchangeably.

CLINICAL SCENARIOS

How would you manage the risk of RABV exposure in the following scenarios?

A 21-year-old male jogger was bitten on the leg by a stray dog in Dublin City.

Ireland is rabies-free and rabies PEP is not recommended. The risk of rabies from a dog bite is negligible. The wound should be cleansed, antibiotics prescribed, and tetanus vaccine given if appropriate.

A 28-year-old female was bitten on the hand while feeding a healthy domestic dog in Cairo.

After review, PEP was not advised. The animal's health and behaviour were observed for 10 days after the incident by authorities in Egypt. The dog remained healthy. Infected animals excrete RABV for only a few days before onset of clinical disease. Therefore, the dog was not infectious at the time of the biting incident. However, if the dog became ill during observation and rabies is suspected, PEP should be given to the person and the dog euthanised with testing of brain tissue for rabies. If the latter is found to be negative, PEP can be stopped.

A hiker was bitten by a wild fox in a mountainous region of the United States.

Rabies PEP should be given promptly following high-risk exposure like a bite from a wild mammal in a rabies-endemic area unless the animal can be tested for rabies.

A bat was found flying around a bedroom in which a toddler was sleeping in an Irish city. The bat escaped and was unavailable for testing.

Rabies PEP should be given. The local Public Health Team should be informed immediately (can be found at www.hpsc.ie/hpsc/NotifiableDiseases/Whotonotify/File,13160,en.pdf).

Bat bites and scratches are tiny and may be unrecognised even after a thorough clinical examination. Also, a sleeping child is unlikely to give an accurate history of contact with the bat. Therefore, direct contact of the bat with the child's mucous membranes cannot be excluded.

Among British Daubenton's bats, lyssaviruses (European bat lyssavirus type 2a) which can cause rabies in humans are endemic, albeit at very low levels *(8, 9)*. It is likely that low-level circulation of lyssaviruses also occurs among Irish Daubenton's bats which is the main species of bat in Ireland. These bats rarely roost in houses and generally avoid contact with people. Sick bats with rabies are usually grounded or fly during daylight or may approach humans. Therefore, the public should not handle sick or dead bats. Although the likelihood of the Irish public being exposed to bat rabies is very small, health professionals should be aware of the need for assessment of rabies transmission.

A dog was seen licking the face of a one-year-old child on the grounds of a hotel in Morocco.

Rabies PEP was not needed after assessment. The concern in this case related to the potential contamination of the child's mucous membranes (mouth) and a small cut on his forehead with the dog's saliva. The hotel owner was phoned and questioned about the status of the dog 10 days after the incident. The dog was alive and healthy and therefore not infectious at the time of the biting incident. Furthermore, the owner had documentation of prior vaccination of the animal. However, as vaccinated animals may rarely develop rabies, the 10-day follow-up for potential exposure is still important.

A person was not compliant with the rabies immunisation schedule for PEP.

If the exposed person misses a dose of rabies vaccine, the scheduled course should be completed and serology testing for rabies antibody performed 7-10 days after the final dose. Contact Public Health for where testing is performed.

A healthcare worker who recently cared for a patient with rabies abroad requested PEP.

Rabies PEP was not needed following assessment of the RABV transmission risk. Healthcare workers are at risk of infection when attending RABV-infected patients if there is direct contact of broken skin or mucous membranes (mouth and conjunctiva) with the patient's saliva, respiratory secretions, tears, cerebrospinal fluid and/or neural tissue when the worker is not wearing personal protective equipment *(10)*. Assessment for PEP is then advised. While standard contact precautions are sufficient during care of patients with rabies, healthcare workers should wear gloves, gowns, masks and eye protection to reduce the risk of mucosal contamination during aerosol-generating procedures such as intubation and suctioning *(6, 11)*. Fortunately, no documented cases of nosocomial transmission have been documented so far.

PREEXPOSURE PROPHYLAXIS

Who should be immunised with rabies vaccine preexposure?

A primary three-dose vaccination course at days 0, 7 and 21-28 should be offered before exposure to individuals who are at risk of acquiring rabies: veterinarians, veterinary nursing staff, animal handlers and laboratorians handling samples from potentially rabid animals *(6)*. Others who should be offered it are travellers who are likely to have frequent animal contact in rabies-endemic areas. Routine serological testing to demonstrate seroconversion is not needed following primary vaccination.

Are booster doses of rabies vaccine needed following preexposure vaccination in Ireland?

Since Ireland is a rabies-free country, veterinarians and their staff are rarely exposed to RABV, so booster doses are not usually needed in these cohorts. Only those working with RABV in research laboratories and who are continuously or frequently exposed to the virus, such as those working with bats, need to have booster doses. For those continuously exposed, testing serum for RABV-specific antibody is done every 6 months and booster given if antibody is below the threshold value while for those with frequent exposure, serological testing should be performed every two years *(6)*.

ADDITIONAL POINTS OF INTEREST ABOUT RABIES

EPIDEMIOLOGY OF RABIES IN HUMANS

How is rabies acquired by humans?

Exposure to saliva from bites from rabid animals is the most common route of transmission from infected animals to humans *(12)*. Transmission from infected mammals occurs by biting of humans or contamination of skin abrasions or mucous membranes with virus-infected saliva. In rabies endemic areas of the world, dogs are the main source (99%) of human rabies but other animal reservoirs of RABV in the wild, including bats, raccoons, skunks, foxes and mongooses, are potential, albeit rare, sources of transmission by animal bites to humans. Sometimes, the bite from a small animal infected with rabies, like a bat, may be unrecognised by the person receiving the bite because of the tiny puncture inflicted by the bat, known as cryptic transmission *(13)*. Infected bats transmit RABV to other members of a colony by biting, grooming and under extreme circumstances in large roosts, virus may be expelled from nasal passages of infected bats through breathing, sneezing and vocalisation *(14)*. Interestingly, there have been rare reports suggesting that human infection may have been acquired by the airborne route in persons visiting caves colonised with extremely large numbers of bats *(15, 16)*. Exposure of an individual to a large inoculum of RABV aerosolised from the nasal passages, excreted saliva and urine may have been the source of infection.

Human-to-human transmission of rabies has been documented only in tissue and organ transplant recipients following transplantation from donors with unrecognised RABV infection *(17)*.

Transmission via inanimate objects is most unlikely because the virus is labile and easily inactivated by sunlight, drying and detergents *(18)*.

PATHOGENESIS AND CLINICAL FEATURES

How does rabies disease develop?

Infection begins with the introduction of virus-filled saliva into muscle at the bite site. The virus may replicate slowly here during the incubation period, usually one to three months, before entering peripheral nerves (19, 20). The virus then travels by retrograde axonal transport via motor or sensory nerves to the spinal cord and ascends to the brain (21). The virus shows a predilection for the cerebellum, hippocampus and limbic system in the brain before centrifugal spread from the central nervous system via motor, sensory and autonomic nerves to many tissues including tear and salivary glands. Therefore, the virus has already disseminated widely before onset of clinical disease (22). Spread to the salivary glands is essential for viral transmission to other hosts through bites, thereby restarting the cycle.

What are the typical clinical features of rabies?

Rabies is almost invariably fatal once clinical disease is evident. Although survivors of clinical rabies are rarely reported, these individuals have serious neurological sequelae. Most survivors had prior immunisation with rabies vaccine (23). While the incubation period is typically one to three months, it can extend to more than a year (24). The first clinical manifestation of rabies is neuropathic pain at the site of infection reflecting inflammation of the dorsal root ganglion corresponding to the site of inoculation due to transmission of virus from interconnecting, infected motor neurons (20). About 10 days later acute neurological manifestations become evident. One of two distinctive presentations occurs: encephalitic ('furious') rabies (80% of cases) and the paralytic form ('dumb') which manifests as paralysis (25). The 'furious' form is characterised by episodic aggression and agitation and other manifestations including hydrophobia, aerophobia, hypersalivation, convulsions and eventually coma (24). Hypertension, cardiac dysrhythmias, fever, sweating and priapism may develop as a result of autonomic nervous system dysfunction (26). Survival time, defined as the number of days between onset of acute neurological disease and death, varies from 7 -21 days with death caused by cardiopulmonary failure (27).

LABORATORY DIAGNOSIS

When would rabies be considered as a possible diagnosis?

A history of exposure to a potential source of infection in a rabies endemic area and the person's clinical presentation, especially with hydrophobia or aerophobia which are unique to rabies, are sufficient to raise suspicion of rabies. An explanation of the source of infection should be sought and public health authorities notified immediately.

Which laboratory tests are used ante-mortem and post-mortem to confirm the diagnosis of rabies?

The local Public Health Director will have information on testing protocol. In general, the following diagnostic approaches are performed.

Detection of RABV antigen in brain tissue is the gold standard for confirming rabies but is usually done post-mortem.

Nuchal skin biopsy can be collected ante-mortem for detection of RABV antigen by direct fluorescent antibody testing.

Saliva, tears or nuchal skin biopsy can be collected ante-mortem for detection of RABV RNA by real-time reverse transcription polymerase chain reaction (rRT-PCR).

Serum and cerebrospinal fluid (CSF) can be tested for rabies-specific IgM and IgG antibody and for rabies-specific virus neutralising antibody but these are likely to be negative early in the disease.

TREATMENT

Is there an antiviral agent of known efficacy available to treat rabies?

There is no proven treatment available currently for symptomatic rabies. Palliation is the necessary limit and standard of care. One approach which has been used is based on the principle that reducing brain injury will allow time for the patient to develop an immune response to eradicate RABV. This is known as the Milwaukee protocol (www.chw.org/display/PPF/DocID/33223/router.asp) but is no longer recommended because of its limited value *(28)*.

REFERENCES

1 A.R. Fooks *et al.*, *Lanc et.* **384**, 1389 (2014)*

2 A.C. Banyard *et al.*, *Viruses.***6**, 2974 (2014)

3 J.S. Evans *et al.*, *Vaccine.* **30**, 7447 (2012)

4 D.J. Dean, G.M. Baer, W.R. Thompson. *Bull. World Health Org.* **28**, 477 (1963)

5 C.E. Rupprecht *et al.*, *MMWR Recomm. Rep.* **59**, 1 (2010)

6 S.E. Manning *et al.*, *MMWR Recomm. Rep.* **57**, 1 (2008)

7 National Zoonoses Committee of Ireland.Rabies Prevention and Control.HPSC. 2015

8 A. Smith, J. Morris, N. Crowcroft. *BMJ.***330**, 491 (2005)

9 S.L. Harris *et al.*, *Biol. Conserv.* **131**, 193 (2006)

10 V.L. Kan *et al.*, *Clin. Infect. Dis.* **60**, 341 (2015)

11 D.J. Weber, W.A. Rutala. *Clin. Infect. Dis.* **32**, 446 (2001)

12 M.Z. Yousaf *et al.*, *Virol. J.* **9**, 50 (2012)

13 S.L. Messenger, J.S. Smith, C.E. Rupprecht. *Clin. Infect. Dis*. **35**, 738 (2002)

14 D.G. Constantine, R.W. Emmons, J.D. Woodie. *Science*.**175**, 1255 (1975)

15 J.R. Kent, M.F. Finegold. *N. Engl. J. Med*. **263**, 1058 (1960)

16 J. Irons *et al.*, *Tex. Rep. Biol. Med*. **15**, 292 (1957)

17 C.E. Rupprecht T. Nagarajan, H. Ertl.*Vaccine*.**15**, 731 (2016)

18 C.E. Ruppreecht, R.V. Gibbons. *N. Engl. J. Med*. **351**, 2626 (2004)*

19 R.E. Willoughby Jr. *Scientific Amer*. **296**, 88 (2007)

20 T. Hemachudha *et al.*, *Lancet Neurol*. **12**, 498 (2013)

21 C.R. Fisher, D.G. Streicker, M.J. Schnell. *Nat. Rev. Microbiol*. **16**, 241 (2018)*

22 G. Ugolini, T. Hemachudha. *Curr.Opin. Infect. Dis*. **31**, 93 (2018)

23 A.C. Jackson. *Curr. Infect. Dis. Rep*. **18**(11), 35 (2017)

24 S.A. Plotkin. *Clin. Infect. Dis*. **30**, 4 (2000)

25 C.S. Mani, D.L. Murray. *Pediatr. Rev*. **27**, 129 (2006)

26 D.M. Greer *et al.*, *N. Engl. J. Med*. **368**, 172 (2013)

27S.J. Udow, R.A. Marrie, A.C. Jackson. *Clin. Infect. Dis*. **57**, 689 (2013)

28 A.C. Jackson. *Antiviral. Res*. **99**, 61 (2013)

A Practical Guide to

Designing
the invisible

by Robert Mills

A Practical Guide to Designing the invisible
by Robert Mills

Published in 2012 by Five Simple Steps
Studio Two, The Coach House
Stanwell Road
Penarth
CF64 3EU
United Kingdom

On the web: *www.fivesimplesteps.com*
and: *www.designingtheinvisible.com*
Please send errors to *errata@fivesimplesteps.com*

Publisher: Five Simple Steps
Development Editor: Simon Mackie
Copy Editor: Bill Harper
Production Editor: Emma Boulton
Production Manager: Sarah Morris
Design & Art Director: Nick Boulton, Mark Boulton
Typesetting: Nick Boulton, Colin Kersley

ISBN: 978-1-907828-06-5

A catalogue record of this book is available from the British Library.

FOREWORD

Mark Boulton

As a designer, you will be asked 'why?' A lot.

Your colleagues will ask you. Your manager, your clients and your peers will too. The answers you give can win or lose work, determine the direction of a design or help win you awards.

Early in my career, I was told several times: 'Tell me, don't show me'. As a commercial designer, explaining your work is a critical part of what you do.

When designing for the web, we're often wrapped up in mechanics. The nuts and bolts of the design process. Browser capabilities, the content, the imagery, the HTML, CSS or Javascript – the *stuff* of our designs. Each of us has a toolbox of design-related tips and tricks that we call upon when similar problems arise. What is often missing from that toolbox however, are the reasons why. The rationale. Why use black for this project? Why not? Why does that sidebar look like wood-grain? Why does this icon look like a fish? Important questions, that demand an answer. And that's what this book will give you: some answers.

So much of what we do is invisible. In fact, someone once said that design is like air: you only notice when it's bad. The subconscious cues, messages and stories are what makes our designs effective; not how pretty they look. To create really great design, you have to understand why; not just for your benefit, but for the person you're explaining it to.

If you're an experienced designer looking for a challenging read on semiotics, then this isn't the book for you. However, if you're dabbling in web design, or just starting out, then Rob Mills has crafted a super-practical guidebook that will give you a few more of those tools to put in that tool box.

A few tools ready for when you need to explain why that icon looks like a fish.

Contents

Part 3

Part 4

Part 5

ACKNOWLEDGEMENTS

This book was far from a solo project, many others offered their time, knowledge and support and these acknowledements go a small way to express my gratitude.

Five Simple Steps
I'm always proud to tell people that I was once part of the FSS team, having been production editor on the very first title. I'm also proud to know join the ranks of their authors. Huge thanks to the whole team:

Mark and Emma: I still think you've both taken a risk by going ahead with this book and I'm so grateful for that risk and for all of the opportunities and support that you have given me, both through Five Simple Steps and through my time at Mark Boulton Design. To say you kick-started my career is an understatement. I sincerely hope that Designing the Invisible is a book that you guys are also proud of and glad to have on the FSS shelf.

Sarah: thanks for the updates, organisation and encouraging words throughout the final stages.

Nick and *Colin*: Thanks for all the hours spent crafting the final book, it was such an incentive to know the book would be in safe hands when handed over and that when it came back it would look incredible!

Nathan, *Dan* and *Alex*: Thanks for all of your hard work in creating the ePub version, the website and for proofing and sense checking the book respectively.

Contributors

Mike Kus: Thanks so much for allowing me to use Carsonified as a case study. Not only was it a privilege to have someone of you calibre willing to share your work so openly but it was a true inspiration to learn about your process.

Matthew Smith: I love the SquaredEye website so was thrilled when you were happy for me to include it in the book and also answer my questions about the site, the story, the process and the decisions behind the final design.

Carolyn Wood: You may say your involvement was small but you still took time to check a chapter and provide some info, both of which made it a better read. I was delighted to be able to have you involved.

David McCandless: Thank you for allowing me to include your infographic for colours in cultures. A picture paints a thousand words and this graphic is the best visual representation I've seen for this subject matter.

Camdon Wilde: Thank you for permission to include the Periodic Table of Typefaces. It's a great resource and one that really complimented the text of my book. Really grateful that you allowed me to share this with my readers.

To anyone else who had a chat with me about the book, shared a link, tweeted words of support and of course bought the book. It means a lot. More than you realise probably.

Editors:

Simon Mackie: There is no doubt in my mind that this book is 100 times better thanks to your input. There's no denying that it was a long road but your comments, feedback and suggestions kept me on track, helped me develop a concise writing style and above all else, made me think about every word that committed to paper. I hope I get to meet you in person one day to buy you a beer!

Bill Harper: I've said it before Bill but I want it written here for all to know, you are truly excellent at what you do. You made me sound like a better version of me! You never put words in my mouth and you always understood exactly what I was trying to say. I cannot imagine releasing this book to the masses without your input. You too are owed many beers!

Family and Friends

Mum, Dad, Rich & Lou: Thanks for letting me talk about the book for about three years and spend many weekends and evenings hidden away working on it. I hope you're proud of the final product.

To all my other friends and family. Thanks for being you, for letting me be me and for buying this book (you had better buy it!!)

Bluegg: I never knew work could be so much fun. I've loved being part of the team in the final months of this book and appreciate the support you've shown by letting me have time off for it and for being behind it 100%. Once you've tried the Bluegg way there is no other way!

INTRODUCTION

I'm fascinated by how much we are influenced by the media and indeed how much they make us think we are in control of our own decisions. Are we really in control though? I'm not so sure because despite being a media savvy species, there are subliminal forces at work affecting our moods, buying habits and emotions.

The layout of a supermarket can cause us to leave with bags of goodies we didn't need. The colour of a hospital wall can stop us from feeling agitated in a stressful environment. A simple icon or sign can quickly tell us if we can proceed or not. The structure of a sentence and words used can convey a mood or tone to us. A logo can reinforce the values of the company it represents.

As we are continually exposed to the hidden messages within the media, we become adept at receiving these messages and the more we are exposed to them the more capable we are at reading them. It's like a continuous circle of exposure, ability to process, exposure, and ability to process etc. This happens to the point where we digest the messages without thinking and that's the fascinating part, how much of the final story are we 'reading' subconsciously? A lot.

This happens on the web of course or else this book wouldn't exist. All of the elements of design communicate to us, either literally through words and images or on a more invisible level. This book is the focus of the latter elements, the invisible ones. Colours, brands, tone of voice, icons, typefaces, they all reveal more of the story and if given the consideration they deserve they will contribute to a more fulfilling user experience for the target audience.

That's a lot of buzz words for one introduction. Let's get on with it and find out how to make the invisible visible.

Part 1

Invisible Communication *101*

What is invisible communication?

The power of invisible communication

Communication in cultures

Who should care and when?

Making the invisible visible

WHAT IS INVISIBLE COMMUNICATION?

'Invisible communication' describes the way we can convey messages, moods and values using more than just words and images. A variety of these methods exist in the design world that can help us tell our stories more effectively and efficiently.

Invisible communication is happening all around us, often on a subconscious level, revealing more of the story being told.

When we talk about the story in the context of invisible communication, we mean the whole package that's being communicated. In the case of a website, all of the page elements – copy, colour, imagery, icons, and tone of voice – contribute to one story, a shared message being communicated.

Here are some examples of invisible communication. More are featured throughout the book, showing invisible communication at work both online and offline.

One well-known example is subliminal messaging. This is where images and sounds within media (such as advertisements) are received and processed by the audience on a subconscious level, or 'below threshold'. It could be the flash of an image or an implied message, and audiences often don't acknowledge them or even realise they've been exposed.

Subliminal messaging has become associated with sexual references and innuendo. This, coupled with controversy around its powers of persuasion, has led to subliminal messaging techniques being banned in several countries, including the USA and the UK.

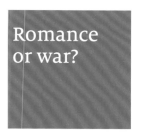

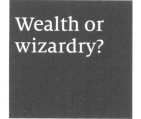

Marriage or
mourning?

Colour is a fascinating invisible communicator, because each
colour has unique connotations. Colours can evoke emotions in
people, guide them when used on signs, and hint at specific moods
such as romance and fear. The meanings communicated by colours
can also vary depending on the culture or context in which they
are used. Red for example may connote romance or war, purple
wizardry or wealth and white can represent both marriage
and mourning

Learn More:
Part 3, 'Using the
right palette', has
more information
and examples on
how colour can
communicate invisibly

Tone of voice is another example of invisible communication.
This isn't what we say but *how* we say it – a significant difference.
We can use tone of voice to express a range of emotions such as
anger, happiness, surprise, and sorrow. The pitch and volume we
speak at influence our tone of voice.

Tone of voice often relates to body language, another form of
invisible communication. With body language we use gestures,
facial expressions and body posture to communicate non-verbally.
Sometimes its message even conflicts with the words we use.

The 7-38-55 rule

The most commonly quoted communication statistics are from
studies conducted by *Albert Mehrabian*. He concluded that
when we communicate, body language conveys the most meaning
(55%), followed by tone of voice (38%) and finally the words
themselves (7%).

Learn More:
See chapter 19 for more information on using tone of voice as invisible communication.

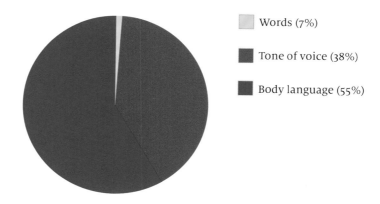

Words (7%)

Tone of voice (38%)

Body language (55%)

Anthropologist Ray Birdwhistell estimated we can make and recognise around 250,000 facial expressions[1]

While the statistics are interesting, they can't be taken literally. Otherwise an email would only communicate 7% of what the author intended, and we would be able understand 93% of what anyone said in a foreign language.

The real value in Mehrabian's studies is that it makes us think about how we communicate, and how much is conveyed in ways we don't always realise or consider.

The few examples I've outlined are all ways to connect with and communicate to an audience beyond words and imagery. Whether you are a designer, a content strategist or a project manager, understanding invisible communication and its uses can enrich your end product through the power of more effective storytelling.

It all comes back to the story.

---

[1] The Definitive Book of Body Language by Allan and Barbara Pease.

A world dominated by the invisible

We live in a world where we are inundated with invisible communication. Billboards, television, films, websites, road signs, adverts and a multitude of media outlets ensure we are rarely left alone. Even supermarkets place products and use specific colours to guide shoppers around a pre-determined route, acting on their subconscious and convincing them to buy items they don't need.

Films are an interesting study of invisible communication because they are littered with codes and references. They're hidden in the narrative or dialogue, and often play on cultural, political and social knowledge. For example, someone packing a suitcase is a 'signifier' – the action alone signifies that person is going somewhere. It doesn't need to be stated specifically in the dialogue exchanged between the characters.

Films use other invisible communication methods, such as colour. In *The Sixth Sense*, for example, the colour red is used as a storytelling device. Red is absent for most of the film, and where it does appear it is significant as it represents "anything in the real world that has been tainted by the other world".[1]

This isn't explained before or during the film. It is left to the audience to notice the use of the colour red and to draw their own conclusions as to its importance. The film is just as enjoyable if the audience doesn't notice, but it does add another layer to the story. An invisible layer, if you like.

This is why colour is one of my favourite invisible communication methods. It can add so much more to a story. Red communicates romance and love, but also danger and war. Green is associated with all things environmental and purple has connotations of royalty, wealth and luxury. Using appropriate colours in the right context can really enhance your storytelling. With invisible communication, the power often lies in how

---

[1] Screenwriter/director M. Night Shyamalan, "Rules and Clues" bonus featurette on the DVD.

audiences can receive and process the messages without realising it. These messages are then reinforced through exposure to media and culture to the point where audiences can get insight and meaning without the message being explicitly stated.

Most people associate the colour red with love, romance and passion. This cultural knowledge means designers can simply use red to create a product or website that screams romanticism.

We learn these associations between colours, symbols and similar devices throughout our lives. The meanings and relevance become reinforced through the continual association between, for example, one colour and its connotations.

Audiences are a clever bunch. They have been exposed to various invisible communication methods (and their corresponding meanings) so often that they learn to read between the lines and draw meaning from them.

The strength of many
While invisible communication methods are useful on their own, they're even more effective when combined. For example, using specific colours, icons, tones of voice, imagery and branding can create an altogether more engaging and successful website.

Invisible communication is just too important to ignore.

What's next?
The rest of this section looks at the power of invisible communication, how it is influenced by cultures, how it can be integrated into design projects, and examples of invisible communication online.

2 THE POWER OF INVISIBLE COMMUNICATION

How we communicate with others can have significant implications on how they perceive us, our business and our products. We have the ability to engage people or offend them, depending on the approach we take.

Good communication is the foundation of successful relationships; invisible communication can help a company build, maintain and preserve a strong relationship with its customers. If your website is a key connection with your audience, then every facet of what and how it communicates will influence your relationship with them.

Why is invisible communication important?
Invisible communication can:

- Provide a more fulfilling user experience
- Communicate more quickly and efficiently
- Make a personal connection with our audience
- Improve our storytelling
- Target the right people in the best way

Thinking about what you say and how you say it will lead to better relationships with your users. Of course the 'what' is the easier of the two – it's the 'how' that needs invisible communication know-how. But if you ignore it, you risk failing to reach the right people.

Was it good for you?

Invisible communication can improve the way users experience our website by making the page elements tell a consistent message that's relevant to them.

The words help them accomplish their tasks through accurate information and clear calls to action. Colours can connote moods and emotions, and the tone we use can make our site feel more personal or friendly.

Good communication will draw users in and show them the way. It should also leave them wanting more, or at the very least let them achieve what they came to do in the first place.

And it should be the same for their entire experience. So as well as the main website it should be in every other touch point between the user and your brand/service, including 404 pages, shopping cart processes and contact forms.

Less haste, more speed

Invisible communication helps us tell stories quickly and efficiently. That's what makes it so powerful.

Icons are a good example of how to communicate quickly and efficiently. If we follow standard conventions, one small symbol can communicate instructions to users or help them navigate our site. The home icon, for example, is a standard way of helping users get back to the homepage. We don't need to state it explicitly with words and copy on the button. A simple icon will suffice. Web users understand an icon vocabulary, which allows designers to say more with less.

They say a picture paints a thousand words. Imagery can quickly convey a story in the same way colour can convey a mood or emotion without needing any supporting content.

Learn more:
Part 2, 'Following the right signs', looks at icons, signs and wayfinding on the web.

Everyone has a story to share

There's that word again! Storytelling has long been used to share information. Telling stories on the web can be a challenge, as we tend to think of it in relation to more traditional methods. By incorporating invisible communication into our design process we can say more to users without being explicit. Invisible communication and storytelling are perfect partners, and their child is a great user experience.

Learn more:
Interested in storytelling? Part 5 is dedicated to this topic!

One advantage of great storytelling is being able to connect to audiences on a more personal level.

By targeting our content at specific audiences we can make our websites more relevant, and therefore more personal. This, along with an appropriate tone of voice and a well-crafted story, can make the difference between great communication and miscommunication.

To tell a great story online we must consider every strand of the story including colour, imagery, copy, branding, information architecture, navigation and tone of voice. We can use them individually to communicate, but combined they create a richer and more fulfilling experience.

Responsible communication

There's a quote from the *Spiderman* comics that tells us "with great power comes great responsibility". This also applies to web design. To design powerful communication vehicles such as websites we have a responsibility to find our story, understand our audience, and then tell that story in the best way possible.

This helps build trust between our users and our brand, product or service. If we don't invest time to plan our story and how invisible communication contributes to it, we risk offending the very people we are targeting. We may even need to change our story depending on the cultural, social and political context we work in.

3

COMMUNICATION IN CULTURES

Our culture encompasses more than just our language. It shapes our perceptions of the world around us. Culture also influences how we communicate and is a key part of telling stories, sharing information and targeting audiences effectively.

While some words and gestures have universal meaning, cultures can vary in their use of language, gestures, and even the meaning of elements such as colour. We need to be aware of these differences when communicating to different groups.

The subconscious culture

Learn more:
If you want to read more about cultural variations of colour, jump to chapter 14. But come back to read the rest of this chapter!

In all cultures, people experience the same emotions: sadness, happiness, anger, laughter, etc. However, each culture also has its own unique qualities, behaviours and messages learnt from birth unconsciously via cultural imprinting.

The environment we grow up in heavily influences our perceptions of the world, as well as the relevance and meaning we place on things like colours, words, language and imagery. For example, in western cultures the colour green represents good luck, but in China good luck is associated with the colour red. As a westerner, you wouldn't make a connection between good luck and the colour red unless you were exposed to Chinese culture.

Cultural meanings and associations are also reinforced via the media and people we interact with, to the point where every time we see a certain colour, symbol or word we immediately understand the meaning behind it.

A good example is the association between a rose and love. In films, books and TV programmes one person will often give another a rose as a symbol of their love. So we're taught that a rose symbolises love, and whenever an example is communicated the symbolism is reinforced. Eventually the knowledge that a rose represents love is processed subconsciously, but only within cultures where this symbolism exists and is relevant.

A cultural message is something everyone within that culture knows that outsiders do not, but which these outsiders can learn.

Changing cultures

As we grow up our interests change. We visit more places, are exposed to different types of media, and our horizons are broadened. Naturally, we attach new meanings to things around us and view the world differently.

Similarly our cultures change over time. Maybe a new political party is elected, or cultures react to environmental issues, and so how we live is affected. Cultures (and their associated messaging) don't change overnight, but over time they evolve, develop and adapt. This means some cultural messages will fade away, others will change and new ones will be introduced. Once these changes and additions have been adopted, they will start being reinforced and eventually become part of the subconscious culture.

Cultural influence

Culture influences all forms of communication, both visible and invisible.

The colour of mourning?

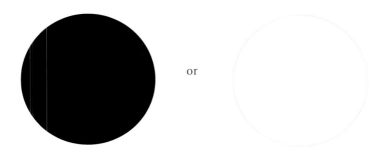

or

Colour is perhaps the best example of how invisible communication varies between cultures. For example, in the western world the colour black signifies mourning and death. But for the Chinese, mourning is historically represented by the colour white.

Communicating effectively and accurately comes down to knowing your audience. Understanding the cultural relevance of colours, signs and other invisible communication types can, in the context of the web, help your site appeal to your users and draw them in.

One symbol, a whole belief system

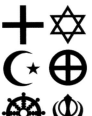

A solitary symbol can represent a whole religious or belief system, as shown here:

Similarly, colours can represent an entire religious or social group. For example:

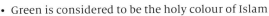

- Green is considered to be the holy colour of Islam
- Judaism is represented by the colour yellow
- In Hinduism, many gods have blue skin
- White is linked to peace across many religions

Used in the right context, colours and symbols can communicate more than the literal shade or visual symbol.

Political parties can also be represented by a colour. In the UK, for example, the following pairings exist:

- Labour – *Red*
- Conservative – *Blue*
- Liberal Democrats – *Yellow*
- The Green Party – *Green*

But these pairings of colour and political party aren't universal. In Belgium, for example, the colour blue represents the liberals, while in Finland it represents the National Coalition Party.

Parties can even be differentiated by different shades of the same colour. In Ireland, for example, the Green Party is represented by light green, while dark green is linked to Sinn Féin. How one colour can stand for such varying values, beliefs and behaviours depending on which part of the world you're in is staggering.

The shrinking world

Naturally, many invisible communication types (such as signs) are more relevant in the cultural context they're meant to be seen in. But thanks to the Internet we have a wider understanding of other cultures and how we can communicate within them.

The Internet is shrinking our world. Not literally – the planet isn't getting smaller. But we can now connect to others more easily than ever before. Through films, websites, music and books, we can learn about other cultures and learn how communication differs between these cultures. The lines between one culture and another can become blurred, but there are still significant differences in what we communicate and how we communicate.

For example, if you avoid making eye contact in the UK or USA you may be perceived as being shifty or rude. But in Japan children are taught to focus their gaze at their teacher's Adam's apple or tie rather than maintain eye contact. Whether or not you look someone in the eye may seem like a small thing, but it can have a big impact if you get the custom wrong.

Do your research

Never assume you know about a culture or group. Things change, sometimes very quickly. It's always worth investing time in researching a culture or audience group. Even if your research confirms and validates your knowledge or assumptions, it is still time well spent.

Don't under-estimate the significance of knowing the cultural, political and religious messages that exist invisibly behind colours, symbols, words, signs and images. Just as you'd probably read up on a particular country's customs (hand gestures, language, ways to act, etc.) before you visit, you should also do your research when communicating via other platforms, such as the web.

Who should care and when?

Invisible communication isn't solely the responsibility of the designer. To achieve the most effective invisible communication the other members of the project team need to be involved during the project cycle.

Who can design the invisible?

It's usually the designer who incorporates invisible communication as part of the overall design. But other members of the team can also get involved, including:

- Copywriters
- Information Architects
- User Experience Experts

Designers

Designers should have an in-depth knowledge of using appropriate colours, icons, typefaces and other methods of communicating through design. And they should consider these methods throughout the whole design phase.

Designers can fuse the design elements together to tell one coherent story. If they take ownership of invisible communication there should be a consistent storytelling approach, as well as a final design that answers the client's brief.

Copywriters

The role of the copywriter is critical when it comes to using invisible communication methods such as tone of voice.

The copywriter shouldn't work in isolation. They should be involved in the project as early as possible to ensure the tone of voice matches the visual design elements. An informal tone of voice will jar when incorporated into a formal design.

Information Architects

The information architect helps to group the information and structure the content (our story). They may not contribute to invisible communication directly by choosing colours or the tone of voice, but they help determine what information should be included and how it should be organised. This will influence not only design decisions, but also what information is shared and ultimately how the story is told. In effect the information architect provides the frame on which the story is hung.

User Experience Experts

User experience (UX) and invisible communication go hand-in-hand. If the invisible communication elements are done right (appropriate colours, brand consistency, appropriate tone of voice and efficient use of signs), then naturally the user experience will be enhanced.

For example the *Threadless* website, which sells t-shirts, has a fun and informal tone of voice, clear navigation and neutral colours that appeal to everyone.

Anyone and Everyone

I'm not saying these are the only people who can or should be involved in invisible communication. A team may have a project manager who is a colour theory expert, or a content strategist who knows how best to communicate to different cultures or audience groups.

But thinking about invisible communication and integrating it into the project process should be a team effort. It should start at the research phase and continue through to the content population and post-launch phases.

The key is effective and accurate communication among the entire project team. If a decision is made about the design, the decision must be passed on to everyone concerned to keep their involvement in line with the overall story. There needs to be a consistent voice telling the story, through both the visible and invisible communication elements. And the only way to achieve that consistency is through a well-managed project.

Invisible communication and the project cycle

Different invisible communication methods will be applied at various points during the project. Exactly what happens when will be influenced by its scope, agreed deliverables and target audience. But despite these variables, most web projects go through certain well-defined phases.

Research and Discovery

This phase occurs after all pre-project meetings have been held, the contract is signed and the project has just kicked off.

Depending on the scope of the project, it may allow time for competitor research, initial design concepts and, most relevant for invisible communication, audience research.

Determining the wider target audience, and then drilling down to specific user groups as needed, will help the project team make design decisions and communicate effectively and efficiently via the invisible. For example, the research and discovery phase can help us learn about the social and cultural worlds our users live in, which will affect not only *what* we communicate but *how* we communicate.

Design

Every project has different requirements and methods, but they all have one phase where invisible communication plays a key role: the design phase. Giving consideration to invisible communication here is fundamental to everything else that follows.

The design stage may involve wire framing, prototyping, designing concepts, generating sitemaps and any number of other design activities. At some point, the team will consider elements such as colour, icons, copy, signage systems and branding. All of which can be used for invisible communication, as we'll discuss later in the book.

How these elements get incorporated into the overall design will be dictated by the designer and project team. But the information obtained during the research phase will point the way and help determine some of these design decisions.

Refinement/Iteration

The refinement phase will include time to ensure all invisible communication is relevant, accurate and complimentary to the overall design and project specification.

At this stage there shouldn't be any drastic design changes (such as a complete colour change), but more tweaking and refinement of the copy, symbols and the design itself.

Targeting the audience

Some methods in our invisible design toolbox (such as colour) may be constrained by the client, particularly if they have already established brand guidelines. If that's the case you'll just have to work within the parameters. But that doesn't mean you can't tailor the rest of the content or design towards a specific audience.

The best way to approach invisible communication is to ask the client a lot of questions about the audience, and the project brief and goals. The project team can then use the answers to make decisions about invisible communication.

Showing, not telling

So far we've identified what invisible communication is, why it is important, how it can be powerful, and who should be involved and when.

In the next chapter I will deconstruct some web pages, and peel back the layers of invisible communication. I want to show it, rather than write about it in detail.

For the rest of the book I'll be talking about how you can design the invisible, using practical examples to demonstrate how the theory works in practice.

5 MAKING THE INVISIBLE VISIBLE

The following websites provide good examples of invisible communication. Although the websites offer different services and target different audiences, they all share common invisible communication techniques that we'll examine in this chapter.

Threadless.com[1]

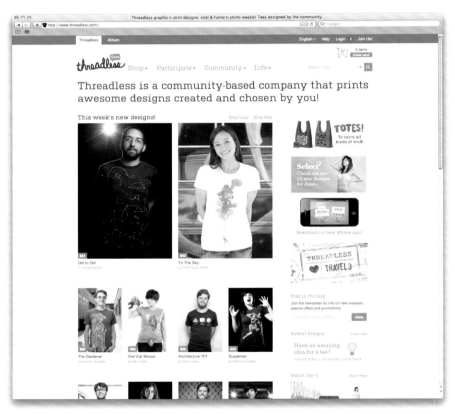

The *Threadless* website sells t-shirts to a young, stylish and slightly geeky market. So it's crucial that it appeals to this specific audience.

---

[1] http://www.threadless.com

Colour

Colour is used to organise content within the site. This is most evident in the Community section, where the forum categories are represented by specific colours.

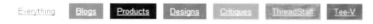

Typeface and tone of voice

Both the typeface and tone of voice on the Threadless site are friendly, informal and approachable.

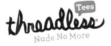

Check out a jillion more designs!

Need help? How may we assist you?

We like you! You should like us on Facebook for exclusive offers and awesome awesomeness!

This fits well with its purpose – selling t-shirts to a young and stylish audience. As the t-shirts are also designed by the Threadless community, the informal tone of voice encourages people to join in and participate.

Invisible communication elements such as colour and tone of voice are used consistency throughout the website. For example, if you click on your empty shopping cart, it says:

> 'I'm so, so hungry! Have mercy and fill my carty belly with delicious Threadless products. You can use the drop-downs above my starving body to get started. Hurry!'

Icons/symbols

The site also makes good use of symbols and icons. The shopping cart icon, for example, serves two purposes. Firstly it can take the user straight to their cart to view any items in it. Secondly, it can indicate whether it's empty or not. The cart has a sad face when it's empty, but as soon as something is added it changes to a happy face.

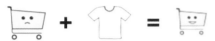

The happy and sad faces have universal meaning, and the predominant US and European Threadless audience would understand them instantly.

These examples of invisible communication, together with the copy and overall design, make Threadless.com a good example of what a website can do for an organisation. It can engage their customers, encourage them to participate, and provide a great user experience.

Nick.com[1]

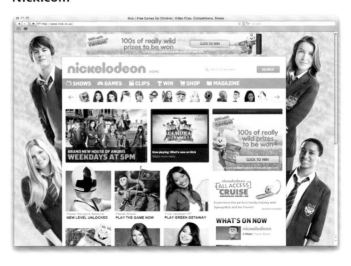

---

[1] http://www.nick.com

Nickelodeon is a TV channel and website for kids. Nickelodeon has brought us some of the most famous kids TV characters, including *SpongeBob SquarePants*. The website offers games, video, and products.

Colour and brand
Orange is Nickelodeon's brand colour, and so is the dominant colour across the whole website. It's used in the main logo, for calls to action and for the navigation.

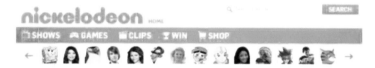

Orange works well for a website aimed at children. It has connotations of happiness and warmth, and it isn't stereotypically associated with one gender or another.

The whole website is a colourful affair with striking and colourful background images, such as on the shows page:

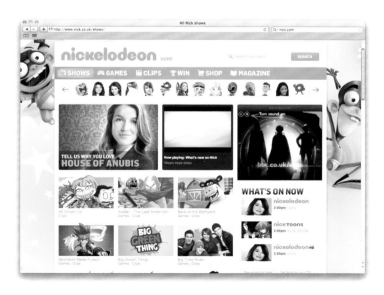

Using colour this way is important because of the website's target audience; more muted tones would communicate a very different vibe and not be as appealing to children.

Imagery

The Nickelodeon website uses very little wording, again due to its target audience. In place of copy they rely heavily on imagery. For example, clicking on the image of SpongeBob SquarePants on the homepage will take you to the SpongeBob page. From here you can click on further images to play specific games.

    Due to the lack of words, the site's tone of voice isn't expressed through written content. Instead, the childlike and friendly mood of the website is invisibly communicated through the heavy use of imagery and bright colours.

Whitehouse.gov[1]

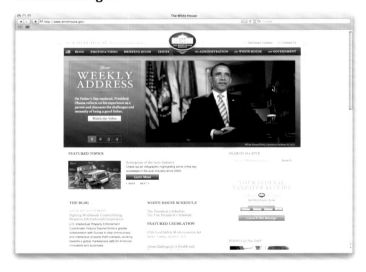

The official website for the *White House* and *President Obama* features photos, videos, news and the White House schedule.

---

[1] http://www.whitehouse.gov

Overall mood

The elements on the White House website combine to give an impression of a serious, formal and professional organisation; three values people would expect of an official government website.

Colour

The main colours of the website are red, white and blue – three colours that communicate patriotism and are quintessentially American. The secondary palette includes brown, a neutral and organic shade.

Typeface and tone of voice

Given who and what this website represents, it is fitting that both the typeface and tone of voice are more formal than we found in the previous examples.

the WHITE HOUSE PRESIDENT BARACK OBAMA

IN THE BRIEFING ROOM

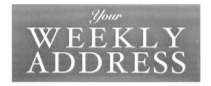

Serif typefaces feel more formal; they are the sort of typefaces found on more high-brow newspapers and in professional contexts.

The tone of voice is very professional, as you might expect. Here's an example:

> 'His story is the American story – values from the heartland, a middle-class upbringing in a strong family, hard work and education as the means of getting ahead, and the conviction that a life so blessed should be lived in service to others.'

There's invisible communication at work here. There is no need to explicitly say this text needs to be read in a serious tone. It is implied through the words themselves, how they look, and the context in which they are placed.

Thinkvitamin.com[1]

![Screenshot of the Think Vitamin website article "How Colour Communicates Meaning"]

Think Vitamin is a blog by *Carsonified*, aimed at those who work in the web industry.

Icons

Icons are a great way to communicate efficiently. Think Vitamin is one of my favourite examples of the power of using icons.
For example, here's how they are used on the main navigation:

While these icons are supported by text such as 'Home' and 'About', they would communicate just as well on their own. Remove the word 'Home', for example, and users would still know the icon would take them to the homepage. 'Write for us' is more specific to Think Vitamin, but the pencil icon is synonymous with writing so even without the words the icon invisibly communicates the content it links to.

---

[1] http://www.thinkvitamin.com

Icons are also used to represent ways users can interact with Think Vitamin:

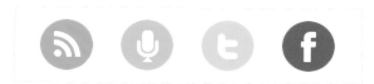

Here they use the brand colours for RSS, *Twitter* and *Facebook* to quickly communicate what each icon does without needing to explain each one.

The green icon isn't standard like the others, and so it isn't as instantly recognisable. But it has still been given its own colour to help users navigate to the Think Vitamin podcasts.

Colour
Colour is used subtly on Think Vitamin. Links are shown in red, and navigation items turn red when rolled over.

Storytelling
Where Think Vitamin excels is in its attention to detail. It weaves a compelling story that draws users in and encourages them to like, comment and share the content. This is achieved through content that is informative, easy to read and relevant. It may not be invisible communication, but it is part of being a good site.

The story is also enhanced through invisible communication methods, with colours and icons adding an extra dimension to the story. They categorise the content, help users navigate the site, and make it easy for users to contribute.

Putting it into practice
Now that we've looked at examples of invisible communication on the web, it's time to look at how we can incorporate these methods into our own designs. The following chapters will show you how to achieve this, and help you appeal to your target audience and improve their user experience.

Part 2

Following the right signs

Showing the way

Context and culture

Wayfinding the world

Warning signs, cultural signs and icons

Case Study: *Guardian.co.uk*

SHOWING THE WAY

Signs help us navigate, communicate danger and explain what we can and cannot do.

We learn the significance and meaning of signs throughout our lives. We quickly become adept at understanding the hidden meaning behind the signs we see, and react to their messages subconsciously.

Carl G. Liungman was born in Sweden in 1938. In 1972 he took an interest in semiotics and compiled an encyclopaedia on Western ideograms. Visit *www.symbol.com* for more information.

"A human being, during his or her childhood, acquires the meanings of the signs used for communication in its culture, as well as a whole series of conventions. Graphic structures rely upon these conventions for their various meanings"

Carl G. Liungman

The web is full of signs: text, icons, images, symbols and website navigation help create a well-understood signage system that can incorporate colour, hierarchy and pointers.

A number of systems exist for classifying symbols and signs. Indeed, the study of signs (known as semiotics) is worthy of its own book. However, we need to understand some fundamental definitions and systems to investigate the importance and significance of signs on the web in the context of invisible communication.

Why signs are important?

Signs are useful because they can help us communicate a great deal of information without having to literally write or show everything.

The benefits of using signs – both online and offline – are:

- They communicate efficiently
- They help people get where they want to be
- They can communicate across languages and cultures
- They can help people achieve their tasks quickly

Signs are useful enough on their own. But when you combine them with other signs or with the physical environment they can become a signage system that leads a person from the start of their journey to the destination.

A good signage system can:

- Stop users getting frustrated with your website
- Increase accessibility of your website
- Lead users down a specified path
- Help users find your content

Semiotics

> "Semiotics is the study of how meaning is socially produced through various languages or codes such as colour, gesture and photography."
>
> (Branston and Stafford)

The field of semiotics is largely concerned with how certain things come to have significance and meaning. It tells us that language is constructed by people and cultures to make sense of the world around them.

A sign on its own has no meaning. It means something when those exposed to it agree on what it defines and represents. Therefore, any language relies on its shared understanding by a specific group of people, and that includes the language of signs and symbols. If a sign meant something different to every person who saw it, then its very reason for being would be invalid.

Some signs, such as a smiley face, are fairly universal. But others are more subjective, and you have to understand its context and convention for its meaning to be effective.

Imagine trying to cross a junction with traffic lights if there was no common definition for what the three colours represented. If the *go* signal was red for one person and green for another it would literally be an accident waiting to happen.

Just as people need to agree on what signs represent, they also need to agree on what words are used to describe certain things. For example, there is no reason why a cow is called a 'cow'. If enough people agreed to it, a cow could well be known as 'sizzlebang'. It is only because we have agreed in our culture that a 'cow' is a cow that the word refers to the animal.

This also happens online. There's a shared understanding that an envelope represents email, and a house icon represents the homepage. If this wasn't the case then the website's navigation would be almost useless.

Classifying signs and symbols

A sign is any object, action, event, or pattern that conveys a meaning. Let's take a look at some different types of signs.

Symbols
A symbol can be defined as an object that represents something other than itself.

For example a rose is a flower, but it can also be a symbol for love.

Ideograms
An ideogram is a character or symbol that represents an idea or a thing without expressing the pronunciation of the sounds used to say it. Examples include '&', '@' and '$', the 'no parking' symbol, and the symbols used to guide people in airports.

Words

Words are signs, too. On a website the word 'Home' can impart the same message as a house icon. But for some audiences the word won't be relevant in their culture, whereas the icon will. We all know what a house/home is; we just have different words to describe it.

Similarly, 'stop' can give the same command as a stopping prohibited sign. Words are important signs, but they need to be used in the right context.

Signifiers/Signified

Ferdinand de Saussure believed that signs consist of:

- A signifier – *the physical form of the sign*
- The signified – *the thing it refers to other than itself; the concept it represents.*

When both the signifier and signified exist, the result is the sign: the whole they combine to form. For example, if there is a sign on a shop doorway that says 'open' then the signifier is the word, 'open'. The signified, however, is that the shop is open for business and you can enter. On the web, an example could be a printer icon. The signifier is the icon itself, while the signified is the suggestion that clicking the icon will allow you to print.

American philosopher Charles Sanders Peirce proposed that signs can be been grouped into three categories:

I. **Icon** – iconic signs that resemble what they signify. One example of this is a photograph. It represents that moment in time and the people in the photo. Icons on your computer are... well, icons, such as the house icon for your homepage, the envelope icon for mail, and the colour palette icon for choosing colours.

Ferdinand de Saussure (1857 – 1913) was a French linguist who pioneered the semiotic study of language as a system of signs organised in code and structures[1]

Charles Sanders Peirce (1839 – 1914) was an American philosopher who produced a classification of different kinds of signs.

[1] Branston and Stafford

Some well-known examples of icons include:

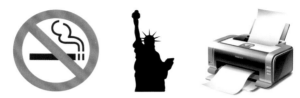

The 'no smoking' sign resembles the object and action it isn't
allowing, the Statue of Liberty silhouette indicates the value
of freedom (as well as the building itself), and the printer icon
resembles a real printer.

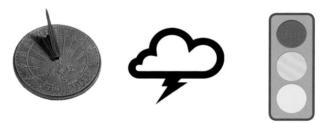

2. **Index** – a signifier that is directly connected to the signified. A
   clockface is an indexical sign of time passing. Smoke indexes
   fire. A hyperlink indexes a webpage. The sign is an indicator of
   something else.

   This sundial indexes time passing. The cloud and thunderbolt
   indicate an imminent storm and the red stop light is a sign you
   should stop your car or risk an accident.

3. **Symbols** – abstractions that use images to represent an object,
   concept or action. For example, symbols of men and women are
   used to communicate gender, and a smoking cigarette is used
   to convey 'no smoking' (when coupled with the red circle
   and strikethrough).

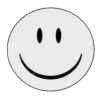 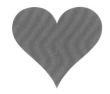 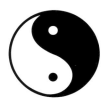

Mathematics is filled with symbols such as addition, subtraction
and the Pi symbol. Copyright and trademarks are also represented
by symbols. A smiley face is symbolic of happiness (although it
also has connotations of drug use), the heart is a symbol for love,
and the yin yang is an old Chinese symbol for the universe now
integrated into Western ideography.

Arbitary signs
Peirce also stated that signs can be arbitrary. These signs have little
or no resemblance to the object, concept or action. Here is the
radioactive sign:

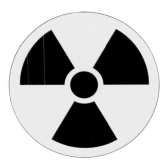

This sign is an abstract representation of radiation with no literal interpretation. Its meaning has been learned over time, having been exposed (pardon the pun) to people over a sustained period. This is what makes it an effective communication device.

This sign is also common in computer flowcharting, meaning external memory or offline storage.

The colour of signs

A sign's colour can help communicate its meaning. Red is commonly associated with danger, and consequently is used on warning signs and, of course, as the traffic light colour telling us to stop.

Red also represents love, but the symbols are given in an entirely different context to when we see road signs so the message is clear.

Similarly, hazard signs are predominantly yellow and black. This has links to nature; bees and wasps use black and yellow markings as a warning. The contrast between these two colours also makes the sign (and therefore the hazard) stand out. This is evident in the radioactive example shown earlier.

Red is linked to 'stop', and green is linked to 'go'. If we changed the colours people expect to see on signs we could confuse them. Let's take a typical sign that tells people not to do something and change the colour.

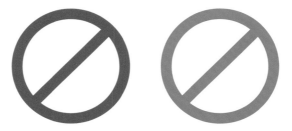

The second sign doesn't feel right because the shape of the sign is telling us 'no' but the colour is telling us 'yes'.

The same applies to other symbols linked to an action or a journey. A tick denotes 'yes' while a cross denotes 'cancel' or 'no'. Swap the colours of these and their meaning is less clear.

A small colour change to a symbol can have big implications for how and what that symbol communicates.

Deconstructing signs

Let's deconstruct some well-known signs so we can see the importance of shape, colour and cultural variations when using signs in design.

No Smoking

- This sign is an icon. It resembles what it signifies: no smoking
- The circle is known in the UK to give an order
- The colour red connotes danger, warning, don't
- The smoke is an index of a lit cigarette. The way it rises from the cigarette represents a lit cigarette as opposed to an unlit one

The line though the cigarette symbol is synonymous with 'no' or 'don't'. This is a meaning that has developed over time with a shared understanding in the western world.

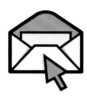

Email

- This sign is an icon, a computer icon for opening email
- In the physical world, mail is received in envelopes. Web icons to represent email have adopted this as the standard icon as users can connect this to something already relevant to them
- Again, this is a shared agreement of the meaning
- The fact that the envelope is open distinguishes it from icons that represent sending or deleting email
- The arrow is a call to action and is representative of opening an email

Speech Bubble

- The speech bubble is a modern ideogram
- It has gained this meaning because it is shown with the point coming out of someone's mouth, representing the words they are saying
- This meaning is far-reaching, with comic books following similar conventions worldwide
- Again, there is a shared understanding amongst audiences and users that a speech bubble represents spoken words

In this chapter we've discussed what signs are, why they are important and the different types of signs. It's now time to look at signage systems in the 'real' world and on the web.

CONTEXT AND CULTURE

Just as body language can have cultural relevance, so too can signs. Signs carry different meanings and significance in different cultures. Some cross cultural boundaries more successfully than others, but often a sign needs to be seen in context for it to communicate effectively.

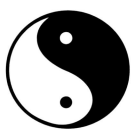

Some signs are born out of one culture but become integrated with others, resulting in a shared meaning and significance. The Yin Yang symbol, for example, is an old Chinese symbol for the universe but is well recognised in western cultures today; it is often used to symbolise opposites or peace.

Many signs used on the web, such as the home, print and email icons, mean the same thing in most places. However, it is never safe to assume this. In certain cultures or contexts, a sign you have used may be communicating the wrong message invisibly.

It's all about the context

As we've discussed, signs only mean something when a group of people agree on that meaning. There may be entire sign systems you aren't aware of, simply because they aren't relevant to your life.

This is where context becomes significant, and an individual sign's agreed meaning moves from just being culturally dependent to being socially, politically and historically dependent.

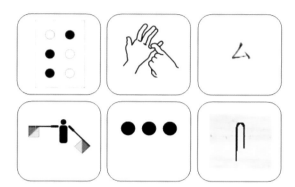

These signs are all for the letter 'S', represented in (from top-left):

- Braille
- British Sign Language
- Chinese Phonetic Alphabet
- Semaphore
- Morse code
- Hieroglyphics

Unless you have learnt how to read Braille, the first sign may look more like a domino. Your knowledge of Braille depends how significant that sign is to your life. For some it is essential, while for others it isn't.

The same applies to the sign language representation. You may have learnt sign language and know how to express the letter 'S', but even sign language can vary from one place to another. For example, British Sign Language is different to other forms, such as American.

The third symbol is the Chinese phonetic alphabet representation of 'S'. You might recognise the character as being Chinese, but unless you speak or write Chinese the sign's specific meaning will probably elude you.

Semaphore is a flag signalling system for communicating from a distance. It is mainly used in the maritime world, and has been around since the Battle of Trafalgar.

Morse code is something most people know about but don't recognise when it's represented visually. The three dots that represent 'S' could also be interpreted as an ellipsis.

The final symbol is an 'S' represented in hieroglyphics. Again you may recognise this as an ancient language, but not necessarily that it represents the letter 'S' specifically.

One sign, many stories

Signs and symbols can have multiple meanings, depending on the culture you look at them in relation to. Whenever you use symbols on the web, it is time well spent to research its origins, just in case you unknowingly tell a story far from the one you wanted.

One example of a symbol used on the web that does not translate across cultures is the podcast symbol from the Think Vitamin website. This isn't as commonly used as symbols for home, email or print, and while some cultures will recognise it others are less likely to do so.

One sign, one story

Generally, however, signs and symbols can work across cultures. The heart symbol is almost universal in its representation of love. A smiley face can represent happiness in several cultures too.

One of the most popular cross-culture symbols is the five-pointed star. This appears on flags for no less than 35 countries, both Western and Eastern. It is also an important military symbol, and so is has significance in a vast group of cultures.

Juxtaposition

Juxtaposition is defined as 'the act or an instance of placing two or more things side by side"

Signs and symbols can also be juxtaposed in their meanings. Even a basic symbol such as a circle can be juxtaposed. It can mean 'everything', but can also represent nothingness, zero or 'no entry'. The same symbol given in different contexts can have different meanings.

But some symbols don't lend themselves to juxtaposition. The heart symbol, for example, is an elementary sign structure that does not carry any opposite meanings.

Understanding signs across cultures

Some signs can be understood outside of the culture they are designed for. This sign is a tsunami warning, which can been seen throughout Southeast Asia.

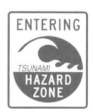

While the UK doesn't have tsunami threats, the sign still has meaning (even without the English text) because we can still recognise the symbol of a wave and the colour blue, which is symbolic of water.

Warning signs in particular are designed to work as visually as possible, with minimal room for misinterpretation. They need to communicate quickly and effectively, hence the minimal text in the tsunami sign.

Similarly, the above sign represents the hazard of kangaroos on or near the road. It is a sign that has utmost importance in Australia where kangaroos are a genuine risk to drivers. In the UK there is no such threat to motorists, but we understand the sign because the kangaroo shape is clearly recognisable as the animal.

Additionally, the colours black and yellow are also used in the UK for hazard signs, so the sign immediately tells us there is a hazard to be aware of. Some signs can only be understood correctly within the culture they are intended for. Others can be interpreted by people from other cultures, but the sign will have no relevance to them.

---

[1] http://www.merriam-webster.com/dictionary/juxtaposition

Changes over time

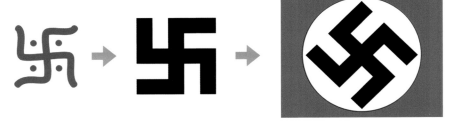

The Hindu swastika   A traditional swastika   The Nazi swastika flag

Signs can have different meanings at different points in time. One example is one of the world's most recognisable and controversial symbols: *the swastika.*

This ideogram is rooted in history. Depending on the era you study, the swastika will have very different meanings and symbolism.

It's an ancient symbol, used by many cultures over the past 3,000 years to represent the sun, four directions, movement, power, good luck and change. Then Hitler revived the swastika and it took on a whole new meaning due to its iconic usage in Nazi Germany.

The swastika became the official emblem of the Nazi party on August 7th 1920, and a symbol that traditionally had positive associations became a sign of hate, violence, death and murder. A far cry from its origins, the symbol now has a stigma attached to it due to its associations with racism, white supremacists and neo-Nazis.

The swastika has had many culturally-dependent meanings, but they have been overridden by the Nazi associations. Whenever this symbol is viewed it can evoke emotions of hurt and anger and conjure up images of torture and P.O.W camps. It is one of the most powerful symbols of the world, but for all the wrong reasons.

Knowledge is power

Making sure you know the different types of symbols and their meaning and place within different cultures is an important part of targeting your work at the right audience. A symbol's meaning can change over time as society, politics and cultures evolve.

Wayfinding the world

Signs exist in our lives to show us the way. In this chapter we'll take a look at signs in the world around us. (In the next chapter we'll look at how wayfinding and signage systems can be applied to the web.)

An obvious example of signs that help us get from A to B are road signs. But the signs in large public buildings, such as hospitals and airports, do the same job. They help us find our way without too much effort, or at least they should.

Various techniques can be used to create a signage system, which combine typefaces, names, colours, sizes, shapes, symbols, positioning and design.

When signage works well it tells us where we are and where we can move to next. When it fails we miss buses, arrive late for appointments, crash cars, get lost, and miss the turn off.

What is wayfinding?

'Wayfinding' is the process of following a system of signs, in places such as airports and hospitals as well as on websites. The term was first used by *Kevin Lynch* in his 1960 publication, *The Image of the City*. Lynch defines wayfinding as:

> *"The process of using spatial and environmental information to navigate to a destination."*

In their book, *Universal Principles of Design*, *William Lidwell*, *Kritina Holden*, and *Jill Butler* state that "whether navigating a college campus, the wilds of a forest or web site, the basic process of wayfinding involves the same four stages: orientation, route decision, route monitoring and destination recognition."[1]

---

[1] Universal Principles of Design, William Lidwell, Kritina Holden, and Jill Butler

1. **Orientation**

   Orientation means knowing where you are in relation to what is around you and where you want to be. The focus is on your current position, where you can move to and how you can get there. You can use landmarks (orientation cues) and signage to make sense of the area around you.

2. **Route Decision**

   Route decision is all about choosing how you will reach your destination. People are more effective at making route decisions if they have limited navigational choices and prompts throughout the route. Signage also helps here.

3. **Route Monitoring**

   As people move though their journey, they need to monitor their route to make sure they're on track to reaching their destination. So as well as showing people the direction of a place, signage needs to regularly tell people where they are so they'll know they are still on track. As Lidwell, Holden and Butler observe, "breadcrumbs are visual cues highlighting the path taken and can aid route monitoring, particularly when a wayfinding mistake has been made, and backtracking is necessary."

4. **Destination Recognition**

   People need to know when they have arrived at their destination.

The Importance of Wayfinding

Wayfinding is essential for people to get from where they are to where they want to be. That includes tourists, drivers and web users alike.

Big buildings such as airports and hospitals can be intimidating, as can the web. Making clear routes for people and helping them complete their task efficiently is an important part of design – and signage is at the heart of this.

Wayfinding is more than just signs

Signs are important, but people will need different types of information at various points in their journey. Signs, colours, typography, words and maps can all contribute to an effective wayfinding system.

Wayfinding problems aren't always due to bad signage, and adding more signs won't solve every wayfinding problem. The key is to create an environment that's easy to navigate, with consistent clues, and where the elements have all been carefully considered with the user firmly in mind.

To create an appropriate wayfinding strategy you need to consider:

- Whom you are directing
- The information they have
- The information they need
- What they want to achieve
- What signs would be most appropriate for them

The journey before the journey

Airports are an interesting example of wayfinding because they need to show people from many different cultures and nationalities how to get from A to B.

A good signage system is important for airports because passengers are often stressed or in a state of anxiety. The last thing they need is the frustration of trying to find their destination. Airports also have many possible routes to choose from – just as there are on the web.

Pictograms
Graphical symbols (or pictograms) are important in airport signage, because they can be understood by more people than the corresponding words. This does depend on the function at hand, as some symbols and pictograms are more universally recognised than others.

Examples of common pictograms

 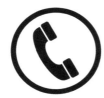

Pictograms were added to the signs in Amsterdam's Schiphol Airport to improve wayfinding for non-English speaking passengers. This airport is the benchmark for all airports following its wayfinding 'redesign' by Bureau Mijksenaar.

Colour
Colour coding areas can be an effective way to help people navigate. They will associate certain places or tasks with a certain colour. It is dangerous to rely solely on colour though – there must also be sufficient information for the colour to reinforce. Amsterdam's Schiphol Airport is held in high regard for its wayfinding and use of colour. Yellow signs provide arrival and departure information, blues signs are used for restaurant facilities, green is the colour for escape routes and anthracite is used in waiting areas.

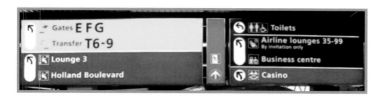

Colour is also a good wayfinding technique for maps. But again, other information is needed to support the colour coding. One example is the map of the London Underground.

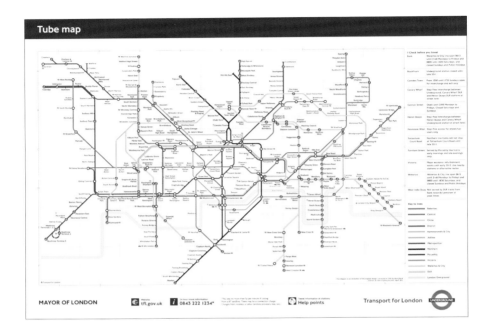

Each route, or line, is represented by a colour – yellow for the Circle line, red for the Central line, and so on. While you still need to know where you are, the station you need to get off at and which direction you need to travel in, the colours make it clear where each line starts and ends.

The colour is important here as this map is a schematic diagram. It doesn't show the geographic information, but rather the relative positions of stations along the lines and the relations and connections between them.

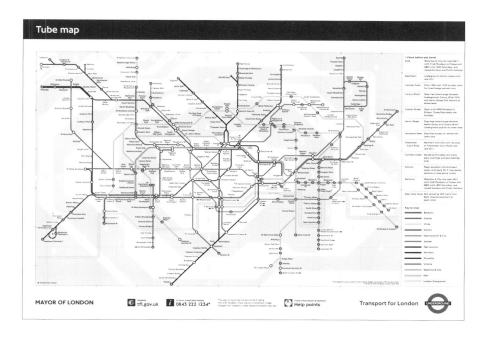

If the colour is removed from the map it is still possible to see each station and navigate. But the distinction between the routes is less clear, and the map's effectiveness as a navigation aid is immediately reduced.

Similarly, the signage uses the same colours, ensuring a consistent system. When you're changing at a station, you can easily find the right platform. It's also used on the screens that display service disruptions.

Naming places

Names on signs have to be comprehensible. If we are instructed to go to gate 28 for boarding then we need a sign that clearly says 'Gate 28'. In hospitals extra attention is given to the names on signs because they are often complex or hard to pronounce medical terms. It is always best to keep it simple. A sign saying 'blood tests' is much easier for most people to understand than 'phlebotomy'.

Avoid jargon. The best way to develop a wayfinding strategy is to assume people or users have no knowledge of the place they are in.

Legibility

Any written information should be as legible as possible, which means paying attention to colour combinations, typefaces and size and placement of signs.

At Schiphol Airport the arrows showing the way are black in a white circle for optimum legibility. Where necessary, signs are also illuminated.

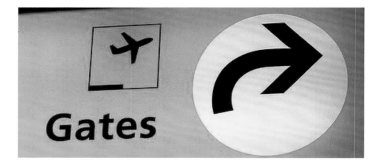

Organising information

How information is organised is just as important as colours, names and signs. The hierarchy of information needs to be considered. What do the users need to know to get going on their journey? What do they need to know along the way? And what do they need to know when they get there?

Information can be categorised numerically, alphabetically or by type, and the choice you make will inevitably affect how the information is presented. Before the redesign at Schiphol airport, the directions were listed alphabetically, which made the signs cluttered and messy.

The size of signs can also hint at the importance of the information they share. Big signs carry more importance than smaller ones. The size of signage can create an information hierarchy, ensuring the most important information isn't relegated to a small sign hidden from view.

Creating a wayfinding strategy

The best way of developing a signage system, whether online or offline, is to put yourself in the position of the user. Ask yourself questions about the journey you think they will be taking.

- Where will they need to go?
- How often will they need to be reassured they are still heading in the right direction?
- What will they need along the way?
- What will they need/expect when they arrive at their destination?
- Will colour coding help?
- How can I make the journey more clear/legible?
- What resources are available if they get lost?

Think about the user and their story, and create a narrative to guide them. Use conventions and signs where necessary, but support it with colours, words and, in extreme conditions, maps.

As Lidwell, Holden and Butler said, whether navigating a forest or a website, the techniques and principles for guiding people are the same. So let's now take a look at wayfinding on the web.

Wayfinding on the web

The web lends itself perfectly to wayfinding strategies. We can form narratives using storytelling, along with practical techniques such as user stories and use cases. Then we can support them with symbols, icons, signs and colour to show the way.

Telling a three-act story

Navigation should tell a story with a past, present, and future:

- Past: *where have I come from?*
- Present: *where am I?*
- Future: *where can I go next/where do I want to be?*

Your users can't answer those questions unless you have a well-signposted website. This is particularly important for the web because you can't guarantee they will start their journey on the homepage. They can land on the path at any point. Information architecture, colour and signposting can show the way, while symbols and icons can communicate specific tasks and calls to action when they arrives at their destination.

Colour coding

As discussed in the previous chapter, colour coding can contribute to a wayfinding system. But never use it in isolation. It must be supported by content.

The Carsonified' website uses colour to clearly distinguish between areas on the site. The homepage is black and white, the jobs page is green, the contact page is orange and so on.

If you spend a lot of time on the site you begin to associate the content with the colours. So if you are looking for job vacancies you will subconsciously head to the 'green section'. But chances are you aren't *that* familiar with the site, so other information is needed to help you complete your journey.

¹ www.carsonified.com

Below are the names of each area along with its colour and icon:

Carsonified uses colour as a navigation tool with the help of clear signposts and symbols. The names given to each page are easy to understand and universally recognised: 'Home', 'Values', 'Team', and so on.

The icons that represent each area are also carefully chosen. The homepage is illustrated with a house icon, for example. Some of the icons have less obvious connotations, such as the soldier for 'Values' and the tree for 'Jobs' (symbolic of growth). They may not be universally recognised symbols, but they are supported by labels that make them clear and concise signs, contributing to an overarching wayfinding system.

Signs and breadcrumbs

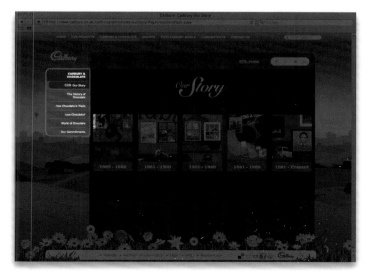

On some websites the wayfinding is subtle. But other sites will literally tell users 'you are here'. This is true of the *Cadbury UK*[1] website.

Visitors are told where they are via a small yellow sign saying 'here' that points to the page they are on. This contributes to a wayfinding system as it helps with orientation.

However, it's not a complete wayfinding system. There are no breadcrumbs, and no other signs for where to go next. The navigation is listed, but there is no way to differentiate between content areas – everything is purple (the deeper into the content you go the lighter the shade of purple becomes), all typography is the same, and there's no obvious hierarchy to the content. The site doesn't lead you on a journey. It just says, 'you are here'.

The same is true on the *Ben and Jerry's*[2] website. They make it very clear where you are, but again there is little clear signposting to further your journey.

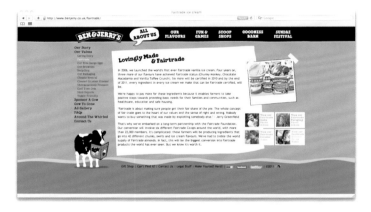

But that isn't to say the site is ruined. Rather, it shows that not every site needs a complete wayfinding system.

The 'All About Us' section is clearly shown. But the navigation down the left-hand side is barely legible, thanks largely to the black text on the site's blue background. If that were a sign in an airport, I'd probably miss my flight.

---

[1] www.cadbury.co.uk

[2] www.benjerry.co.uk

An example of a website that gives users a clear path, in terms of both where they came from and where they are on the site, is that of user experience blog, UX Booth'.

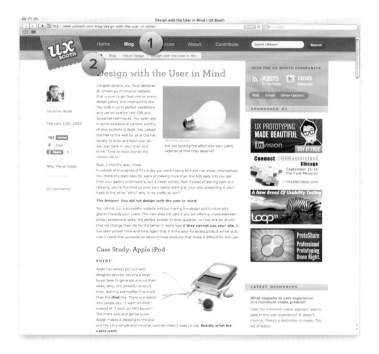

As we can see from the screenshot, the site marks the user's current location by making the 'Blog' section title more prominent in the main navigation (*1*). And the breadcrumb trail shows not only where they are but also how they got there (*2*): Home −> Blog −> Visual design −> Design with the user in mind.

UX Booth uses arrows to show the journey that was made between these four pages. Arrows are the most obvious symbol for this as they show the way, point forward and have a universal meaning.

¹ www.uxbooth.com

Some sites are also good at showing the journey a user is yet to take. This is particularly important when they need to complete a specific process, such as when purchasing goods or searching for a holiday.

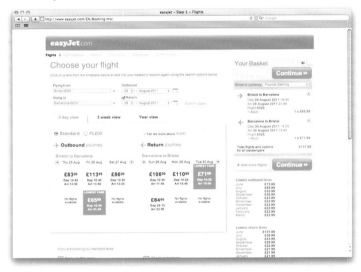

This page is from low budget airline, *Easyjet*[1]. As you can see, when users have been through the search process and would like to book a flight the steps to follow seem relatively clear. But it's also a good example of how small improvements could have a big impact.

The path ahead is shown to users but it is somewhat discrete in the top area of the page. The image above shows us that we are on the flight search page and that the journey ahead of us will include flight options, hotels, car rental, checkout and finally confirmation.

But is this enough? Easyjet have tried to discern the different steps to the process but it feels like a wayfinding system that could be improved. Perhaps if the stages were numbered or there was more distinction between current step and those that follow. They could even make it tabbed.

[1] www.easyjet.com

The stage you are on is made bold in the breadcrumbs and you can also click on any of the future stages to jump straight to those, but this isn't exactly clear.

For those who do get lost or stranded, there is no call to action available for help or more information. Which may result in users simply leaving the site without booking anything. Not good for Easyjet and not a good experience for their users either.

Information Architecture

Information architecture can also contribute to a wayfinding system. Even designs with little or no wayfinding in terms of signs can help users achieve their task if the information is in the right place. After all, words are also signs.

The *Apple* UK site is a good example of how information architecture can guide users without needing any colour coding or signs. The simplicity of its navigation makes it easy for users to get where they want to be.

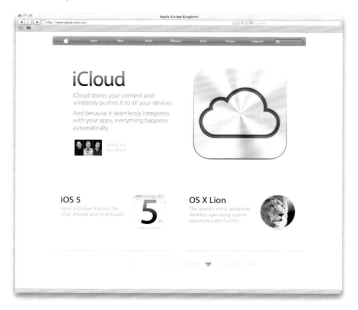

For example, there is no 'products' section. Instead, each product has its own main navigation item. Then when you click further into the site, such as by selecting 'iPod', the information architecture continues to show the way:

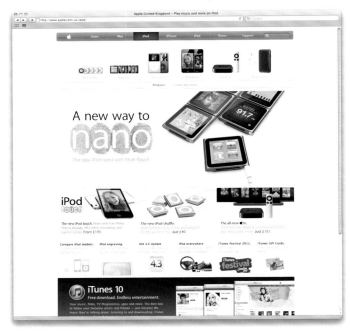

The iPod sub-menu for shows the available products and accessories. Again, the way the information is organised helps users achieve their goal, find the information they need, and also lets them know what area of the site they are in.

Icons

Icons can help users find their way. They are commonly used as calls to action and to represent tasks that users can complete. The meanings of these icons are, as previously discussed, learnt over time and agreed on by a culture or group.

Most websites support their icons with text to reinforce the meaning. A blog called *Fresho1*[1], from a South African design agency, uses only icons:

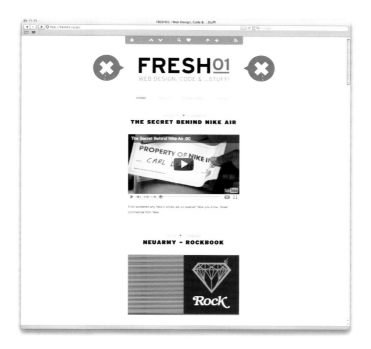

We can see that the Fresho1 homepage uses standard icons to represent 'home', 'search', 'next post', 'previous post', 'to top' and 'to bottom'. While this works reasonably well, having two different sets of arrows does make it somewhat confusing.

Relying on icons alone is challenging, so most websites support icons with minimal text anchors. Here's an example from the website of Tesco, the supermarket giant.

---

[1] http://fresho1.co.za/

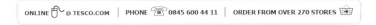

From the image above we can see three icons being used to communicate three tasks:

- A computer mouse is used to show that orders can be taken online
- A phone is used to tell customers the number for phone orders
- A shopping basket with an arrow inside is used for in-store orders

These are relatively common icons for representing the corresponding tasks, but the accompanying content helps clarify them.

Wayfinding on the web

A wayfinding system on the web can consist of:

- Colour coding
- Icons and symbols
- Information architecture

To design a successful wayfinding system you must be clear about the journey your users will experience. Ask questions about where they are, where they need to go and what they need to get there. The Guardian website is a good example of how to design a successful wayfinding system, and it's the subject of the next chapter.

10

CASE STUDY: *GUARDIAN.CO.UK*

To better show how a signage system can be applied to the web, I want to look at a site that's content heavy, with many layers and different categories of content. *The Guardian* newspaper website is the perfect example.

Here's the homepage:

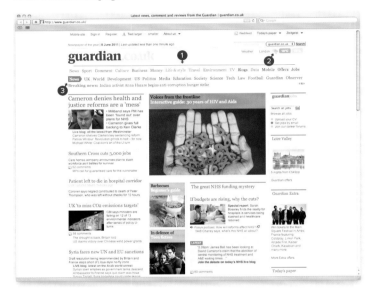

Several wayfinding points of interest are at work here:

1. **Colour coding**

   The Guardian site is content rich. The website creates additional structure and wayfinding support by colour coding the different sections. News is red, sport is green, money is purple, and so on.

   You might argue they chose the colours to represent the sections they classify, such as green for environment. But ultimately the main purpose is to distinguish between different content areas within the site.

   For example when the lines, navigation and header are red, users should be aware they are in the main 'News' section. 'Sport' and 'Environment' are both green, though they are different shades. (Green represents sport due to the colour of pitches, so it is also relevant to this section on the Guardian website.)

2. **Icons**

This isn't an icon-heavy website. The most obvious icons used here on the homepage are for the weather.

This means users don't have to dig deep to get an update on the day's weather. Just by glancing at the homepage they can see what the forecast will be (in this case, rainy).

3. **Signs**

Arrows are used in conjunction with colour coding to show the way. In this example we are clearly in the main section because of the colour red, the word 'News' and the arrow. This arrow shows we are on the main page but also points us towards deeper content where we can look specifically at UK news, world news, political news, US news, and so forth.

Navigation = wayfinding

Let's look closely at how the Guardian website's navigation clearly shows the way.

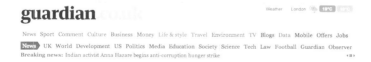

1. When users arrive at the Guardian site the navigation appears as shown above. They can select a top-level item such as 'Comment', 'Culture' or 'Travel' or delve deeper into the 'News' section.

2. When a top level item is chosen, for example 'Culture', the navigation changes:

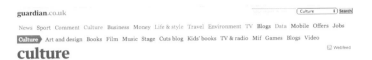

culture

As you can see, the colour of the arrow has changed to pink. It also shows us we are now in the 'Culture' section, and points to further subcategories such as 'Art and design', 'Books', and 'Film'.

There has been a subtle but distinct shift in the information we are presented with. As we move further into the site the wayfinding becomes ever more clear:

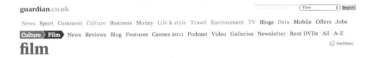

film

Here we are reminded we are in the 'Culture' section, thanks to the consistent pink colour. The navigation above shows us where we came from ('Culture') and where we are ('Film'), which is marked in a different shade from the same palette . And it shows us where we can move to within the 'Film' section: 'News', 'Reviews', 'Features', and so on.

This is a clear past, present and future structure, as well as a clear signage system.

As we move to a particular article under the 'Film' subcategory we see one more sign showing us where we are:

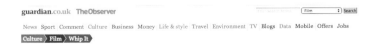

As you can see, 'Whip It' has now been added to the mix. This shows us we are on a feature about 'Whip It', that sits under the 'Film' category that is part of the 'Culture' section. Clear wayfinding supported by clever and considered use of colour.

Colour

The way the Guardian site uses colour is one reason it's such a good example of wayfinding.

As we discussed earlier, they use it to identify the different sections on the site, such as pink for 'Culture', blue for 'Business', green for 'Sport' and purple for 'Money'.

Users may not immediately know which colour represents what section, but those who use the site heavily make the connection almost subconsciously.

In fact colour plays such an important part in distinguishing between content areas they include a colour guide on the site.

A guide to colours and sections:

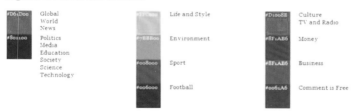

Even on their experimental 'Zeitgeist' section, which shows trending news, topics and articles from the Guardian, they use colour to show what category the trending content belongs to.

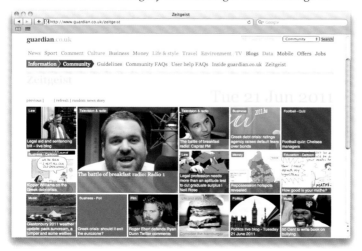

Icons

The Guardian site also uses icons to communicate quickly and efficiently, particularly in areas where users interact and generate content.

Here are some of the icons that pepper the Guardian site:

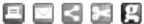

The icons are also supported by words, but differently to the Tesco example in the previous chapter. The words on the Guardian site aren't anchored to the icons, but rather appear when you mouse over them:

- The print icon is a well-understood online icon. Even without the words 'printable version', most users will know what it represents given its common use and shared understanding
- The mail icon for 'send to a friend' is relatively easy to decipher. Envelope icons are used to show that something can be emailed
- The 'share' icon is one point leading to two others. This represents one person sharing with two others, and hints at a network
- 'Clip' is shown with a scissor icon. Scissors are symbolic of cutting so the relevance here is self-explanatory. The clip function lets you send the article to your clippings file
- As there are numerous ways to get in touch with the newspaper, the Guardian has opted for a smaller version of its logo for the 'contact us' icon instead of the usual phone, email or pen icons

Any comments or content that users contribute to the Guardian site are shown using a speech bubble symbol, unless the users add their own avatar.

 Comments (148)

We associate the speech bubble icon with commenting and conversation. So when users see this icon they know it's somewhere they can share their opinions.

This convention makes it clear the content is user-generated, and not something written by a Guardian journalist. It also makes it clear the site is encouraging interaction. While we may take this icon and its use for granted, its meaning is only achieved by using it consistently in similar contexts. (It's also supported by text-- 'What You're Saying' at the top.)

Another content area where the Guardian site uses icons to communicate effectively is the weather page:

United Kingdom	London (Five-day forecast)		18°C	64°F	Sunny with showers
	Cheltenham (Five-day forecast)		15°C	59°F	Sunny with showers
	Edinburgh (Five-day forecast)		14°C	57°F	Sunny with showers
	Manchester (Five-day forecast)		16°C	60°F	Sunny with showers
	United Kingdom				
Europe	Paris (Five-day forecast)		20°C	68°F	Mostly cloudy, some showers
	Berlin (Five-day forecast)		23°C	73°F	Mostly cloudy
	Istanbul (Five-day forecast)		31°C	87°F	Sunny
	Europe				
North America	New York (Five-day forecast)	HOT	36°C	96°F	Hot
	Mexico City (Five-day forecast)		25°C	77°F	Sunny with showers
	North America				

These icons quickly give users an overview of the weather, but are also anchored by more detailed information if it's needed.

Organising information

Despite the many signs, clues and cues to help users navigate and complete their required task, the Guardian site also has a detailed and well-designed site index.

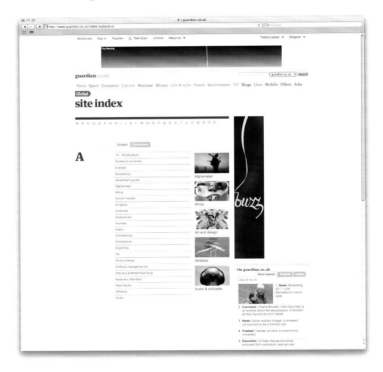

Here, the information is organised alphabetically, and then by subject or contributor. This is a good example of how to present vast amounts of information to users and give them clear pathways. Users need a quick and easy way to find what they want. If they use the site index to do so then breaking it down this way helps plot a route for them to get what they want.

Mobile wayfinding

The conventions the Guardian has employed on its website also translate to its iPhone app. The wayfinding components are similar, but given the nature of the platform they've put more emphasis on icons and symbols across the user interface.

The sections are coloured in the same way as the website. As we can see from the main page below, the search function and settings are symbolically represented. (These are *Apple* standard icons.)

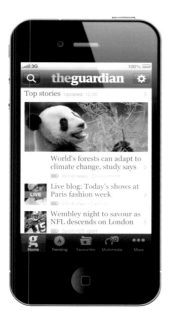

The arrows at the right of the news title make it clear that tapping the news story will take us to the actual article with more information.

The menu at the bottom of the screen uses icons effectively, making it clear what each one will lead to.

If we move to a content page the wayfinding system is even clearer:

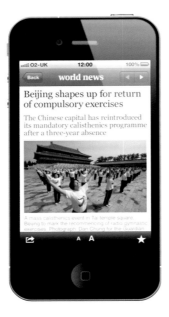

Here, red tells us we are in the 'News' section. Again, arrows show the route back and the route forward. The different sized letters in the footer show us that we can view the content with different font sizes, and the star lets us mark the page as a favourite. The star is a good choice for this icon because they are associated with good things, such as rewarding good behaviour in children.

The use of icons and symbols on the menu is the perfect example of where graphics can communicate, while contributing to a wayfinding system.

A wayfinding system

Whether on the homepage, a main topic or a specific article, there is a clear signage system at work. It shows users where they've been, where they are, and the options for where they can move to next.

Symbols and icons communicate calls to action and tasks quickly and efficiently, with the support of colour coding.

But don't forget that the content on the Guardian site is as much a sign as anything else. The information is organised sensibly and understandably so users will instinctively know where to go for certain content types.

The content is supported by a wayfinding system that, while it may well be dominated by colour, also uses icons effectively. And this wayfinding is consistent on the website, the mobile site, and even in the print edition.

The Guardian website succeeds by combining the value of all these signs and pointers. Collectively, they form a clear and useful method for users to find their way. The Guardian website has a lot of content to navigate through, so having an effective wayfinding system is vital.

Part 3

Using the right palette

The importance of colour

The colour of life

Connotation and Denotation

Colour in Cultures

Case Study: *Carsonified.com*

11   THE IMPORTANCE OF COLOUR

Colour is an important element in design. Each colour brings with it psychological associations, cultural significance, and an influence that can affect our mood.

In this section I'll focus on the messages and values that colours can communicate subliminally through design. I won't be looking at colour theory, but will explain how there's more to colour than just the shades we perceive.

To discover how colour communicates invisibly we need to look beneath the surface. We'll start by looking at some basic notions of what colour can bring and its importance as a communication tool, both on the web and in our everyday lives.

Understanding the power of colour helps with design decisions and choosing the most appropriate colours for the task in hand. It's only when we appreciate the power and importance of colour that we can discover how it enhances the user experience.

Colour and evolution

Throughout evolution, colour has become a part of our genetic code. From the time the first humans began hunting and gathering, the varied colours of our surroundings helped them to survive. (For example, they quickly learned not to eat the red poisonous berries.) These days colour is used to teach us where to go and where to avoid, such as the red on road signs communicating the no-go areas.

Humans crave stimulation. As we receive most input visually, a lack of colour jars with our fundamental needs. Our world is full of colour, and we have evolved to use it to survive and communicate.

Communicating through colour

Colour can communicate meaning in two ways: natural associations and psychological associations.

Natural associations come from the associations we draw between colours and our surroundings. Psychological associations, however, are learned through life experiences and influence how we react to colours on a personal level.

Some of these associations cross cultures, while others are culture dependent. For example, the association between the colour blue and the sea is probably about as universal as we can get. But blue also has more specific meanings in different cultures, which I will talk about later in this section.

Often these associations and reactions to colour happen on a visceral level; we don't consciously realise we are doing it. But these associations are important from an invisible design perspective, because colours can evoke certain emotions in us. And it's those emotions that influence our opinions, buying decisions and user experience.

Storytelling

Colour associations can vary between gender and age. They can also be influenced by social and political ideologies. While single colours tell stories (such as using red in stories of love and green in environmental stories), colour combinations do the job even better.

Here's a perfect example: think of a red, white and blue combination. Those three colours combined are patriotism personified, thanks to flags such as the Stars and the Stripes or the Union flag, which represent a whole nation. Those flags embody complete cultural, political and social systems.

People connect colours to their everyday experiences. Colours add narrative to any text they read, and can help guide them down a specific path. Colour is just one variable in your story, but it's perhaps the one that will grab their attention and help them form immediate opinions about your product, service, or website.

Visual judgement

People make a subconscious judgment about a person, environment, or product within 90 seconds of seeing it. And between 62% and 90% of that assessment is based on colour alone. (Source: CCICOLOR – Institute for Color Research).

Despite my best efforts, I do judge a book by its cover. I also form opinions of products, including websites, within seconds. For branding and marketing, visual impressions are extremely significant.

A study carried out by the Seoul International Color Expo 2004 showed that 92.6 percent of participants placed the most importance on the way a product looks when buying things. Another 5.6 percent said how it felt when they touched it was most important. Hearing and smell each drew 0.9 percent.

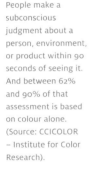
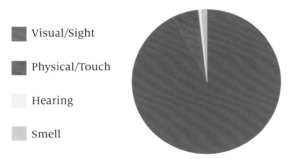

Visual/Sight

Physical/Touch

Hearing

Smell

With our eyes doing nearly all the work, colour clearly plays a part in our decision making process when shopping for physical products. Colour is just as significant online, if not more so, because we don't use the other senses on the web.

The art of communicating visual information is all about getting and retaining your audience's attention. And what catches the eye's attention in the first place? Colour.

My favourite colour

I wanted to learn more about the power of colour as a
communication tool and what it means to people. So I used my
blog and Twitter to conduct some lo-fi research, asking what
people's favourite colours were and why.

Here are some of the answers I received:

- Orange: *warm, associated with holidays and the sun*
- Red: *warm, and the national colour of Wales*
- Purple: *associated with wealth and gorgeous sunsets*
- Yellow: *a happy colour*
- Black: *simple and understandable*
- Blue: *reminds me of the ocean and I love the ocean*

These answers show how important a colour can be to someone
because of how it makes them feel. We're drawn to colours because
of the places, seasons, objects, nationalities and brands we
associate them with. Not to mention the emotions, behaviours and
moods they evoke in us.

With colours communicating such an array of messages,
there must be implications for design. Choosing colours is not a
decision to be made lightly.

Uses of colour

Colour can help us to achieve a variety of design goals, both online and in the real world. They can:

- Improve memory
- Influence buying decisions
- Tell stories
- Communicate cultural and political messages
- Evoke emotions and influence moods
- Bring static content to life
- Attract attention
- Indicate meaning
- Group elements
- Help with navigation

In the next chapter we'll take a deeper look at how colour influences us.

THE COLOUR OF LIFE AND THE WEB

To discover how we can use colour online to affect moods, influence buying decisions and improve navigation, let's look at just what colour gives us.

Colour vs. Black and White

The differences between black and white and colour images seem obvious at face value, but the different ways they communicate aren't quite as clear. Why is colour so powerful? It's worth looking at an example to emphasise the importance of colour and help answer this question.

Here is a scene shown in black and white:

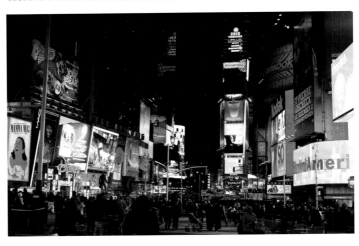

This image has its own charming qualities; indeed some images can be more striking without colour. Black and white photos, for example, hint at worlds gone by and conjure up feelings of nostalgia. The photo above may be charming, but it doesn't convey the atmosphere or energy of the place it depicts.

Here is the same scene shown in colour:

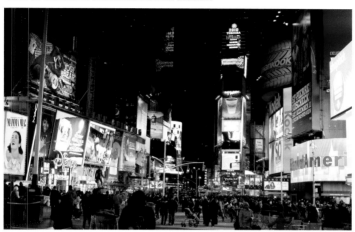

As you can see, colour adds atmosphere to the scene. It brings the static content to life, and emphasises the bright lights of the neon adverts, the shop signs, and even the movement at street level. We get a sense of just how bright, frantic, overwhelming and urban the place is – even if we don't know a thing about Times Square.

This doesn't mean you should always choose colour over black and white. There is a place for monochromatic design, such as *Khoi Vinh*'s beautiful Subtraction website'.

12 percent of people dream only in black and white.

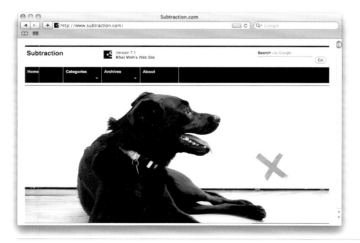

---

¹ www.subtraction.com

However, I find it harder to communicate through black and white because I can't connect a monochrome colour scheme to many emotions and life experiences beyond the feeling of 'retro'. Having missed the black and white television era I've always been surrounded by colour. So I immediately associate black and white with the past – a world I was never exposed to.

Colour brings things to life

Colour can affect every level of the user experience. It brings things to life and gives a sense of dimension and depth. It also creates a stronger connection between the user and what they see on the screen, as they can more easily relate it to something in the 'real' world.

Scott McCloud touches on this in his excellent book, *Understanding Comics: The Invisible Art*. McCloud teaches us that:

> *"Another property of flat colours is their tendency to emphasise the shape of objects, both animate and inanimate, as any child who has ever colored-by-numbers knows instinctively. These colours objectify their subjects. We become more aware of the physical form of objects than in black and white."*

While McCloud was talking specifically about comic book art, his point can be applied across other communication platforms, including the web.

Here's another benefit. Adverts, comics, websites, and other visual media usually have a lot of content that can't be processed all at once. Colour can give one area or specific piece of content more prominence over another. It can help us group content, and lead the user's eyes to specific areas by adding an 'invisible' hierarchy of importance to the content.

Colour aids memory

We've evolved to remember the colours of things that can help us (such as edible fruit in trees) and harm us (such as wasps and bees). It's an innate human ability to associate colours with feelings, danger, cultures and the world around us. So it's no surprise that we remember things better if they are in colour.

Studies have been conducted to test the theory that colour improves memory. While I won't be discussing the research in detail here, the conclusions are relevant.

A study in the Journal of Experimental Psychology: Learning, Memory and Cognition, published by the American Psychological Association (APA)[1], reports how the visual system exploits colour information. Adding colour to a scene is like adding extra data that helps the brain process and store images more efficiently than those in black and white. And that in turn makes them easier to recall.

With that in mind, here are two sequences of symbols, with one sequence in black and white and the other in colour. In theory you should remember the sequence of colour symbols more readily than the black and white ones. (Don't worry, I'm not going to test you later.)

Here they are in black and white:

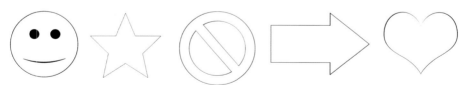

---

[1] May 2002 issue of the Journal of Experimental Psychology: Learning, Memory and Cognition, published by the American Psychological Association (APA)
"The Contributions of Color to Recognition Memory for Natural Scenes,", Vol 28. No.3., 5-May-2002

And now with a splash of colour:

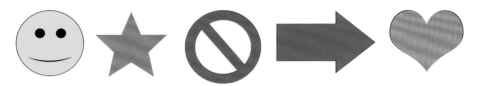

Just as Scott McCloud stated, adding colour brings these symbols to life. It helps us relate them to our world, and improves our ability to recall them in test situations.

Pink and red connote love, so a pink heart is easier to remember than a black and white one. Similarly, we know red can also represent danger, which is why the third symbol is easier to recall than its black and white counterpart. We can link the red version to signs we see regularly.

Green has come to communicate the process of moving forward, such as green for go on traffic lights. So an arrow pointing the way in a green colour lets us join the dots between the symbol, the colour and a real life example. A black and white arrow pointing in the same direction has fewer (if any) links to our world so we can't digest it as easily, making it harder to recall later on.

Colour influences us

Colour influences our moods and our spending habits. Let's look at how important colour is when trying to influence the latter.

Apple

Apple produces iMacs and iPods in a variety of colours. These colours say a lot about the item's owner, and they influence our decision on what product to buy.

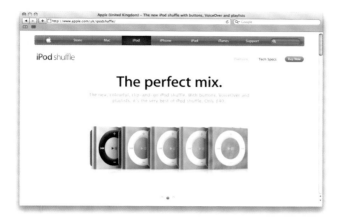

The colours that iPods come in influence our decision over which product to buy. I would never buy a pink iPod for myself because it is stereotypically a girl's colour. Blue and black, on the other hand, are top of my list. For me, the fact such a choice even exists speaks volumes. As consumers we can now buy a music player that best reflects our own personalities.

This colour preference stretches beyond Apple products though. I'd never buy a pink t-shirt, but I have plenty of blue, black and grey ones. And it's not just because I prefer those colours. I'm also influenced by what different colours communicate and how they are linked to genders in particular. Call me stereotypical, but these are associations many succumb to and it has weaved itself into my subconscious.

Colour affects our mood

As we've already discussed, colour evokes emotions in us and affects our moods. A simple shade can make us feel happy. This is invisible communication, and while we may not enter a yellow room and think "That colour is making me feel cheery", it does influence us subconsciously. And the colours we see online will likely have a similar affect.

Let's now look at a real world example where colour is used to influence our moods.

Hospitals and surgeries.

Doctor's surgeries often have green or blue walls, as these tones are said to help people relax. Blue helps the muscles to relax and so the heart beats slower, thus inducing a sense of calm. It also causes the brain to secrete tranquilising hormones. Green creates an environment of emotional balance where the eyes relax and concentration increases. In many cases the uniforms for surgeons and nurses are also green for the same calming reasons.

It also happens at mental health units, where the walls are often beige with a pink tint. Combined with mint green floors, it creates a soothing, harmonious and calm area--important in an environment where unpredictable behaviour can be commonplace.

Hospitals and surgeries avoid using strong colours. Instead they use neutral tones, which help create a sense of wellbeing. Red in particular can make the heart beat faster (not advisable for people with high blood pressure) and so they avoid it. Similarly too much yellow is said to cause headaches, and studies have shown that babies cry more in yellow-coloured rooms.

Bright and bold for the young

In stark contrast, schools and play areas favour strong and bold colours as these are more appealing to children and create happy, bright environments for them.

Research has shown children don't like the colour green as they associate it with vegetables. In his book *Color Psychology and Color Therapy*, Faber Birren learnt that yellow is popular with children but as we move into adulthood it shows less popularity.

Birren found that:

> *"with maturity comes a greater liking for hues of shorter*
> *wave length (blue, green, purple) than for hues of longer*
> *wave length (red, orange, and yellow)"*

Colours will influence our moods differently as we mature. We also gain more life experience, and so have a greater range of colour association.

Colour idioms

Another example of how we associate colours with moods and emotions is in common sayings. I'm sure you've heard most of these:

- He was green with envy
- I'm feeling blue
- She saw red
- They were green around the gills
- We found him black and blue
- The black sheep of the family
- I caught her red-handed
- We were tickled pink
- She told a little white lie

We can use colours this way because we know the associations. For example, 'She saw red' works because we have learnt that red can represent anger and rage. Green is a colour that represents being envious. (It even appears in the Skype emoticon for 'envy'.)

In the next chapter we'll take a closer look at the connotations – the implied meanings – of various colours.

13

CONNOTATIONS OF COLOUR

One thing that fascinates me is the connotations – the meanings –
we associate with colour.

It's worth looking beyond the literal and investigating the
hidden meanings of colours. Doing so can teach us valuable
lessons, and help us create websites that not only look the part,
but also target their audiences perfectly.

Connotation and denotation

The denotation of something is its literal meaning – the most
specific or direct meaning of a word, as opposed to its associated
meanings, or connotations. For colour, then, the denotation of red
is the literal shade of red.

Let's look at this symbol:

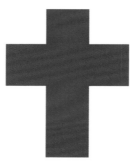

The denotation here is a brown cross. It is a cross and it's brown.
But the connotation is that it's a religious symbol or, more
specifically, the symbol of Christianity.

Connotation is the implied or suggested meaning. For red, the
connotation varies depending on the context, but the two most
common connotations for red are danger and love.

Take this rose, for example:

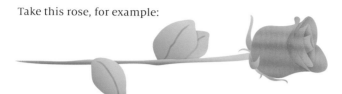

The denotation here is a red rose with a green stem. The connotation, however, is passion and love. A red rose is a symbol of these emotions, and that's what it has come to represent.

Red has many connotations, including stop, danger, and warnings. That's why it's commonly seen on road signs.

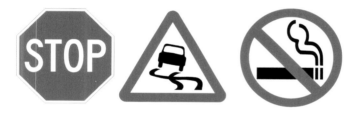

Is this a black circle?

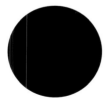

Yes, if we look at it literally. The denotation here is the absence of colour. It is simply a circle that is black.

The connotation, however, could be any number of things: fear of the unknown, a black hole, the dark, a void, or even space (a natural association often reinforced in media such as films, particularly science fiction).

Thinking of colours in relation to their connotations can help us make the right decisions when choosing colour in website design. Instead of choosing colours just because they looks good, we start asking ourselves whether they tell the right story, or represent the most appropriate mood.

I've already given some examples where colours can create a particular mood, such as in hospitals. But now we'll look at this aspect of colour theory in more depth, and across a wider range of colours.

The expert opinion

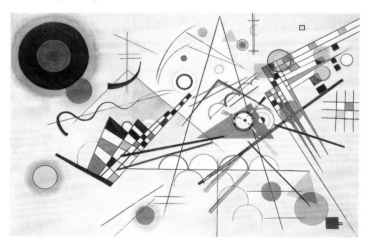

Wassily Kandinsky was one of the first pioneers of colour theory. A renowned Russian painter and art theorist, he is often considered the founder of abstract art. As an authoritative voice on colour, Kandinsky believed colours could have both emotional and physical effects on people. He thought that – alongside other formal elements, such as line, shape, and form – colour is a language that communicates to all.

As part of his theory, Kandinsky associated the following colours with certain qualities:

Warm, cheeky, exciting, happy
Deep, inner, peaceful, supernatural
Stillness, peace, hidden strength, passive
Harmony, silence, cleanliness
Grief, dark, unknown
Soundless, emotionless
Alive, restless, glowing, confident
Dull, hard, inhibited
Radiant, healthy, serious
Morbid, grief, sickness

The qualities Kandinsky describes aren't necessarily obvious connections. But they do show us how colours can connote emotions, temperatures, seasons, and moods, as well as make us think of specific objects, places, and animals.

But here's a question: Do we immediately associate the colours with the emotions when we see those colours in our world and online?

Colours and their connotations
Let's delve a little deeper and take a look at various colours and how they can motivate us emotionally.

Red

Connotes: *love, passion, desire, danger, war, blood, strength, power*

Red is an intense colour that raises blood pressure and increases respiration rates. Its high visibility makes it ideal for hazard and warning signs, as well as fire protection equipment.

Red can stimulate people, and lends itself nicely to 'Buy it now' or 'Click here' calls to action. It's also common in eating establishments because it's an appetite stimulant.

Yellow

Connotes: *sunshine, happiness, energy, cheerfulness, spontaneous*

Yellow is a cheery colour that many people associate with being happy. It stimulates mental activity, and also has a warming effect. In its brightest form yellow is an attention grabber, and objects in this colour certainly stand out from the crowd (such as the iconic New York taxicabs). It can be a very effective way to highlight the most important elements of your design. However, it also has connotations of spontaneity, so its suitability may depend on the story you are trying to tell.

It's also used with black for hazard signs, as it stands out against black more than other colours do.

Yellow is a contradictory colour. It's often associated with happiness, and yet using it too much can have negative effects, such as inducing headaches. Studies have shown that babies are more likely to cry in yellow rooms. Yellow is also said to increase metabolism and enhance concentration.

Blue

Connotes: *cool, icy, sea, sky, trust, loyalty, wisdom, heaven, truth, intelligence*

Blue has a calming effect, and so is commonly used in hospitals and surgeries. It also has connotations of purity and cleanliness, and its obvious association with the sea and sky make it an ideal choice for promoting airlines and cruises.

But blue can be cold and unwelcoming, depending on the tone. It also suppresses the appetite, so avoid it if promoting or designing food-related products and sites. And it's a stereotypically male colour.

When combined with other colours, blue can connote patriotic messages and political statements. People recommend wearing blue to interviews as it symbolises loyalty.

Green

Connotes: *nature, relaxation, growth, harmony, fresh, wealth, fertility*

Green is restful and harmonious, and is a recommended colour for improving concentration. Because of its connotations of growth and nature it is commonly used for topics such as recycling, organic, and being environmentally friendly.

Brides in the Middle Ages wore green to symbolise fertility.

Darker greens are usually associated with wealth and money.

Purple

Connotes: *royalty, luxury, wizardry, power, nobility, ambition, mystery, magic*

Fewer links exist between purple and the natural world than the other colours, and so it is often considered to be artificial. This may be why it is often linked to fantasy and magic.

Purple can also be a more feminine colour (depending on the shade), while brighter purple is used for children's products. (Let's face it: Barney the Dinosaur is about as bright as they come.)

Orange

Connotes: *warmth, sunshine, joy, citrus, Autumn, enthusiasm, success, stimulation*

Orange, like red, is a hot colour. So it's no surprise that it's used for fire and heat. It is said to increase the oxygen supply to the brain and therefore stimulate mental activity.

Brown

Connotes: *reliable, stable, earth, nature, natural, genuine, dirty*

Brown is warm and comforting. It can stimulate the appetite, and because of its associations with the soil it symbolises being down to earth.

Black

Connotes: *death, evil, mystery, power, elegance, space, voids, grief, mourning*

Black is associated with fear and the unknown. It usually has a negative connotation, although it can also connote strength and authority.

White

Connotes: *peace, elegance, innocence, purity, clinical, sterile, icy, light, virginity, transparent*

White is an innocent colour, linked to purity and neutrality. White 'goes with everything'. Doctors and nurses wear white to imply sterility.

It is also the most common colour for brides to wear. Bridal white is associated with being virginal, though red is usually the colour people associate with love.

Colours on the web

Let's take a look at some websites to see how they use colours to
tell their stories:

La Senza is an underwear store and as expected the website
is predominantly pink and black. Pink (along with red) has
connotations of love and romance. Combined with black this then
adds a sexy feel to the site.

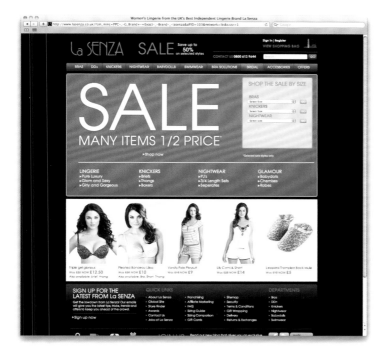

For seasons you can be sure that wintry websites will be blue and
white, colours that connote coldness, ice and freezing. Autumnal
websites will go for brown, red and orange to reflect the shades
of trees during this time. Spring themed sites will use green, blue
and yellow. Spring is all about growth. Green communicates
that value.

But what if you could change the colour of a website?
Would that also change the feeling it imparts, in line with the
connotations discussed previously? Well, the *BBC* homepage
allows users to change the colour, and the results are rather
insightful.

The Users Decide
We choose colours all the time when buying clothes, decorating
and designing. Now you can choose from 13 colours on the BBC
homepage, or even have them on rotation. Users rarely get to make
these decisions online.

Here is the BBC homepage. You can see the sections where
you can change the colour. (You can't have one section blue and
another one red. They all have to be the same colour.)
When these block colours change, the colour of the text links also
change to the user's choice of page colour.

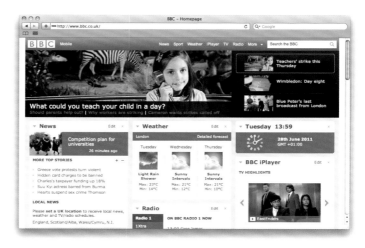

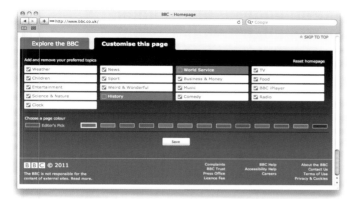

Everyone will have their own colour preferences. Personally I would select from the first five or the last five colours, and ignore the ones in between.

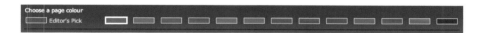

Why? Because to me the three middle colours connote feminine qualities. Pink tones are seen today as stereotypically girl's colours. The fact I am more likely to choose the blue shades or brown and black options is echoed in my choice of iPod colour, clothes and general colour preference in everyday life. Why should it be any different online?

People's choices could also be linked to how they perceive the BBC brand. For some it may always be the traditional red they think of, while for others it might be pink as per the BBC3 TV channel.

A simple colour change may seem insignificant. But it's amazing how different the homepage can not only look but also communicate and connote varying messages just by changing the colour.

Let's look at the BBC Homepage in six different colours and see how each one makes the site feel.

Red:

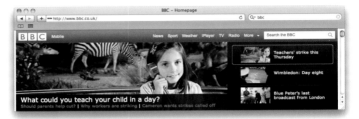

Red is the staple colour for the BBC. In this context it connotes trust and tradition, (values commonly associated with the corporation) rather than love and romance.

While the page does hint at romanticism it isn't screaming that message to us. For me the choice of red for the BBC homepage is the safest of all the colour choices.

Green:

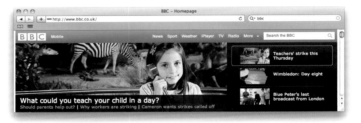

The change in colour immediately shifts the tone of the site, making it look more like a nature website.

It's natural, earthy, and friendly – all connotations of green because most colour symbolism is linked to nature.

It also adopts a fresh feel and, more so than the other colours, makes me feel calm and relaxed.

Purple:

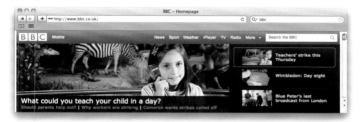

Purple makes the site more futuristic than the previous two colours, perhaps because there are few associations between purple and the natural world.

It gives the site a more feminine touch and reminds me of websites for cosmetic products, but also the sites of specific brands such as Cadburys.

Black:

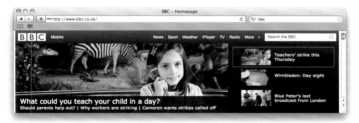

This page tells a different story altogether. Using black instead of the other brighter options makes it look more traditional and less friendly.

It also seems more masculine, and instils a sense of nostalgia in me. It also reminds me of a newspaper, which does fit the BBC's reputation of being a reliable news source.

For those reasons I struggle to feel comfortable with this option. I can't quite connect to it in the same way I can with the other colour options.

Orange:

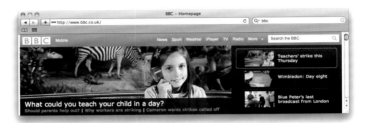

Fresh, summery, bright. These are the messages I'm getting from this page. This is definitely one of the more eye-catching colours out of the six selected. It is warm and inviting, and has a happy vibe about it. It also feels quite energetic and youthful, though I wouldn't normally use those adjectives to describe the BBC.

Blue:

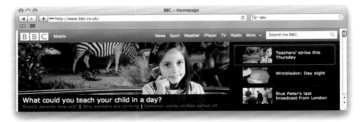

This is my favourite of all the colours. It feels fresh and relaxing, and I find it easier on the eyes than some of the other options.

I feel at ease with blue in general, so it's bound to influence my colour choice here. It hints at the ocean and blue skies, which both make me feel more positive.

What this little experiment shows us is that each colour hints at different qualities. They each tell a different story. The content is the same on all these pages, but changing the colour has changed the whole feel of the page.

Now let's look at how colour connotations can vary between cultures.

Colour in cultures

Many of the colour connotations we've discussed so far have been UK-centric and focused more on Western tradition. But some meanings are culture dependant, and a given colour can send very different messages in different places around the world.

As a designer you need to know your audience when choosing colours, or you risk conveying an entirely different message from the one you intended.

Worldwide differences

The most notable difference in colour connotations is between the Eastern and Western cultures, although this boundary is starting to blur. The differences can range from one colour representing opposite values to more subtle variations.

How a culture perceives a particular colour will influence its use as a communication tool. The branding on specific products can provide the best insight into this area. Green, for example, is seen on products targeted at Austrian or Turkish audiences. However, green is an unpopular colour in Belgium and France, and so wouldn't be an effective way to influence people's shopping habits in those countries.

Here's another example. Orange is the national colour of the Netherlands, and so often connotes patriotism there. In the UK, however, orange is the brand colour for corporate giants such as *Orange* and *EasyJet*.

This shows how the core message of one colour can vary between locations (and often does).

One of the best examples of a location where colour choice has a profound impact on the companies selling there is China.

Spotlight on China

Product and web designers can fall into a trap if they overlook the cultural differences between Western markets and China.

In China, red is a symbol of good luck and happiness. It's a powerful colour for branding and consumerism in China because of its positive effect on people's moods – ideal for subliminally influencing people to buy something.

Bright colours are used to great effect on food products in China. But personal care items tend to be dominated by pastel and diluted tones. In keeping with these values, *General Mills* changes its packaging for the Chinese market, opting for brighter colours. (For those not familiar with General Mills, its worldwide brands include *Betty Crocker*, *Old El Paso* and *Cheerios*.)

Kleenex, the tissue manufacturer, use bright colours on its US branding and packaging but favours pastel colours for the Chinese market.

Neutral – welcome to all

If there's one colour that can cross cultural boundaries, it's white. White is pure and clean. While it can have cultural relevance (such as being the symbolic colour of weddings in the UK), it's also used to appeal to the masses due to its inoffensive and calm connotations.

Official tourism websites often avoid using any strong signature colours in favour of white. Maybe it's because white is peaceful, neutral and inoffensive, and so will appeal to everyone.

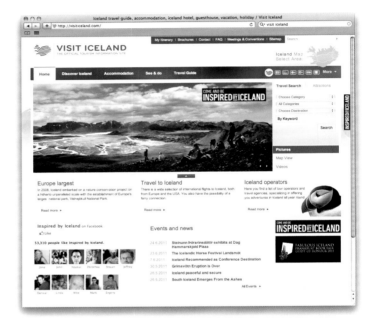

http://www.visiticeland.com/

With other colours anchored to certain messages, it would be difficult to target different cultures with the same colour as they would each read it in different ways. For that reason, white seems to be a safe bet.

However, to better understand why white transcends cultures let's look at colours in relation to their cultural significance.

Colouring by cultures

In the next few pages I will look at several colours and give examples of how they are interpreted in different countries around the world. I'll also provide examples from the East and the West, and show instances where they match.

- China – *good luck, marriage (it's worn by brides), celebration ("paint the town red")*
- India – *purity, danger, symbol for a soldier*
- South Africa – *mourning*
- Russia – *communism. (Red means beautiful in Russia. The Bolsheviks used a red flag as their symbol when they overthrew the tsar in 1917, and so red became a symbol of communism.)*
- UK – *danger, passion, love, stop, Christmas*

Perhaps the most universal use of red is signalling stop on traffic lights. It's a colour that draws attention, highlights important objects, and is commonly associated with danger, no entry and stop – an association reaffirmed through road signs.

Red first became connected with stop signs in the 1830s when used for railroad signalling. Then in 1954 the *US Federal Highway Administration* (FHA) published *The Manual on Uniform Traffic Control Devices* (MUTCD). It was in this manual that the stop sign was standardised as red with white type.

Red is also the most common colour in national flags.

- Japan – *courage*
- Egypt and Burma – *mourning*
- China – *royalty*
- India – *the symbol for a merchant or a farmer, Hindus wear yellow to celebrate the festival of spring*
- UK – *hope, hazards*

Yellow is highly visible, and so is often used to warn of hazards (especially when combined with black).

- China – *exorcism, cheating, disgrace*
- India – *Islam*
- UK – *spring, St Patrick's Day, good luck (four leaf clover), national colour of Ireland*
- USA – *wealth*
- Spain – *perverseness*
- North Africa – *corruption*

Perhaps the most universal association for green is nature. Trees are the same colour around the world, and so everyone can make the same these association.

- Thailand – *mourning, orchid, royalty*
- UK – *magic, royalty, luxury*
- USA – *The U.S. military decorates soldiers wounded or killed in battle with a "Purple Heart"*

Purple is hard to deconstruct because it has so few associations to the natural world. (I can only think of beetroot.) Therefore its symbolism is learned through cultural association. It is often cited as being a plush colour with connotations of royalty, luxury and wealth.

In the late 1960s, purple became a symbol of gay pride, supported by the "Purple Power" catchphrase.

- UK – *Conservatism*
- USA – *Liberalism*
- Iran – *mourning*
- Ancient Rome – *public servants wore blue. Today police and other public servants wear blue*

Blue is very popular because of its association with the sea and the sky – representations that are certainly more universal than others. It is also most commonly linked to boys in the western world.

Regarding its political significance: Blue in the UK is associated with the Conservative Party while in the USA it's associated with the Democratic Party. This clearly shows how one colour can have a completely opposite meaning from one culture to another. The fact such a dichotomy even exists shows how much you need to think about colour choices in design.

- Netherlands – *Royalty*
- India – *Hinduism*
- Northern Ireland – *Protestantism*
- USA – *cheap goods, Halloween*

Orange is an appetite stimulant, so it's a useful colour for restaurants. Like red, it increases oxygen supply to the brain and stimulates mental activity. As it becomes brighter it also becomes more energetic.

It also gives the sensation of heat due to its connotations of fire and flames.

- India – *sorrow, unhappiness*
- UK – *marriage, angels, peace*
- China, Korea, Vietnam, Japan – *traditionally a colour of mourning*

White is commonly linked to marriage, as it's the colour most brides choose to wear. (This tradition dates back to Ancient Greece.) It is also symbolic of peace, due to the white flags of surrender.

- UK – *mourning (funerals), intelligence (graduation robes)*
- *China – black is for little boys*
- Thailand – *unhappiness, bad luck*
- Kenya and Tanzania (tribes) – *black is associated with rain clouds and therefore symbolises prosperity and life*

Black, while often perceived as a negative colour, can also have connotations of sophistication, technology and gadgets.

It's also linked to elegance due to formal black tie events and little black dresses. (It's even said to make people appear slimmer)

Information is Beautiful is a website by *David McCandless* that 'visualizes information – facts, data, ideas, subjects, issues, statistics, questions – all with the minimum of words."

On his website David produced a stunning infographic that shows what colours mean in different cultures.

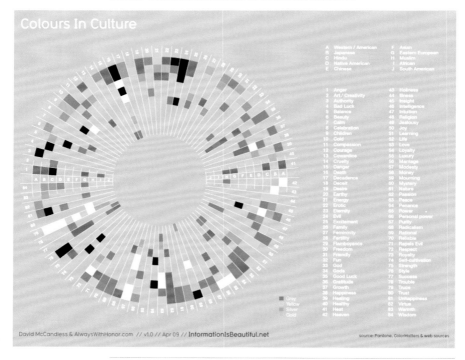

[1] http://www.informationisbeautiful.net/visualizations/colours-in-cultures/

Politically correct colours

A by-product of culture, politics can be represented through colour too. In the UK, each political party is associated with a specific colour. Labour are red, Conservatives are blue, Liberal Democrats are yellow and the Green Party are, well, green.

The political connotations of colours could be significant (depending on your target audience), and knowing the political conventions will help support your message rather than contradict it.

For example, if you were designing a website for a left-leaning think tank then you probably shouldn't use a lot of blue, as this is associated with the Conservatives (the right wing).

Changes through time

The cultural significance of colours can change. Never assume that what a colour represents now is the same as 10, 50 or 100 years ago. Cultures evolve, and the cultural significance of colours can also shift over time.

For example, white has traditionally been the colour of mourning in China. But young Chinese brides are now wearing white gowns to emulate the Western tradition. White was also the colour of mourning in Japan many centuries ago, but it has since changed to black.

Colour selection

You could spend days researching the meaning of every colour throughout the world. The key is to focus your attention on the audience you're targeting, and determine the significance of colours to them in relation to their culture.

Some projects bring with them brand guidelines, and you may well be tied into a certain colour or combination of colours. Even then it is still worth conducting your own research to ensure the colours you have been told to use support the brand, company, or story you are designing for. Be informed, and your designs will be relevant.

15 — CASE STUDY: *CARSONIFIED.COM*

So far we've established:

- Why colour is important
- How it can communicate to us
- What it tells us
- How the messages it communicates can vary between cultures

Now let's look at a real-life example of just how powerful colour can be.

While researching this book I got to speak with *Mike Kus* (one of my favourite designers) about the role colour played in the redesign of the Carsonified website. What followed was a fascinating insight into the power of colour, and why it is so important in design.

The brief

The new Carsonified site had to:

- Express the company's character
- Communicate what they do on the homepage (Carsonified is an events company)
- Include links to the 'Home', 'Events', 'Mission', 'Jobs', 'Contact' and 'Team' pages
- Communicate the specific message, "We are passionate about what we do"

Carsonified also has a popular online blog for designers and developers called 'Think Vitamin'. This was being removed from its own domain and included in the new Carsonified site. But still had to retain its own identity.

The aim of the redesign was to express the feeling of Carsonified, make a statement with the holding page and provoke a reaction in the audience.

I talked to Mike in some detail about the redesign process, and he confirmed that from quite early on in the project he wanted to use colour effectively to show Carsonified's bright personality. But it also had to communicate the organization's serious side.

And that was the challenge Mike faced – striking the right balance between designing a colourful website and keeping it simple. The redesign process came up with a number of different concepts. Many were rejected because they didn't fit with the story that needed to be told. Some of the earlier designs were also too personal and more sketchbook – they didn't have a strong message.

Storytelling and colour

They decided to bring more colour into the design, and to use the content itself to communicate the desired message. By working on storytelling and the use of colour, they turned designs that weren't hitting the mark into the final concept.

With this goal in mind, they created these options:

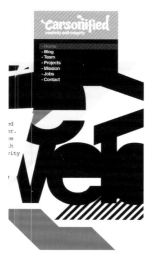
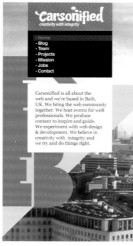
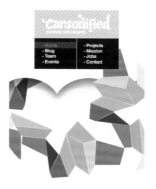

That last concept illustrates the problem Mike was trying to solve. Wanting the site to be bright and bold, Mike opted for a multi-colour approach. But the simplicity was lost, as the two don't go hand in hand. The multi-colour option does connote playfulness, but it was too fussy.

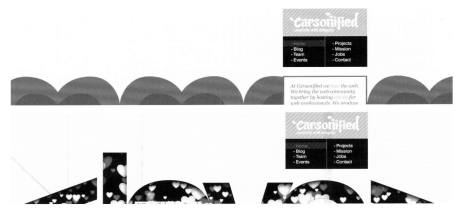

As you can see, the designs became bolder and the use of colour more important. But these are still a long way from what the finished site looks like. The use of pink, red, the word 'love' and the heart shapes all reinforce the notion of passion. But while Mike had the story nailed, he felt he needed to inject Carsonified's personality into the design.

That personality came in the form of illustrations. Mike added them to one of the concepts centred around passion, and produced two options for the homepage:

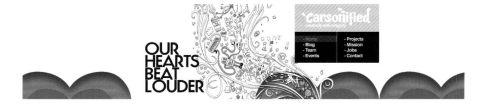

As the design was refined the use of colour was honed, which led to an unlikely source of inspiration.

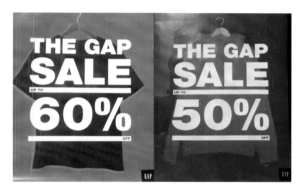

Mike explained how he saw these for sale posters in the window of a Gap store and was immediately hit by how simple they were.

> "The posters were brash and in your face and you wouldn't necessarily associate this style with beautiful design. But I realised how powerful bold simplicity could be when used in a creative way."

This triggered another inspiration. The United Colours of Benetton advertising campaigns relied heavily on colour, but in the form of simple, flat colours. According to Mike, "You need to think outside the box when designing for the web as you are more likely to come up with something original and apt."

With these posters firmly in mind, they tackled the redesign with a new approach: include bold colour in a simple way, and keep the colours used on each page to a minimum.

This concept evolved to become one colour per page. Within hours the final iteration was completed and Mike knew it was the one that would go live. He continued producing illustrations to tell the story in combination with the copy and the colours.

The homepage

When we chatted about the homepage it was interesting to hear how Mike consciously chose black to make it different from every other page.

Here's the homepage how it looked when the site was launched:

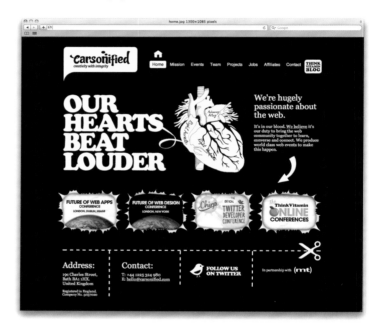

Black and white can have negative connotations. But Mike's goal was to make a statement, and so he chose to make the homepage "an anti-page" in the sense that every page would feature a bold colour except the homepage. If users landed on the homepage they would see a black and white site, but as they moved further into the content the colours would reveal themselves page by page. (The white was also an off-white colour, to give it a retro feel.)

And here is the most recent version as of June 2011:

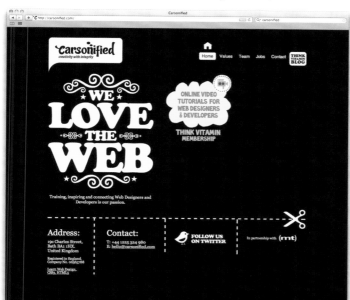

The lack of colour here does indeed jar with the other pages, but that was the whole point. When users landed on the homepage it was meant to provoke a reaction (good or bad), which would hopefully lure people in to explore the rest of the site and reveal the colour and story beyond.

Showing the way

A conscious decision had clearly been made about what colour each page would be, and I wanted to know if the selection was random or influenced by the meanings that colours communicate. I was pleased to hear the colour choices were not random, but purposefully used as a way finding technique. As Mike explained:

> "The top level navigation is bright, and no two pages have the same colour. Then, as we move to the team pages the colours become less bright and more dull, but also more personal."

Top-level navigation:

Carsonified
creativity with integrity
Home Values Team Jobs Contact
THINK VITAMIN BLOG
OUR CORE VALUES
At Carsonified we hold our core values close to our heart. They're what we're all about. Let us take you through them.
Ryan
Founder
Ryan loves web tech, coffee and movies. (Is it wrong to see The Matrix seven times at the cinema?) He's got a degree in Computer Science and is passionate about connecting and encouraging people - which is why he's passionate about running events for the web community. He loves his wife and can't believe he's a dad.
ryan@carsonified.com
Ryan on Twitter
Ryan
Gill
Jo
Lou
Tash
Cat
Guy
Allison
Alan
Nick
Jim
Michael
Jon
Will
Pete
GROW
Sorry no vacancies at the moment
Working at Carsonified
The Benefits
The four day week
Your very own iPhone
MAKE CONTACT
Your Name
Your Email
Your Message
Send Message

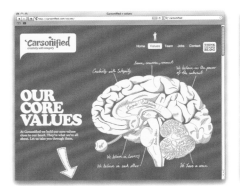

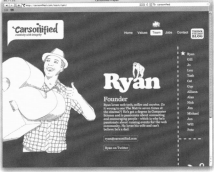

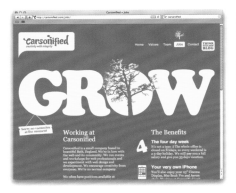

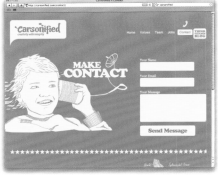

Secondary Navigation:

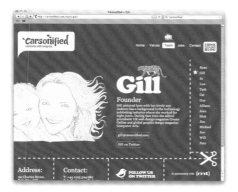
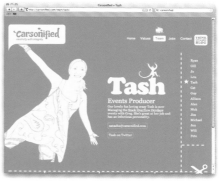
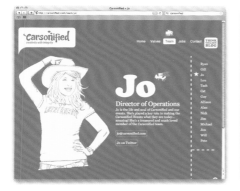
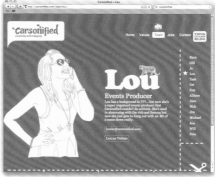

The clever use of single-colour pages leads the user through the site. There is no colour merging between content, and users will instinctively know where they are by the page colour alone.

Matching content to colour

A fundamental part of choosing the right colours was to look at the content of each page. As you can see, the colours chosen support the copy and echo the story on each page.

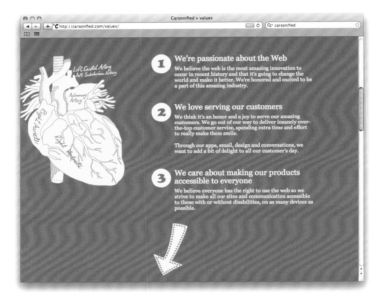

The 'Values' page does this by using the colour red. The content is all about Carsonified believing in what they do and having a passion for their work. And no colour connotes these values better than red.

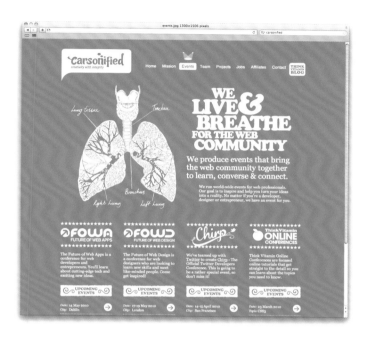

Similarly, Mike chose blue for the 'Events' page because 'it is centred around the notion that we live and breathe what we do. I chose blue because of its associations with air and breathing.' This page is no longer live on the current Carsonified site.

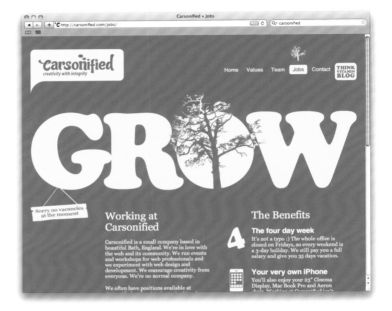

The 'Jobs' page is all about the team expanding and growing. This is communicated through the colour green because of its associations with nature. The word 'grow' dominates the top of the page, along with an image of a tree. These three elements all emphasise the notion of growth and new beginnings – the perfect message for a jobs page.

People often take colour for granted when it's used correctly. And that's the beauty of colour – peopledon't think about it unless we break a convention that makes them notice.

Here's Mike's perspective on it:

> *"If you challenge peoples preconceived notion of colour it makes them talk. We believe the jobs page wouldn't have worked on dull grey."*

The original version of the contacts page featured a dull, muted colour. A user noticed this, and contacted Mike to say it was out of place with the other top-level navigation pages. As a direct result, Mike changed the page to its current orange shade.

Team Pages

On generic pages and pages about the company, a single colour was used to communicate the desired message. Selecting a colour for the team pages was more difficult because each person couldn't be defined or represented by one colour alone. According to Mike, the colour choices in this section were made more with a sense of fun.

The final design definitely offers a solution to the problem presented in the brief. In particular, using one colour per page allowed the site to be bright and full of the Carsonified personality, but also simple – something the earlier designs failed to achieve.

Knowledge is colour

I was impressed by Mike's knowledge of colour and how important it was in his designs. It was never a secondary thought or a passing idea – it was a fundamental part of his design process.

I asked Mike what his best colour tip for other people would be. His response? "Keep it simple."

The Carsonified website couldn't use any fewer colours – it's as simple as it could be. Yes, colour does dominate and is a major reason the site works so well. But it uses only one simple, solid colour per page. Mike summed it up perfectly:

> "The simpler you keep colour, the more you can say to everybody. You don't want to have to get users to work things out if they are only on your site for a few seconds. I believe colour has helped me create a design for Carsonified that people will remember in just those few seconds of seeing it."

Part 4

Using the correct language

The invisible side of language

How the words look

The Periodic Table of Typefaces

Tone of voice

Case study: *Innocent Drinks*

THE INVISIBLE SIDE OF LANGUAGE

How can language be invisible?

When we talk to someone in person, our words are supported by body language, tone of voice, pitch, volume, accent, expression and cues – all forms of invisible communication. By using these invisible cues, we can convey emotions and moods such as sarcasm and anger without having to say we are being sarcastic or feel angry.

When writing for the web, we can still communicate invisibly through the tone of our writing voice, the look of our words, and the overall design of our website.

Some common definitions of 'language':[1]

1. A body of words and the systems for their use common to a people who are of the same community or nation, the same geographical area, or the same cultural tradition.

2. Communication by voice in the distinctively human manner, using arbitrary sounds in conventional ways with conventional meanings; speech.

3. Any system of formalized symbols, signs, sounds, gestures, or the like used or conceived as a means of communicating thought, emotion, etc.

How language communicates invisibly depends on the words we choose and how we use them. We can't convey pitch or volume when we write, but our writing can still convey tone of voice, pace and mood.

[1] http://dictionary.reference.com/browse/language

Why written language is an important part of your invisible communication toolbox

While the written word is obviously valuable because it's the most literal way to tell your story, it's also important because:

1. The words that you choose can communicate the personality of your company/brand

If you want your company to come across as approachable, fun and passionate, your language needs to express those values.

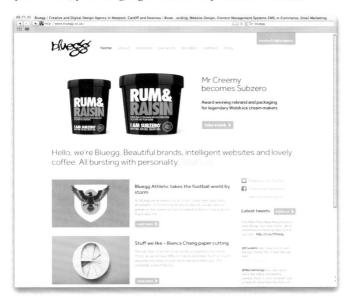

At *Bluegg* where I am Studio Manager, we often get comments relating to how we accurately market ourselves through our website as we use language that expresses our personality, such as:

- Hello, we're Bluegg. Beautiful brands, intelligent websites and lovely coffee. All bursting with personality. That's us
- Come see us, the kettle's on and the Wii is loading
- Still use a fax? Really? Fair enough

As you can see, the language is chatty and friendly. But it also communicates that Bluegg are passionate and approachable, reinforcing the branding and visuals on the studio website.

Humans use around 370 million words in an average lifetime. (Source: BBC Focus Magazine, October 2009)

2. Certain words and phrases are more effective for engaging your audience

For example, the most effective headlines for engaging readers often start with phrases such as 'How can you...', 'The secret of...' and 'Your guide to...'.

Asking questions is a good way to draw people in. *Yahoo* does it on its homepage with news items and feature articles:

- 'Dying hair grey is becoming a hot new trend among celebs - but how well do they pull off the "granny' look"?'
- 'Plan a trip to these European locations that inspired some of the most iconic film scenes. Where are they?'

See no evil, hear no evil

With written language, the reader has to make assumptions about the context and tone of voice the words are implying. This is why you must carefully consider your copy, as readers can easily misinterpret what you've written.

This problem is made worse by the fact that readers expect web copy to be concise and to the point, which means every word counts.

When we write for the web we need to keep in mind user behaviour; users tend to scan pages rather than read them in detail. We have to adapt how we communicate on the web and that includes our use of language.

When writing for the web our copy should be concise, objective and an aid for users rather than a distraction. Using invisible communication methods to augment our copy will help us say more with less.

Supporting the words

Using other forms of invisible communication (e.g. symbols, colour, typeface, branding and imagery) can support the written copy and help you tell your story.

For example, a dating website would likely have specific words in its copy that helps to tell the story of the site: 'companion', 'relationship', 'match', 'love', 'partner', 'search' and so forth. The copy could be supported by images of happy couples and the colour red, which represents passion, love and romance.

Targeting the words

In real life, we talk to with all sorts of people, both verbally and in writing. How we communicate varies from person to person, depending on the relationships we have with them. An email I write to a friend will be far more informal and chatty than one I write to a client.

To communicate effectively you need to appreciate and understand the relationship between you and your audience, so you can you make informed decisions about the written language you will use.

HOW THE WORDS LOOK

When we communicate in person, our body language, facial expressions and gestures all reveal our true thoughts and feelings. We can provide similar cues when we write through our handwriting and typefaces.

Online, the way your words look – the typeface, essentially – will communicate invisibly to your audience, as people associate different typefaces with different sets of values.

Serif versus Sans-serif

A serif typeface is one that has 'serifs' – smaller lines used to finish off the main stroke of a letter. Examples of serif typefaces include Times New Roman, Georgia and Garamond. Here is the letter 'm' with serifs:

A sans-serif typeface is one without any serifs. Examples of sans-serif typefaces include Arial, Helvetica and Tahoma:

Tip from UX Booth[1]

"Whereas an ornate font may make you stand out, if your users are unable to read your content, there is no point having it. A good sans serif, like Helvetica, is easy on the eyes and won't make your readers strain to decipher your information. Unique fonts work well in banners or graphics, but the actual content should be simple and not tiny".[2]

---

[1] UX Booth is a user experience and usability blog
[2] http://www.uxbooth.com/blog/11-quick-tips-for-more-usable-content/

In most cases, serif fonts tend to look more formal than sans-serif fonts. So if your website is aimed at professional corporate bodies, a serif font may help convey your message.

Typeface Tales

As well as the sans-serif and serif categories, it is also worth looking at specific typefaces to better understand how they can communicate invisibly and reinforce specific sets of values.

For more on different typefaces and their stories, see chapter 18, The Periodic Table of Typefaces.

Comic Sans, for example, is often bemoaned for being a hideous font. But it serves a purpose: the way it looks hints at an informal, friendly and fun set of values. With that in mind, it's no wonder typefaces like Comic Sans find themselves on so many items aimed at children.

Because so many businesses use Comic Sans on products aimed at young audiences, the values associated with that typeface become reinforced, and it will keep being used in that context.

Here is one example:

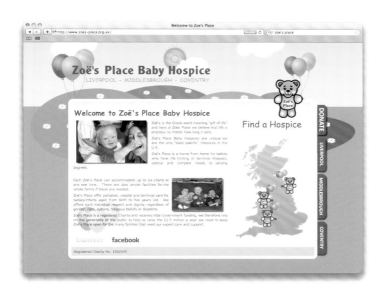

Similarly, we often see historical texts and periods represented by an Olde English or calligraphic typeface. (Films and books in particular reinforce this representation.)

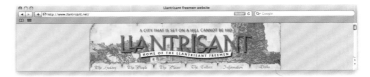

If a website was being designed for a medieval banqueting event company, a calligraphy-style typeface would be suitable. It communicates quickly to the audience by using knowledge and expectations they already have.

Context is key

To decide what typeface would be most suitable for your story, you have to know your audience. The words themselves are key, of course, but knowing certain groups of typefaces communicate certain values will help improve the user experience you are creating.

Part of this decision-making process comes down to genre and context. Let's look at some examples from the web.

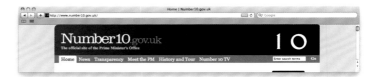

Here the designer has opted for a serif typeface for the headings. That's a suitable choice for an official government website, as it would want to be seen as intelligent, professional and formal. The site may come across as being stuffy, but would you have any faith or trust in your government if its site were set in Comic Sans?

Let's look at a site aimed at a completely different audience to the Downing Street site:

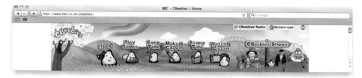

This is the website for the BBC's *CBeebies*, a television channel produced by the BBC for children aged 6 years and under.

As you can see, the typeface is bubbly and rounded. It comes across as fun and informal: a good choice for a website aimed at children who want to learn and have fun. If this website were in Times New Roman or a similar serif typeface, it would immediately conflict with the character of the site and the target audience.

This isn't to say that sans-serif typefaces can't look sophisticated. This website for London tourism adopts a sans-serif typeface, but thanks to the colours and design it still manages to look trustworthy, reliable and appealing.

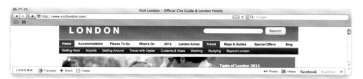

Start at the top

I think website headers act in the same way as newspaper mastheads. They can represent the values and tone of the content that follows, largely due to what the header's typeface communicates.

By communicating the right values in the header through the typeface, it sets up the user experience that follows.

Here are a few examples:

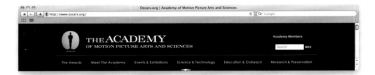

The Academy of Motion Picture Arts and Sciences has adopted a serif typeface with gold, black and white colours. These elements combine to communicate sophistication, professionalism, intelligence and formality – all perfect connotations for such a prestigious organisation.

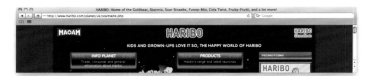

Haribo is a sweets manufacturer. Its homepage header is brighter, and the sans-serif typeface connotes fun, informality, and being childlike and approachable – values that sit perfectly with its products and the target audience.

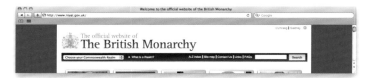

The official website for *The British Monarchy* is one example of where a serif typeface is a must. The typeface and colours communicate sophistication, luxury, formalness, wealth and (perhaps less obviously) freshness. (The latter is thanks largely to the connotations of the colours blue and white.)

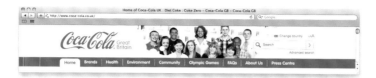

The *Coke* header is bright, rounded and fun. The typeface for the navigation is approachable, clear and simple. It immediately communicates a message about the brand, and sets the tone for the rest of the content.

These examples all show typefaces we would expect to see. If the British Monarchy were presented in a less formal typeface, you can clearly see how it would invisibly communicate the wrong messages: In Comic Sans, the header looks inappropriate.

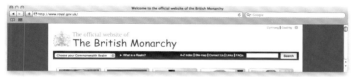

Following the rules

Whether copy is bolded, italicised, underlined or a different size also communicates to your users. They may make assumptions based on common practices, such as underlined words being links or bolded words being headings. Make sure you make it clear what the rules are within your site, and be consistent.

Making the right decision

If the typeface you choose doesn't sit with your company's values and brand, or if it conflicts with other design elements, the messages your site communicates will be inconsistent. And it will have a negative impact on the user experience.

Choose typefaces carefully, and remember they also have to be legible. This isn't to say the importance shifts from the actual words to their aesthetics – what you say is still crucial. But consider how the words look, as they will help you tell your story on a subconscious and invisible level.

18

THE PERIODIC TABLE OF TYPEFACES

The typeface you select can really add another layer of communication to your design.A great visual reference tool for selecting an appropriate typeface is the *Periodic Table of Typefaces*.[1]

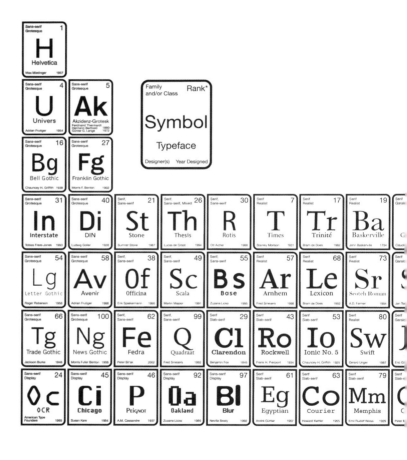

Sans-serif Geometric 2 F Futura Paul Renner 1927
Sans-serif Humanist 8 Gs Gill Sans Eric Gill 1930
Sans-serif Humanist 9 O Optima Hermann Zapf 1954
Sans-serif Humanist 14 Fr Frutiger Adrian Frutiger 1977
Sans-serif Humanist 18 S Syntax Hans Eduard Meier 1968
Sans-serif Humanist 20 Me Meta Erik Spiekermann 1991
Sans-serif Geometric 22 Ag Avant Garde Herb Lubalin 1968
Serif Didone 3 B Bodoni Giambattista Bodoni 1790
Sans-serif Humanist 32 My Myriad Robert Slimbach Carol Twombly 1992
Sans-serif Humanist 65 Fo Formata Bernd Möllenstädt 1984
Sans-serif Humanist 71 Pr Prokyon Erhard Kaiser 2002
Sans-serif Humanist 72 Mt Metro William A. Dwiggins 1929
Sans-serif Humanist 74 Ao Antique Olive Roger Excoffon 1962
Sans-serif Geometric 47 E Eurostile Aldo Novarese 1962
Serif Didone 13 D Didot Firmin Didot 1799
10
Serif Garalde 11 M Minion Robert Slimbach 1990
Serif Garalde 12 L Lucida Charles Bigelow Kris Holmes 1985
Serif Garalde 15 Fl Fleischmann Erhard Kaiser 1997
Sans-serif Humanist 75 Da Dax Hans Reichel 1995
Sans-serif Humanist 78 Ts Today Sans Volker Küster 1988
Sans-serif Humanist 87 If Info Erik Spiekermann 1996
Sans-serif Geometric 60 Go Gotham Tobias Frere-Jones 2000
Serif Didone 44 W Walbaum Justus Walbaum 1800
28
Serif Garalde 34 J Jenson Robert Slimbach 1995
Serif Garalde 35 Gr Griffo Classico Franko Luin 1993
Serif Garalde 36 Gc Garamond Classico Franko Luin 1993
Serif Garalde 37 Ch Cheltenham Bertram G. Goodhue Ingalls Kimball 1896
Sans-serif Humanist 90 Am Amplitude Christian Schwartz 2003
Sans-serif Humanist 91 Bc Bell Centennial Matthew Carter 1978
Sans-serif Geometric 96 N Neutraface Christian Schwartz 2002
Serif Didone 48 Ma Matrix Zuzana Licko 1986
42
Serif Garalde 52 K Kis Nicolas Kis 1690
Serif Garalde 64 Pa Palatino Hermann Zapf 1950
Serif Garalde 76 Cb Cooper Black Oswald B. Cooper 1920
Serif Garalde 88 Sp Spectrum Jan van Krimpen 1943
Serif Garalde 89 Po Proforma Petr van Blokland 1988
Sans-serif Humanist 94 CG Copperplate Gothic Frederic W. Goudy 1901
Glyphic Inscriptional 25 TA Trajan Carol Twombly 1989
Serif Didone 50 Ce Century Morris Fuller Benton 1919
33
Blackletter 39 Gf Gebetbuch Fraktur Hans Schönsperger ca. 1514
Blackletter 56 Uf Unger Fraktur Johann F. Unger 1793
Blackletter 59 Mg Manuscript-Gotisch Wolfgang Hopyl 1514
Blackletter 67 Bf Breitkopf Fraktur Johann G.I. Breitkopf 1793
Blackletter 82 Ff Fette Fraktur Johann C. Bauer 1850
Blackletter 85 Wg Wilhelm Klingspor Gotisch Rudolf Koch 1925
Blackletter 86 Wr Weiss Rundgotisch Emil Rudolf Weiss 1936
Blackletter 93 Fs Fette Deutsche Schrift Rudolf Koch 1910
Script 51 Z Zapfino Hermann Zapf 1998
Script 69 Mi Mistral Roger Excoffon 1953
Script 70 Ha Hands LettError 1991
Script 77 Sn Snell Roundhand Matthew Carter 1966
Script 81 Rc Robert Granjon 1652
Script 83 Bi Bickham Script Richard Lipton 1997
Script 95 un uncial Victor Hammer 1923
Script 98 Bo Beowulf Peter Baker 1996

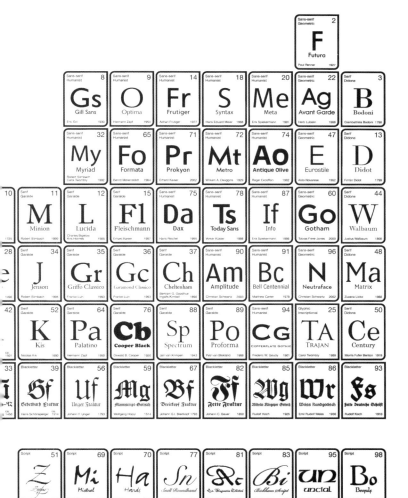

What is the Periodic Table of Typefaces?

Created by Camdon Wilde of Squidspot.com, the table brings together the 100 most popular typefaces and categorises them in a similar way to the periodic table of elements used in chemistry.

The table groups typefaces into families and classes, such as sans-serif, serif, script and glyphic. Each cell lists a typeface, a one or two-character symbol, the designer, the year it was designed, and its ranking out of 100.

Here are the sites used to determine the rankings:

- The 100 Best Fonts Of All Time – *www.100besteschriften.de/*
- Paul Shaws Top 100 Types survey – *www.tdc.org/reviews/typelist.html*
- 21 Most Used Fonts By Professional Designers – *www.instantshift. com/2008/10/05/21-most-used-fonts-by-professional-designers/*
- Top 7 Fonts Used By Professionals In Graphic Design – *justcreativedesign. com/2008/09/23/top-7-fonts-used-by-professionals-in-graphic-design-2/*
- 30 Fonts That ALL Designers Must Know & Should Own – *justcreativedesign. com/2008/03/02/30-best-font-downloads-for-designers/*
- Typefaces no one gets fired for using – *www.cameronmoll.com/ archives/001168.html*

A quick glance at the table clearly shows there are differences in how different typefaces communicate. Some are traditional, while others are more informal.

Alluding to time gone by

Typefaces such as Manuscript-Gotish and Unger Fraktur hint at times gone by, as they are derived from the calligraphy we see on ancient scrolls and manuscripts.

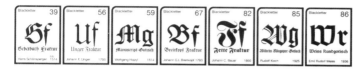

Formal and traditional

Other typefaces are more formal and traditional, such as the examples below.

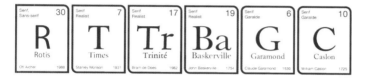

These typefaces are often used in broadsheet newspapers and their corresponding websites. They hint at sophisticated, high-brow and professional content.

Informal and modern

Many sans-serif typefaces feel more informal and modern. They are clean, less 'fussy', and approachable.

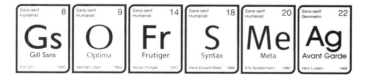

These typefaces would complement a friendly tone of voice, and hint at something more casual.

Context specific

Other typefaces are so strong in their visual appearance they
would only work in a limited number of contexts.

Thanks to its rounded edges, Cooper Black connotes values of
playfulness and child-like qualities. It would work well on a
website aimed at youngsters, but would be completely out of place
on a news or other 'serious' website.

Oakland, Mistral and OCR have such specific looks they would
be detrimental to most design contexts on the web.

As we discussed earlier, while the words we use are crucial,
how they look can also communicate to audiences. A particular
typeface may work well in some contexts, but in others it may well
communicate values that contradict the subject matter or even the
words themselves.

Next we'll look at tone of voice, which is also more about how
we communicate than what we are saying.

TONE OF VOICE

When writing for the web, tone of voice is an important tool you can use to communicate beyond the actual words used. But getting the tone of voice right can be challenging, even for experienced writers.

What is tone of voice?

Tone of voice isn't what's said but rather how it's said. When we speak to people, we can use the tone of our voice to express emotions such as happiness, seriousness, sarcasm and anger. We can use the tone of voice in our writing to express those same emotions.

Studies by *Albert Mehrabian* show that when we converse with others in person, only 7% of what we communicate is through our words. The other 93% is made up by our body language (55%) and our tone of voice (38%)

Why is tone of voice important?

The right tone of voice will draw users in, connect with them, and give them a better user experience. It can also create an identity that sets you apart from everyone else.

But choosing the wrong tone of voice can create conflicting impressions of your business. You wouldn't want to create an informal and visually friendly website and then use a formal and corporate tone of voice.

While your tone of voice should be consistent, it can vary slightly depending on the context. For example, your blog may be more chatty and informal than the copy on your main website. But you still need to make it clear that both platforms are from the same organisation.

How you 'speak' to your audience will affect their overall user experience. If your tone of voice is friendly and personable they may feel more comfortable using your site.

Picking the right tone

When writing for the web, the tone of voice you adopt depends on:

- Your product/service
- The personality you're trying to convey
- Your audience

The decisions you need to make about your tone of voice include:

- How formal/informal will it be?
- How much jargon will you include?
- How friendly or amusing will it be?

Before you can make any decisions about the most suitable tone of voice, you need to understand those three points. What is your story, who is it for and how should you tell it?

For example, the tone of voice used on the website of *The Sun* (a UK tabloid newspaper) is significantly different to that used on the website of *The Times* (a UK broadsheet newspaper), even though both websites are owned by the same parent company.

Why? Because they have different target audiences, values and positions within the news market.

The Sun's website has an informal, chatty and less sophisticated tone of voice than The Times' website, where the tone of voice is more formal and professional. But this is to be expected, as these newspaper websites are mirroring the tone of voice used in the print editions.

One thing to remember: whatever tone of voice you choose, you still need clear and accurate content, usability and SEO.

If a company has brand guidelines to follow they should outline the tone of voice used for the website, including the language used (and not used) and who the audience is.

You need to make sure your copy still does its job, whether it's providing information or getting users to register.

When writing for the web you should be concise and accurate as possible, as users scan the pages rather than read them. This means every word counts, making it even more difficult to get the tone of voice right.

Doing some audience research beforehand will help you decide on the tone of voice to use. You can ask simple questions, such as:

- Can I use humour?
- Should I use jargon?
- Can I use slang?
- What punctuation should I use?

Getting answers to questions like this will help you set your boundaries and how you should pitch your tone. Let's look at two websites and discuss the tone of voice they use:

Vimeo[1]

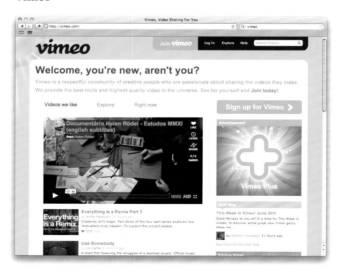

---

[1] http://www.vimeo.com

The tone of voice here is friendly and informal. Sentences such as 'Welcome, you're new, aren't you?' are inviting and sound like they're coming from a friend. Similarly, Vimeo has chosen 'Videos we like' rather than something like 'Recommended videos'.

This creates a feeling that your friends are suggesting something they think you'd enjoy, whereas 'Recommended' would feel much more impersonal.

Vimeo uses this tone of voice throughout their site, both in the navigation (the option to 'Explore' as well as search) and in their calls to action ('Join' rather than 'Sign up').

When you click to join Vimeo you are asked, 'which Vimeo is right for you?' The site talks directly to you, which makes it feel like a one-on-one conversation that draws you in. All of this complements the community feel of the website and service it provides.

After signing up, you see this:

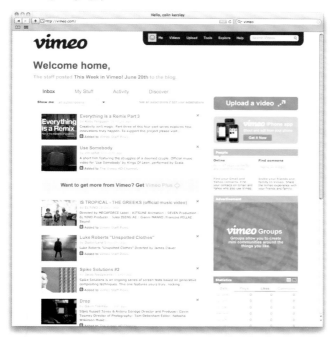

'We're glad you're here' is, again, friendly and approachable.

A large part of Vimeo is user-generated content and interaction, and it has chosen the perfect tone of voice to achieve this. It appeals to its target audience, and encourages them to join the community, share videos and interact with others.

Here's some of my favourite copy from across the Vimeo website:

- 'We are the staff. These are the videos we like the bestest.'
- 'Uh oh, wait a sec' (when an email address is not verified)
- 'Vimeo + awesomeness = Vimeo Plus'
- 'You have no recent activity and that makes us sad'

Vimeo has successfully considered its audience and created a tone of voice that makes it almost impossible not to get involved or move deeper into the website.

The second website we'll look at uses a more formal tone of voice.

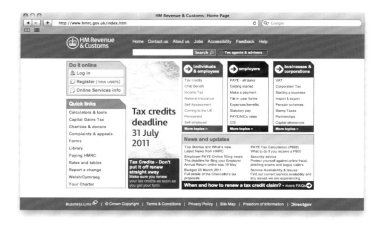

The website for HM Revenue and Customs (HMRC) needs a different tone of voice to Vimeo because it serves a far more serious purpose, and has a very different target audience.

In fact, it has a few different audiences: individuals and employees, employers, and businesses and corporations. The site uses colour to segment these audiences on the homepage, but the tone of voice is consistent throughout.

HMRC has opted for standard navigation and traditional titles such as 'Contact us', 'About us' and 'Help'. The tone is professional, clear and approachable – no quirky alternatives here.

The distinct lack of jargon makes the often complex information easier to digest, partly helped by the tone of voice. It has to be professional because of the services it provides, but it never becomes intimidating or too corporate.

While the tone of voice is professional, it lacks the personality that other sites (such as Vimeo) are able to use.

Both Vimeo and HMRC have pitched their tones of voice perfectly. The sites communicate their content in the most appropriate manner, making them more effective at promoting their services. Different tones of voice, but both equally important.

CASE STUDY: *INNOCENT DRINKS*

Innocent Drinks is a UK-based company that produces smoothies, fruit juices and veg pots. Founded in 1999, the company pioneered the informal, chatty and friendly tone of voice other brands have been quick to adopt.

Innocent is a particularly interesting example because its brand is far more than just its visual identity. In fact, the way it uses words on its website, advertising and packaging is a major contributor to its success. The copy is as much a part of the brand as any visual elements, and this coherent storytelling sets the Innocent brand apart from its many competitors.

The Innocent Typeface

The first thing to note about Innocent's marketing material, both online and offline, is the typeface. As we talked about in chapter 17, an appropriate typeface can communicate certain values and create a specific mood.

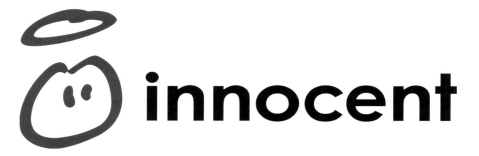

Innocent uses a very informal, sans-serif typeface. It's rounded and fun (much like their logo) and reflects the values they want the brand to portray. A more formal typeface (such as Times New Roman) simply wouldn't work. We'd still be able to read the content clearly and find what we wanted, but it wouldn't have the same feel or reflect Innocent's brand values.

The Innocent brand is playful. The company can have fun with both how it presents its brand visually (such as with its typeface) and how it uses words in its copy.

In his book 'Building a Brand from Nothing but Fruit', John Simmons asked Will Awdry, one of advertising's finest writers, how he would describe the Innocent tone of voice. Awdry answered:

> *"Innocent's great power is its consistency of voice.*
> *The accents in the voice are innocence, truth, fun,*
> *wholesomeness, wit, spirit, lack of pomposity, honesty and*
> *lightness of touch."*

Awdry hits the nail on the head with that description. Let's take a look at some examples and find out why.

The Innocent tone of voice – offline

Before we look at how important Innocent's tone of voice is to its brand and to invisible communication, let's look at some examples of how it uses tone of voice in its offline marketing materials and on its product labels.

Innocent's marketing copy is simple, which is why it's so effective. One poster advert from 2006 said:

> *"Easy as pie. Tasty as pie. Healthy as mung beans. Innocent*
> *smoothies. Nothing but nothing but fruit."*

The copy is friendly and chatty, but also communicates a serious message that anchors the Innocent brand: Innocent smoothies are healthy with no additives, just fruit.

In 2003 Innocent ran a series of adverts with simple imagery and short messages that set the tone for future ad campaigns. Here are the visually simple yet high impact adverts:

sometimes we feel like sitting in the woods with no clothes on. but then we have to come home and make the drinks.

they grow on trees

made from freshly squeezed cows*

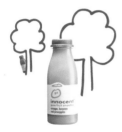

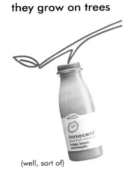

(well, sort of)

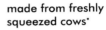

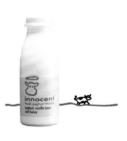

*no cows were harmed during the making of this drink

Even as early as 2003, Innocent's tone of voice was one of fun, humour and playfulness. It's also a little bit cheeky at times.

Innocent recently embarked on an advertising campaign featuring rabbits and more of the friendly, informal statements they have become known for.

Here are some examples:

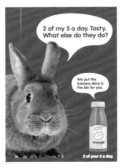

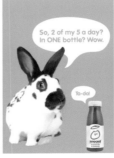

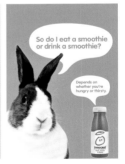

These adverts stand out thanks to the single bold colours, the imagery of the rabbits, and the statements they make. 'We put the banana skins in the bin for you' is a great way of telling consumers the hard work is already done so they can just enjoy the healthy drinks. These statements start a relationship between supplier and consumer, but it's a relationship framed more as a friendship.

You can see some of the previous labels, complete with their stories, in the label gallery on the Innocent website: *http://www.innocentdrinks.co.uk/bored/gallery/labels/*

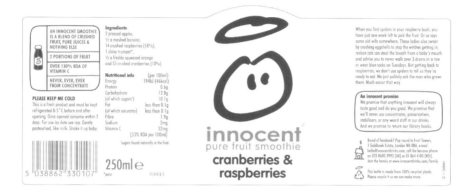

The labels on the bottles continue the approach, but with a greater emphasis on storytelling. Even on its labels, where space is limited, Innocent has mastered the ability to tell stories that promote and reinforce its own brand values. Innocent also give each label a name such as 'communal showers', 'charades' and 'Thai bus drivers'. It's almost like a story title.

The labels all have the same quirkiness and playful writing, such as 'never, ever, ever from concentrate', 'This bottle is now made from 50% recycled plastic. We're still working on the rest', and 'Shake it up baby'. But some stories also change over time as more labels are produced.

Here are three labels, each with a story to tell:

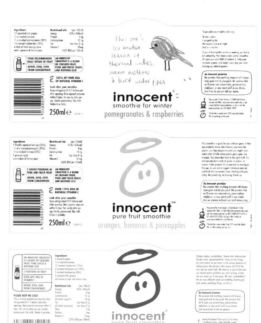

Here are some more examples of their copy, taken directly from Innocent smoothie labels:

> '*My mum's started buying our smoothies (and that's after 5 whole years, the skinflint).*'

> '*This means that I've got to behave and not say anything too rude or controversial. So, mum, they are really good for you. They are made with 100% pure fresh fruit. They contain loads of vitamin C (a day and a half's worth). They are as fat-free as an apple or banana and that's because they are just fruit. Is that good enough for you mum?*'

'Right, I'm off to smash some windows and have a fag.'

'... and step away from the desk 2 3 4, come on, really work it
... now, off to the shops, oh yes, keep those knees up, keep it
working 2 3 4 ... stop at the lights, mind the cyclist ... and into
the shop, just grab the bottle 2 3 4 ... feel it in the triceps, oh
yeah ... you're feeling good now ... stepping to the till, ignore
the chocolate, keep stepping, let's see those glutes shake 2 3 4
... and we'll finish with the unscrew, pop those wrists 2 3 4 ...
looking good ... and relax.'

Innocent's copy is humorous, light-hearted, fun and a talking
point. It's also very clever, because people will buy another
smoothie to read a new story.

It doesn't end there, though. The Innocent tone of voice is also
evident on its website.

The Innocent tone – online

The Innocent website is a fun place to visit. Sure it has information
about the company, the brand and the products, but the way it
shares this information with users is a joy to read. Innocent has
nailed it again.

Let's see how Innocent has achieved a tone of voice online
that's consistent with its offline marketing activity. We'll start at
the homepage, and then move on to examples within the site.

The Homepage

The homepage immediately creates a sense of fun. This is down to
the graphics, the typeface (as discussed at the start of this chapter)
and the words themselves.

Here's an example of the homepage from June 2011:

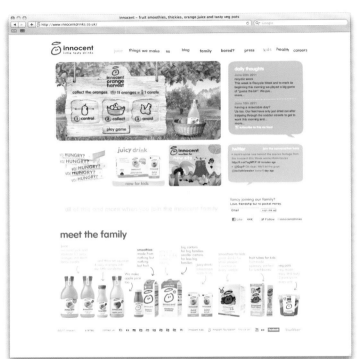

What you can't see in this static image is the words moving in the navigation. They wobble from side to side, which adds to the fun factor.

If we look specifically at the words, we can see how the navigation again adopts a playful, informal and friendly approach. Innocent could have used the word 'products' in the navigation, but instead opted for 'things we make' – a much friendlier way to lead users to that area of the website. Similarly, instead of 'fun stuff' the site poses the question: 'bored?' It's a more effective call to action.

The Innocent tone of voice is evident throughout the homepage, with copy such as:

> 'Fancy joining our family? Love, friendship but no pocket money.'

It really does make it sound like a fun place to work. The 'Us' page contains my favourite examples of the Innocent tone of voice. Again, these examples are taken straight from the page:

> 'Our vehicles. Some of our vans are cows and some are grass-covered ones that dance. Obviously.'

> 'Call the banana phone or just have a look at some bad pictures of us.'

> 'We had good jobs before we started Innocent. Why did we change?'

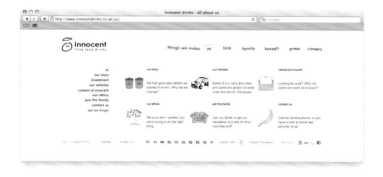

The way these sentences are written, and their tone of voice, adds another layer to the storytelling. The tone of voice is friendly and playful, which also hints at the Innocent brand values and ethics.

This playful tone continues on the 'Family' page:

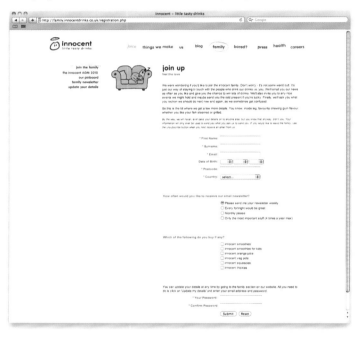

This is where users can sign up to the Innocent newsletter. But rather than the usual 'sign up here to receive our newsletter' copy, Innocent has come up with a much more imaginative way to get users to sign up. Again, the content is gold:

> *'We were wondering if you'd like to join the innocent family. Don't worry - it's not some weird cult. It's just our way of staying in touch with the people who drink our drinks i.e. you.'*

> *'So this is the bit where we get a few more details. You know, inside leg, favourite chewing gum flavour, whether you like your fish steamed or grilled.'*

How could you resist after reading that?

There's more to Innocent than just the humour, though. It's now a large and successful organisation, so it has a duty to be responsible and professional. Its copy is both of these things, but in the Innocent way.

For example, by law the website needs to tell users that if they sign up to the newsletter their details won't be passed to third parties and they can unsubscribe at any time. This is how Innocent lets their users know:

> 'By the way, we will never, ever pass your details on to anyone else, but you knew that anyway, didn't you. Your information will only ever be used to send you what you ask us to send you. If you would like to leave the family, use the unsubscribe button when you next receive an email from us.'

Innocent can still be playful and friendly, even when addressing more serious issues.

Innocent's invisible communication

Invisible communication plays a key role in the highly successful way Innocent builds a relationship with its audience. Ultimately, Innocent is just a manufacturing company. Yet the way it tells its story makes it more than just a manufacturer, and demonstrates the power of words in communication, branding and marketing.

The words in the copy, and the tone they are written in, portray Innocent to the world as a friend. While Innocent might well be the pioneers of building a brand largely on the strength of language, many have since followed in its footsteps.

Let's remind ourselves of the three elements of Innocent's invisible communication methods:

1. Typeface – *how the words look*
2. Language – *the actual words on the page/screen*
3. Tone of voice – *how those words sound*

But there's one more element at work here. One that ensures the other three invisible communication methods work. One that we've already touched on in this chapter.

Consistency.

Consistently friendly

The consistent tone of voice, typeface and language used across their adverts, labels and website are paramount to Innocent building and maintaining a brand with strong values that appeals to consumers.

The correlation between tone of voice and consumer appeal is explained by *John Simms* in his book *Building a Brand from Nothing but Fruit*. As Simms explains:

> *'Perhaps a brand's 'tone of voice' could not only help differentiate it from competitors but also create bonds of affection and loyalty with different audiences.'*

And that's why Innocent is so successful: its tone of voice is consistent across all consumer touch points, including the website.

The Innocent personality is communicated not only visibly in its imagery and marketing materials, but also invisibly through its typeface and tone of voice. It's a two-pronged approach to storytelling where both conscious and subconscious elements combine to tell a complete story.

Part 5

Telling the best story

Introduction to storytelling

Storytelling conventions

Storytelling on the web

Storytelling through brands

Case Study: *Squaredeye.com*

21

INTRODUCTION TO STORYTELLING

From the day we are born we hear stories. At first they are simple nursery rhymes and fairytales. As we mature so to do the stories we hear, bringing with them added meaning, hidden messages and subliminal communication. This exposure to stories makes our ability to understand them practically innate.

We've all learned the conventions of storytelling, and so we recognise story structures, events and characters almost instantly. And absorbing information from those stories happens almost subconsciously. We quickly piece together the story, make assumptions about the characters (based on whether we see them as a hero or a villain), and create expectations of how the story will end.

We can also use storytelling on other platforms, such as the web. The challenge is to understand storytelling methods enough to apply them so users can digest the story easily. We have to carefully construct a story and use our narrative to make the story seem natural.

Each storytelling platform brings along certain conventions. Some apply to several media, while others are exclusive to a particular platform. We can apply traditional storytelling techniques to the web, but we need to adapt them for the new parameters that online storytelling brings with it.

But before I discuss how we can use storytelling on the web, I want to look at the advantages of using it as a communication tool and how it works in the invisible sense.

What is storytelling?

In storytelling there are three strands to consider:

- Narrative – *A term referring to a sequence of events organised into a story with a particular structure*[1]
- Story – *All of the events in a narrative, those presented directly to an audience and those which might be inferred*[2]
- Characterisation – *The method used to develop a character*

---

[1][2] Branston and Stafford. The Media Student's Guide.

Let's examine these concepts using a story with a familiar structure: *the fairytale of Little Red Riding Hood*.

The story is the events that occur, the little girl in the red cloak meets a wolf in the woods. The wolf later pretends to be the little girl's grandmother and eats them both up. The hunter cuts the wolf open and both the girl and the grandmother emerge unharmed.

The narrative is the way these events are told. For a fairytale, the most common method is starting the story with, 'once upon a time', presenting the events in chronological order and concluding with, 'and they all lived happily ever after'.

Characterisation reveals information about the characters in the story, how they look, the things they say, their thoughts and speech.

The story is the elements or events that make up the tale, while the narrative is how it is told. This is a key distinction to keep in mind when telling stories online because there will often be a number of ways to tell a particular story. Knowing what you want to say (your story) is the first thing to understand. Only then can you address how to tell that story in the best way for your audience.

Where do we find stories?

Stories are told all around us. We hear them during our daily commutes, in the workplace, in the media we consume and in our social interactions. We don't always recognise them as stories because they are such an integral part of how we communicate.

Offline, storytelling is evident in:

- Books and magazines
- Films and TV programmes
- Adverts
- Chatting with friends
- Photos

Online, we can share stories through:

- Blogs
- Tweets
- Forums
- Social media status updates
- Websites as a whole

Storytelling is an integral part of our communication.

Why do we tell stories?

Storytelling is a valuable and useful communication tool, both online and offline, for two reasons.

I. Finding order in the chaos

Storytelling can help us make sense of the world around us. The pace of our lives is increasing, and information overload is a problem for many people. We need a way to organise the information we receive.

Stories are frameworks for interpretation that help us find meaning and understanding. We can process information more efficiently by organising it in a way that is familiar to us. By bringing structure to our lives we can position ourselves to cope better during times of hardship or drama. We can anticipate the next part of the journey and act accordingly.

The web often has more information than we need. Websites can target a range of people, each with their own needs or task to complete. Users need to discover the information relevant to achieving their goal. If the website's story incorporates symbols, key words, calls to action and well-crafted copy, finding order in the chaos will be much easier for the user.

2. **The emotional connection**

Stories can induce emotional responses in people. They make us laugh, make us cry and sometimes even shock us. This ability to make us respond emotionally is useful because it can help us engage with the story.

Stories have a unique ability to appeal to our emotions, motivate us and persuade us. Our brains are seemingly wired to understand and enjoy stories, and as people we have a predilection for storytelling.

The emotional relationship between stories and their audiences can transcend platforms. Admittedly, we aren't as likely to be as involved in a website as we would a film or a book – it's a different kind of relationship. But good storytelling through colour, symbols, and text can still evoke emotions in web users, or at the very least help them engage with a website.

How can stories be invisible?

If we're surrounded by stories, how can they be invisible?

Many stories are invisible because the person hearing it doesn't realise it is one. Magazine adverts, for example, are carefully constructed stories, but most readers wouldn't see them that way. And a story in a website will also be invisible a lot of the time because the person visiting the site doesn't see it as one.

That doesn't mean invisible stories aren't important. In fact, they can be more important than traditional stories because they help the audience or user engage and achieve their goal more efficiently. They just doesn't realise they're being guided by a narrative or a well-considered story.

22 STORYTELLING CONVENTIONS

In the last chapter we defined story and narrative, looked at why it's such a valuable communication tool, and how it works on a subliminal level. Now it's time to talk about storytelling conventions that will help us design stories relevant to our target audience.

Media studies textbooks usually discuss narrative theory as it relates to film. We can also use it on the web, but we need to keep in mind that:

> 'Narrative theory suggests that stories share certain features, regardless of media and culture. Particular media are able to 'tell' stories in different ways."

This means that while we can learn from the narrative theory of other media, we have to modify it to suit the web. Our goal – engaging an audience with our story – is the same, but we must tailor our stories to suit the media we're telling them with.

Narrative Theory

Traditional narrative theory came from studies into folk tales and fairytales. These types of stories are primarily concerned with character function and plot development. We can't just take these and apply them to the web: when would we ever design a website with a clearly defined hero and villain?

What we can take from these stories is how a set of conventions exist for each media. This consistency will help audiences engage with, and understand your story.

For example, if you go to see a disaster movie you probably know enough about that genre to have certain expectations about what will happen. Similarly, many users these days know different types of websites, and so will have a level of expectation about how they will function.

---

[1] Branston and Stafford. The Media Student's Guide.

Learning from other media

Narrative is evident in many media including photography, comic strips, and films. We can learn from these to improve our online stories.

Photography

Narrative is usually thought of in relation to movies and books. But it is also present in photos. A photo captures a moment of time, but a great photo makes us imagine what happened before the moment was captured, or what happened soon after.

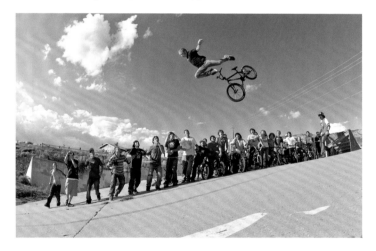

Narrative is signalled here, depending on the content of the photograph. Don't underestimate the power of imagery as a contributor to your story.

Film

The power of film is how much it can communicate at once through visuals, costume, cinematography, dialogue, character function and story.

Films can teach us the art of slowly revealing a story, piece by piece. They can also teach us the value of deciding what to show (and not to show), what adds to the story, and what is simply 'noise'.Like film, the web is really visual storytelling. A great example of visual storytelling in film is the *Disney Pixar* production, *Wall.E*. The movie has relatively little dialogue, with emotion conveyed through expressions and gestures.

The Director of Wall.E, *Andrew Stanton*, knew the story had to be engaging for the film to work without dialogue. He says "action is more generally understood than words. The lift of an eyebrow, however faint, may convey more than a hundred words".[1]

Online, we don't even have the luxury of expressions and gestures. That means we have to focus on the details. Great storytelling doesn't come from dialogue alone.

The lack of dialogue in silent movies, Wall.E and on the web, forces the creator to tell the story in other ways: through visuals, colour, hierarchy of information, content and so on. As Stanton says, "simplicity and clarity give the visual storyteller room to grow".

On the web we can't just throw in some dialogue to explain everything. It has to be inferred and laid out by carefully choosing:

- Imagery
- Tone of voice of the copy
- Symbols, icons and colours
- Hierarchy of information
- Navigation

As you can see, we need to bring together a number of elements to tell stories online.

The lack of dialogue is also a limitation of the web as a storytelling medium. We need to consider what the web can do that other media cannot, as it will have a significant impact on our story and how we tell it.

---

[1] The Art of Wall.E, Tim Hauser

Storytelling constraints online

In many ways the web is an ideal storytelling platform because it's largely concerned with presenting information. But there are some constraints you need to be aware of when storytelling on the web.

Truncated communication

Sometimes the web restricts the amount of information we can give. (As I said in chapter 19, every word counts.) This, along with it needing to be scannable so users can find the information they need, means we need to tell our stories quickly and efficiently.

Non-linear narrative

There's no guarantee that users will land on your site's homepage. They could land anywhere on your site, which means they may be joining the story partway through. Your site need clear signposts and well-considered navigation to let them know not only where they are, but also where they can move to next (and how they can get there).

You need to decide where your story begins. This will have a profound impact on the story that follows. Thinking back to Little Red Riding Hood, imagine how different the story would be if it began with the wolf eating Little Red Riding Hood.

Communicating the tone of voice

As we discussed in chapter 19, you can achieve tone of voice through the words you choose – informal or formal, full or jargon or easy to read. Even the sentence structure can influence the tone and pace of the voice.

Finding your story

Before you can know what conventions will help you tell your story, you need to know what that story is and, just as important, who it's being told to.

Once you understand that, you can start applying the conventions. Who are the characters? What codes will be useful? What will the tone of voice be? Learn from other media, but don't forget to adapt the conventions to suit the online environment.

23   STORYTELLING AND THE WEB

We've looked at storytelling techniques in other media, and how some of those techniques can be carried over to the web. Let's now look at some practical examples of storytelling techniques on the web.

Use Cases

Use cases are different to personas. A use case helps you understand the interaction between the user and your web site: their story. A persona is more to do with generating characters based on behaviours, data and assumptions.

Use cases can help you define the stories within your website. By focusing on the users, how they interact with your site and its content, you can discover the best ways to help them.

A use case is 'a methodology used in system analysis to identify, clarify, and organise system requirements. The use case is made up of a set of possible sequences of interactions between systems and users in a particular environment and related to a particular goal." In other words, they bridge the gap between the needs of the user and the site you are designing by listing their intentions and the website's response to each one.

 To put it another way, use cases focus on the journey the user will take, whereas personas use data to create people representing the audience.

Incorporating use cases into the project is a practical way to express its requirements, and can help you design your story.

As well as your overarching story, specific stories underneath will relate to certain groups of users. Use cases let you explore these stories, and determine what a group of users will want to achieve. This will help you design to their story using copy, imagery, icons, colour, hierarchy and navigation.

How to write use cases and define your story

No two people will write use cases the same way, and no two projects will be alike. But here are some pointers for writing use cases with storytelling in mind.

---

[1] http://searchsoftwarequality.techtarget.com/sDefinition/0,,sid92_gci334062,00.html

1. **Don't be a perfectionist**

   Use cases can be refined through iterations. It might take a few attempts before you find a method that suits you, but that's okay. Don't overthink it, just get going.

2. **Define your use case actors**

   Who will use your site? Depending on the scope of the project, you may need several actors. Try to focus on the core actors first. For example, if we were creating use cases for *eBay* or a similar auction site, our actors could be bidders, sellers, suppliers or wholesalers. But the core actors would be buyers and sellers.

   For sites where there could be a lot of actors, focus on the main roles. This will help you define the most important stories within your site and content.

   Don't give the actors names. Instead, focus on the role they will play when carrying out their tasks (in this case, buyer and seller). If we name them John and Jane then we're straying into persona territory.

3. **Define what their goals are**

   What will our buyers and sellers want to achieve? They may have several goals, so again focus on the core behaviours. An eBay buyer might need to create an account, log in, search for an item, place a bid, and purchase an item. They may also need to carry out a few smaller tasks , but it's the core behaviours that will power the story.

4. **Consider the crossovers**

   If two or more characters have many shared goals as well as individual ones, then it might be worth creating a generic actor for those shared goals. We can then eradicate any duplicate behaviours by streamlining the story.

   For our eBay example the buyer and seller both need to create accounts, but after that their stories are quite different so we don't need a generic actor.

5. **Prioritise use cases**

Once we have our list of behaviours (creates account, searches listings, places bid etc.), we can prioritise them according to the scope of the project. What tasks are essential for getting your site live? What tasks will have to be part of your story? What tasks can wait until a phase two? Number each use case, name it and include a short description.

Both the buyer's and seller's behaviours are crucial, and would be high priority before our eBay site could go live.

6. **Create the basic flow**

Outline the site's story when everything goes to plan. What stages will the user go through to complete their task if there aren't any problems along the way? (Think of it as linear narrative.) For our eBay buyer the flow could include creating an account, searching for an item, comparing items, selecting one, bidding for it (or buying it immediately), moving through the checkout process, and leaving feedback when the item is received.

For our seller, the flow could include creating an account, adding a listing and entering information, defining a price, adding an image, and so on. It could finish with either removing or re-listing the item (if it isn't sold), or invoicing for a sold item, receiving payment and dispatching the item.

7. **The alternate flow**

This is the non-linear narrative. Here we need to outline the story when things don't go to plan. These problems may never occur, but it doesn't hurt to plan for them. In our eBay example, the user may be forced down an alternate flow if their session times out, or their payment is refused. Perhaps they've been outbid at the last minute – what are their options now?

8. **Present your data**

Once you've determined your use cases and their stories, you can represent them either graphically or by writing a simple outline. In any case, you now understand your users and their stories, which will in turn help you figure out the best way to tell your own.

Telling stories to your clients

Use cases are all about your users and their needs. We can also tell stories to our clients, and the best way to do this is through personas. (You can also use them to make design decisions, but here I'll just be discussing them in terms of informing clients.)

Personas give both the project team and your clients a shared understanding of your end users or audience groups. The information can be used to create coherent stories to help clients understand more about their users and what they need. It will also help them understand the design process.

Here are some guidelines that have helped me generate personas on past projects:

1. Have around six key personas. If you have too many you'll lose focus. Have too few, and you could leave out a vital audience segment

2. Personas should be based on actual data (from censuses, surveys or audience research). This adds credibility, and ensures your personas are representative

3. Consider what people say – this reveals their goals and attitudes. You could run focus groups to hear what people think, or maybe you have questionnaires or data where they share their thoughts with you

4. Consider what people do. Actual behaviour reveals more than what people say. Depending on the project at hand you may want to look at online shopping habits – what they buy, where they buy it from, and so on. Or perhaps you need data on specific habits to cross reference with other research. Do people actually do what they say they do?

5. What people say isn't always what they do. When placed in a research situation, people often say what they think you want to hear rather than being honest about what they do

Here's some anecdotal evidence of that last rule from *Steve Mulder*, author of *The User is Always Right*. Mulder often uses this story at his seminars to emphasise the gap between what users say, and what they really do.

> 'An electronic company were testing for a new boom box they hoped to start selling. Their research included focus groups where they showed the two colour options, yellow and black. The participants were in agreement that yellow was the best colour because it is a vibrant and energetic colour. At the end of the focus group they were each allowed to take a boom box home, and could choose yellow or black. They all chose black.'

Your personas (preferably generated in conjunction with the client) will help the client see users as real people with real needs. It moves the discussion from 'User A will need to book a ticket online' to 'Sophie needs to buy three tickets for herself and two friends as a birthday present'. There's a lot more of a story included with Sophie than with User A, which will help your clients better understand their site, their goals and their content.

A little story goes a long way.

Understanding your audience

The best way to tell an immersive story and connect with your audience is by understanding them and knowing what their goals are. This concept is known as qualia.

Qualia is to put yourself in someone else's position to experience what a situation is like for them. If you do this through use cases and personas, you'll understand your audience much better. The more you understand your audience, the easier it will be to tell a story that engages them.

Knowing the conventions

Films can be classified into genres: horror, science fiction, romantic comedy, and so on. Each genre has its own conventions – a set of criteria that helps audiences recognise the genre and better understand the story. A film that opens with a spacecraft whizzing through space will give the audience a totally different expectation to one that opens with a man proposing to his girlfriend.

While I'm not suggesting websites can be classed by genres, they do share some conventions that can influence and inform your story. A social networking site, for example, will need to let users interact, comment on each others' lives, share photos, and so on.

Of course there are no rules, and to blindly follow convention is to risk diluting creativity. But being aware of conventions will help you include elements in your story that will let your users engage quickly and set their expectation level.

Planning the story

Films have scripts that dictate the order of events, who says what, when, to whom, and so on. They provides the structure for the film. Books have outlines and a table of contents, which act as a structure for the content. Websites have sitemaps.

Sitemaps seem to be waning in popularity, but they serve an

important purpose: they outline your site, which ultimately is an outline of your story. Even if you don't want one on the finished site, generating a sitemap in the early stages of the project will help you understand the site's needs, goals and content: the story. It will also help the client understand, and to focus on the most important needs of their site.

Linked to the sitemap is the navigation, as discussed in chapter 9. There's no guarantee users will land at your homepage so you need to show them where they are, where they have come from and where they can move to next (the beginning, middle and end of the story).

A few simple signposting techniques and breadcrumb trails will act as narrative to guide the user through their story to the desired result. If they get lost along the way, the sitemap and well-considered navigation should get them back on track.

Designing the story
Designing the story is a very involved process. It takes on board all the planning and research, the many hours with the client, and the many days of preparation.

Here are a few elements that can not only contribute to the story design process, but also help create an all-encompassing story:

- Your elements need to be consistent – the tone of voice, the images that anchor the copy and the colour palette, and so on. You also need to consider how to structure the information and present the hierarchy to best tell the story

- Each design element – information architecture, content, colour, typography, branding and so on – may not be relevant to every story. It really depends on the project at hand. But when they come together the story becomes most effective and clear

Evaluating your story before the launch

Before you launch the site, you can evaluate how relevant and accurate your story is through user testing.

You need to test two elements:

1. What story did the users really experience?
2. Is your story still relevant?

The first question is important. Even though you've worked hard to understand your user's stories, in practice testing may reveal processes and needs you didn't consider.

This leads to the second point of assessing what parts of your story are still relevant (based on the test findings) and removing anything you no longer need.

Evaluating your story after the launch

The work doesn't end when the site has been launched. Client and user needs will change, changes in society and culture may influence the story, and things simply stop being current. Keep your story accurate and relevant – otherwise what purpose does it serve?

Tools such as *Google Analytics* can show us how users move through the site, what content they look at, how they interact with it and how long they stay. We can then use this information to make any necessary changes to our story.

That's one of the web's greatest advantages over films and books. We can change the story *after* we've released it.

STORYTELLING THROUGH BRANDS

While most people think of a company's brand as just its logo, it's actually a lot more than that. By considering all the elements that make up a brand – logo, colours, tone of voice, typefaces, etc. – we can tell a coherent story.

How brands communicate invisibly

What is a brand?
A brand is a name, sign, symbol, slogan or anything that is used to identify and distinguish a specific product, service or business.[1]

In our lives we become familiar with various brands, and we grow to understand the experience and values those brands represents. This recognition comes down to storytelling, consistency and reinforcement.

When a company decides on a brand story, that story is consistently communicated and referred to whenever the brand is used. Audiences soon develop an understanding and expectation of the brand, and every time they come into contact with it the story is reinforced.

But you don't have to be a big corporation to use a brand to tell a story. The key is to make sure the brand story is told consistently.

How do brands tell stories?

A brand represents the values of a company or product. It tells its story through slogans and visual elements (such as logos), and communicating invisibly using colour and icons. Here are some brand elements that contribute to the overall story:

- **Values**
  A brand should be born from carefully chosen values. They may not be explicitly written on the product or in its marketing material, but any brand worthy of success will be underwritten by a mission statement and values that represent the company.

[1] Aaker, David (1991). Managing Brand Equity.

- **Mission statements**

  These summarise everything a company is striving for and should tell its story succinctly.

- **Slogans**

  The short snappy text that anchors a logo or adorns a company's printed materials adds to the brand's story. In fact, the slogan can encapsulate the story, just in very short form (for example, *Nike's* 'Just do it' and Apple's 'Think different'). Successful slogans work independently of the logo – the few words selected for the slogan communicate a lot about the brand story and bring added context to the logo.

- **Colour**

  Colours have hidden meanings and can connote certain values and messages. So choosing the brand's dominant colour, in its logo and elsewhere, is important in telling the right story.

- **Logo**

  While a logo represents the brand, it isn't the sole vehicle for it. It just happens to be the most visual and widely-used way for many companies to communicate their brands.

Brands by colour

Here's a chart showing some common brands and the colours they use. You'll notice that both *BP* and *Friends of the Earth* have adopted green as their brand colour, most likely due to the natural associations of that colour.

Google, eBay and *Windows* have multicoloured logos. This might be to demonstrate they are about communities, and appealing to many people in more than one culture.

Services such as *AA Motor Rescue* and *Yellow Pages* are yellow and food manufacturers such as *Coca-Cola* and *Walkers Crisps* are red.

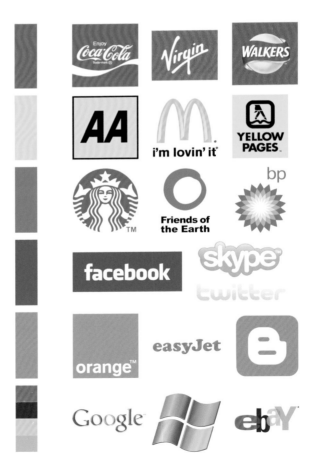

Different types of story

Brands can tell their stories in a very literal way or a very
subtle way.

Drupal's' branding, for example, is quite literal. The name Drupal,
'derives from the English pronunciation of the Dutch word
druppel, which means drop'.
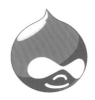
    The logo (more fondly known in the Drupal community as
the Drupalicon) looks like a droplet of water, and is blue – a colour
synonymous with water.

FedEx however has a more subtle storytelling approach, especially
when it comes to its logo.

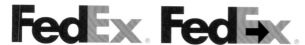

Here is the same logo but with a certain section highlighted
in black. This very clever and subtle use of white space creates
an arrow inside the logo, which represents the notion of moving
forward, progression and delivery.

Telling a story

In branding, there has to be a story to tell. But how you tell the
story is almost as important as the story itself. You may never
explicitly reveal your brand values or mission statements your to
users/customers, but they will influence (and provide the basis of)
your story.
    If you're creating a new brand, think about your story as early
in the process as possible. If you're refreshing a brand, ask yourself
if the story is still relevant or whether it needs to be re-imagined.
    It all comes back to two things: knowing your story, and
knowing your audience. This is something *Matthew Smith* of
SquaredEye does know, and his website is one that tells the right
story in the best way to the target audience, as we'll discover in the
next and final chapter.

[1] Drupal.org

25   CASE STUDY: *SQUAREDEYE.COM*

I'd like to finish with one of my favourite examples of storytelling: the website of design studio Squared Eye.

As you will see, Squared Eye paid a lot of attention to detail while knitting it all together. This, along with the imagery, copy and colours, have all been combined to reveal a well-crafted and rounded story.

This case study focuses on a redesign of the Squared Eye website in Spring 2009. You will learn not only about a website that tells a story, but also about the story discovery process itself (which is just as important).

Squared Eye is a design studio headed by Matthew Smith, and based in Greenville, South Carolina. Matthew gave me permission to include Squared Eye in this book, and his answers to my questions reveal a great deal of the subtleties of storytelling, the ability to tell stories on the web, and how one image can tie it all together.

This chapter was written in early 2011. Since then SquaredEye has joined forces with Zaarly. Fear not though, the SquaredEye website discussed in this chapter can still be viewed here: *http:// old.squaredeye.com/*

I asked Matthew to define the Squared Eye story

"A monstrous appetite for the tiniest details. We love to provide the magic moments for our clients customers, and even for our clients during our design process. We're craftsman in every sense of the word. It even gets worked out when we make mistakes, we want to learn from our mistakes with care and detail. Nothing gets swept under the rug. I think a big part of what gets passed via word of mouth from client to client, is the fact that we understand business, not just visual design. This keeps surprising our clients in the best ways, and when we finish their projects, they often tell us that they could immediately start another - just to keep working with us. It's amazing, but I think it's all about people feeling taken care of, and understood, and provided for professionally. I don't think it's magic or rocket science, it's just good work."

That's quite a detailed answer, and communicating it all through
the website without reams of copy is no easy task. Matthew thinks
the company has captured the entire story in a solitary brand
mark: *the whale*.

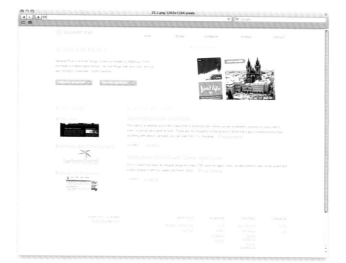

Then.

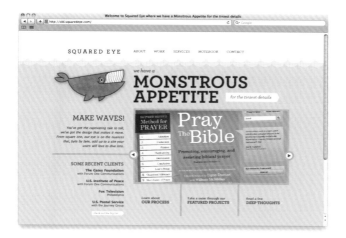

Now.

Then and Now

The motivation behind the redesign was simple: Matthew wanted Squared Eye to grow and earn a reputation for producing wonderful work. And he didn't think the branding – such as it was – did justice to his hopes for the company.

When I asked Matthew about the motivation behind the redesign, his response was quite clear:

> *"I knew it was time to be surer of what I was doing with my freelancing. I have been raised to offer clear expectations and follow through on them, and that's what I felt was missing in what I was doing with Squared Eye prior to re-branding."*

What Matthew realised was that to successfully tell a story, you need to fully understand it. He continues:

> *"Re-branding would be a research project into knowing better who I am. My goal wasn't to nail it down perfectly, but to make a clear mark in the sand – from this point forward, I'm going this way."*

Despite being quite a capable designer himself, Matthew trusted the redesign of the brand to an external company: *Able*, led by *Greg Ash*.

Able came up with the entity that would bring the brand and the story together, and later communicate it in one lone image: the whale.

It was created for the logotype and business cards. But the website implementation and everything else Squared Eye achieved was all completed in-house.

Finding the story?

Matthew is often asked why he outsourced the creation of his own brand. Surely he knew his story better than anyone else could? Matthew admits others were sceptical of his decision. 'When I started the re-branding process with Able, many of my colleagues, and even some clients, were confused. Why would I hire someone to design the Squared Eye logo and help me think through an identity, when I am a perfectly capable designer?

Before you can decide how to tell your story, you need to know what that story is, inside and out.

> *"The answer was clear. I've learned that, in my personal life, external counsel is the most effective way to get to know myself, so why would business be any different?"*

When researching and planning your story, look beyond your own knowledge. This will help you develop the story, and sense-check your own opinions.

Finding the story, fine tuning it and then presenting it via the website took several steps. Here's the process Able used, which can be applied to other web design projects.

Able began their research by speaking to Squared Eye's clients, families and colleagues. This is where they learned Squared Eye's current story. Matthew saw this step of the process as "the equivalent of good user testing, but for identity rather than interaction."

This part of the process really delved into the finer details of the Squared Eye story. Just as importantly, it helped them discover the company's identity, its audience, its competitors, and the companies it aspired to. This became invaluable for Matthew as he 'knew more about Squared Eye than ever before. By simply listening well, Able helped us start to become what we wanted to be, not just ease into what daily business would make us.'

Able also helped Squared Eye choose a mood. Matthew spent several weeks with Able to work out the 'particulars of the brand rationale and from there, the brand's visual presence and identity.'

It was at this stage that Matthew really felt confident about the Squared Eye brand and how to "articulate to clients just how Squared Eye was going to help them bring their sites to life – and give them products their users could really dive into."

Even when your story is clear, you need to keep your audience in mind, as they will have an impact on how that story is told. Tools such as use cases and personas can help you understand your audience.

By the end of this discovery phase, the Squared Eye story was well and truly mapped out. Even though the words 'story' or 'storytelling' hadn't been discussed, Able and Squared Eye had already defined the current story, researched and analysed the company, and started to visualise the new version of the story.

Telling the story

The one element that ended up binding everything together was Levi, the whale.

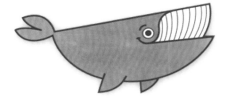

Levi is short for Leviathan. For Matthew, "he perfectly represents the Squared Eye presence and everything we want to be. In Levi, Able helped us articulate our appetite for detail. Just as the Blue Whale chows down on 250,000 pounds of tiny krill a year, so Squared Eye thrives on the little nuances that change a simple interaction into an experience, and a regular user into a believer."

That's the Squared Eye story they would eventually tell on their website. But while Matthew felt the whale perfectly encapsulated that story, it soon became apparent that for users to make the connection the storytelling needed to be a bit more literal.

Levi was not only a character in the story, but also embodied the story itself. His role was integral to communicating what was needed.

Matthew believes 'the whale says it all' but Levi alone wasn't enough to tell the story. The name 'Squared Eye' doesn't immediately suggest whales, and so they needed the copy on the site to tell the story about what the whale represented to their audience.

The tiniest details

If we focus on the Squared Eye homepage and the 'About' page, we can see clear storytelling elements at work, all combining to tell one coherent story.

The homepage:

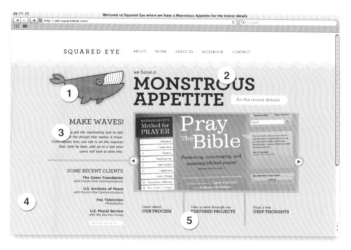

Five key areas on this homepage tell the Squared Eye story.

1. Levi the whale. The image is a pleasing one that captures the user's attention. It immediately sets a tone for the website, and its presence on other pages lets the story unfold as users move through the site
2. The attention-grabbing headline: 'We have a monstrous appetite for the tiniest details'. This is where the whale starts to make sense. You don't need to be an expert on whales to know they too have a monstrous appetite. Through this headline we are starting to learn about the brand values of Squared Eye
3. Some of the site's copy was written by *Carolyn Wood* of *Pixelingo*, in response to specific needs Matthew discussed with her. More than copy, she helped by bringing critical questions to Matthew – questions that informed his story and helped him think through issues ahead

As well as writing for a few other sections, Carolyn wrote the paragraph on the home page to help Matthew tie together all the visual images and words on the site for his visitors: squared, eye, appetite, a grid image, details, waves, and an invitation that uses the word, 'You,' to speak directly to them.

This is where the storytelling becomes more literal. 'Make waves!' has obvious ties to the whale and the sea. The copy beneath this says:

> *'You've got the captivating tale to tell, we've got the design that makes it move. From square one, our eye is on the nuances that, byte by byte, add up to a site your users will love to dive into.'*

That one paragraph explains the connection between the whale and Squared Eye, the needs of the clients and Squared Eye's services, as well as a little about their work process.

While a strong brand shouldn't need a detailed explanation, the copy hints at the story and brings a slightly subtle narrative to the homepage. Once users are familiar with the brand they won't need to read the copy to get the full story. They'll get it all from Levi instead.

4. The colour blue and the ocean themes are the most graphic and immediate elements of the story. They both have close obvious ties to the whale. But even without the wave shape between the header and the main content area, it still has connotations of the ocean, especially as they use a marine blue throughout the website. (If you look closely, you'll see the blue background is actually a tightly woven grid of tiny squares.)

5. The copy further down the page has two important functions: a call to action that leads the user further into the site, and adding to the story. The three areas are:

- Learn about our process
- Take a swim through our featured projects
- Read a few deep thoughts

The 'About' page

The 'About' page reinforces the story first told on the homepage, and also reveals a little more detail. As we learn more about Squared Eye and the people who work there, we also learn more about their work methods and the importance they place on paying attention to the finer details.

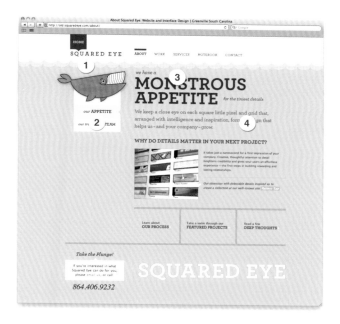

1. Once again the story is reinforced by consistently using and positioning both the Squared Eye name and Levi the whale
2. The copy continues the theme from the homepage. For example, instead of using 'our process', Squared Eye have used 'our appetite'. A small difference, but think how much more the word 'appetite' tells the Squared Eye story than 'process'
3. The 'monstrous appetite' headline is again used to full affect here, along with the blue ocean-inspired background

4. The copy in this area explains the story in a little more detail. I'm not convinced it needs to be so descriptive or laid out so literally, as the more subtle stories are often the most enjoyable. But it's the last chance to tie everything together before the user moves to deeper pages that focus on the company's work and services. Here the copy tells us:

> 'The whale keeps a sharp eye on tasty, tiny creatures that together make him colossal as he glides through the big, blue sea.'

> 'We keep a close eye on each square little pixel and grid that, arranged with intelligence and inspiration, form a design that helps us – and your company – grow.'

The story unfolds

It would be easy to have a whale and a few chunks of copy explain everything on the homepage, then revert back to the typical copy you see on this type of site – 'this is how we work', 'look at some of our projects', etc. But as we have discussed earlier, there is no guarantee your users will start your story at the beginning.

Squared Eye allows for this by using the same tone of voice, choice of words and theme in all of its copy and supplementary content throughout the site. Here are some examples:

Here is the copy from the 'Team' page. I've highlighted the words that continue to tell the story:

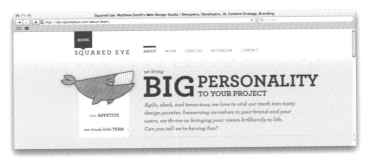

'We bring the **big** personality to your project. Agile, sleek and tenacious, we love to **sink our teeth** into **tasty** design puzzles. **Immersing** ourselves in your brand and your users, we thrive on brining your vision brilliantly to life. Can you tell we're having fun?'

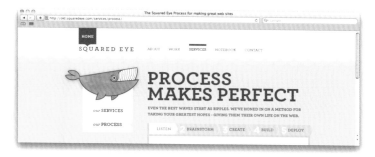

The copy on the 'Our Process' page tells us:

'Even the best **waves** start as **ripples**. We've honed in on a method for taking your greatest hopes – giving them their own life on the web.'

On the 'Services' page the most obvious story connection sits at the bottom of the page.

'Now that you've seen what we can do, **come swim with us**, and see how we do it.'

The 'Services' page also tells the story, with '**Take the plunge**' having an obvious connection to both the ocean and the whale.

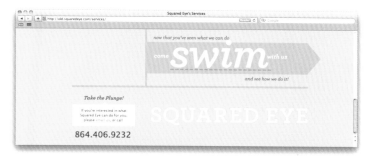

The story within the story

The beauty of this website isn't just how it tells the Squared Eye brand story, but also how it tells stories within that story. Specifically, how the company works on projects and what the end results are.

Case studies are stories, too. They have clearly defined narratives, leading the reader step-by-step through a specific process. Sometimes they have characters and, depending on the project, may even have twists in the tale.

The case studies on the Squared Eye site are great examples of simple storytelling on the web.

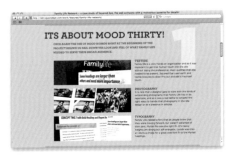

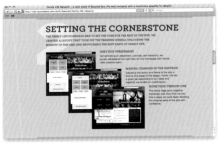

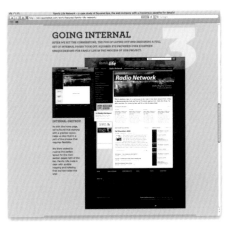

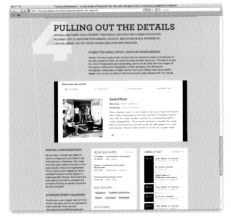

This case study shows how a story can be segmented, provided the order is clear. Simply adding the numbers 1-4 here immediately create a narrative to tell the story of this particular project.

I was particularly impressed with the storytelling on the Squared Eye site, and asked Matthew if this was a conscious part of his redesign process.

It wasn't.

The focus was on defining Squared Eye, and then communicating it in the best way possible. He may not have called the process 'storytelling', but that's exactly what Matthew was doing.

The success of the story

I was particularly interested about whether the website redesign produced any tangible results for Matthew. He told me the new brand turned him from an outsider to an insider within the design community. Matthew also believes "the story of Squared Eye really compels people to think differently about design, and for that matter, about freelancing and business."

The situation speaks for itself. Matthew's business has tripled in just two years, leading to bigger and more challenging projects for the team. The stats also show the redesign attracted more potential customers as they went from an average of 40 visits a day to around 530 a day.

Almost there

We've now reached the end of not only the Squared Eye story, but also my own.

Along the way we have looked at a broad range of topics including signs, colour, tone of voice, typefaces and branding. Broad, yes, but all ways we can communicate invisibly. And they can all be used as storytelling devices to improve and enhance how we communicate on the web.

Stories are a vital part of how we share information, preserve cultures and communicate with others. As the web becomes more and more a part of our everyday lives, we would be silly to ignore the power of storytelling. We should try and tell great stories online in the same way we have done offline for centuries.

Everyone has a story to tell, and the web lets us share them with a much wider audience.

This has been my story.

I look forward to reading yours.

Attributions *In order of appearance*

1. Invisible communication 101

7-38-55 rule - *http://en.wikipedia.org/wiki/Albert_Mehrabian#7.25-38.25-55.25_rule* || Religious symbols - *http://makeready.wordpress.com* ||

2. Following the right signs

Definition of semiotics - **The Media Student's Book** - *Gill Branston and Roy Stafford* || Statue of Liberty icon - *http://www.123rf.com/photo_3452242_white-silhouette-of-the-couple-doves-on-sky-background.html* || Printer Icon - *http://www.iconarchive.com/show/dragon-soft-icons-by-artua/Printer-icon.html* || Sundial - *http://ccphysics.us/henriques/a105l/Sundial.htm* || Podcast icon - *http://thinkvitamin.com* || Tsunami sign - *http://yourtown.pressdemocrat.com/2010/03/bodega-bay/why-no-tsunami-warning-signs-on-sonoma-coast-2/* || Hindu Swastika - *http://photobucket.com/images/hindu%20swastika/* || Swastika flag - *http://www.clipartguide.com/_pages/0512-0709-1217-2411.html* || Photograph of Schipol Airport Signage - *Robert Mills* || **London Underground Map** - *http://www.tfl.gov.uk/assets/downloads/standard-tube-map.pdf* || Photograph of Schipol Airport Signage - *Robert Mills* || **Carsonified** icons - *http://carsonified.com/* || **Apple UK** - *http://www.apple.com/uk/* || **Tesco** icons - *http://www.tesco.com/groceries/* || **Guardian** - *http://www.guardian.co.uk/*

3. Using the right palette

Photograph of Times Square – *Glenn R Carter* || Illustration of rose - *Gareth Strange* || Stop sign - *http://www.clker.com/clipart-6863.html* || Slippery road sign - *http://en.wikipedia.org/wiki/File:Singapore_Road_Signs_-_Warning_Sign_-_Slippery_road.svg* || No smoking sign - *http://en.wikipedia.org/wiki/File:No_smoking_symbol.svg* || **Kandinsky** painting - *http://marialaterza.blogspot.com/2010/10/wassily-kandinsky.html* || **La Senza** - *http://www.lasenza.co.uk/* || **BBC** - *http://www.bbc.co.uk/*

4. Using the correct language

Bluegg - *http://www.bluegg.co.uk/* || **Zoe's Place Baby Hospice** - *http://www. zoes-place.org.uk/* || **Llantrisant Freemen** - *http://www.llantrisant.net/* || **Downing Street** - *http://www.number10.gov.uk/* || **CBeebies** - *http://www.bbc.co.uk/cbeebies/* || **Visit London** - *http://www.visitlondon.com/* || **Academy of Motion Picture Arts and Sciences** - *http://www.oscars.org/* || **Haribo UK** - *http://www.haribo.com/ planet/uk/startseite.php* || **The British Monarchy** - *http://www.royal.gov.uk/* || **Coca-Cola** - *http://www.coca-cola.co.uk/* || **HMRC** - *http://www.hmrc.gov.uk/index. htm* || **Innocent** - *http://www.innocentdrinks.co.uk/*

5. Telling the best story

Photograph of biker - *http://www.officeforward.com/the-moment-just-before-the-pain-begins/* || **Coca-Cola** ©2011 The Coca-Cola Company, all rights reserved. || **Virgin** ©2011 Virgin, all rights reserved. || **Walkers** ©2011 Walkers, all rights reserved. || **The AA** ©2011 The AA, all rights reserved. || **McDonald's** ©2011 McDonald's , all rights reserved. || **Yellow Pages** ©2011 Yellow Pages, all rights reserved. || **Starbucks** ©2011 Starbucks Corporation, all rights reserved. || **Friends of the Earth** ©2011 Friends of the Earth Trust/Limited, all rights reserved. || **BP** ©2011 BP p.l.c, all rights reserved. || **Facebook** ©2011 Facebook, all rights reserved. || **Skype** ©2011 Skype Limited, all rights reserved. || **Twitter** ©2011 Twitter, all rights reserved. || **Orange** ©2011 Orange, all rights reserved. || **easyJet** ©2011 easyJet Airline Company Limited, all rights reserved. || **Blogger** ©2011 Google, all rights reserved. || **Google** ©2011 Google, all rights reserved. || **Windows** ©2011 Microsoft, all rights reserved. || **ebay** ©2011 ebay Inc, all rights reserved. || **FedEx** logo - used with permission by it's creator - *Lindon Leader* || **SquaredEye** – All imagery supplied by and attributed to - *Matthew Smith* - *http://old.squaredeye.com/*

Index
*The letter **n** after a page number indicates a mention in a marginal note.*

J

K

L

M

N

O

P

Q

R

S

Y